SKIN AND WOUND INFECTION

SKIN AND WOUND INFECTION

Investigation and Treatment in Practice

David V Seal,
Roderick J Hay and
Keith R Middleton

With guest chapters by
Jackie Middleton and Philip A Thomas

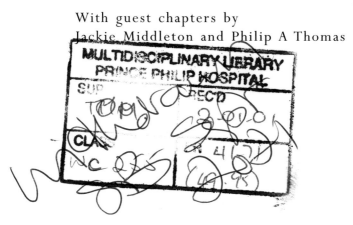
MARTIN DUNITZ

First published in the United Kingdom in 2000
by Martin Dunitz Ltd, The Livery House, 7–9 Pratt Street, London NW1 0AE

A CIP record for this book is available from the British Library.

ISBN 1-85317-735-0

Distributed in the USA by:
Blackwell Science Inc.
Commerce Place, 350 Main Street
Malden, MA 02148, USA
Tel: 1-800-215-1000

Distributed in Canada by:
Login Brothers Book Company
324 Salteaux Crescent
Winnipeg, Manitoba, R3J 3T2
Canada
Tel: 204-224-4068

Distributed in Brazil by:
Ernesto Reichmann Distribuidora de Livros, Ltda
Rua Coronel Marques 335, Tatuape 03440-000
São Paulo
Brazil

Composition by Scribe Design, Gillingham, Kent
Printed and bound in Singapore by Kyodo Printing Pte Ltd

CONTENTS

CONTRIBUTORS

Roderick J Hay DM FRCP FRCPath
Professor of Cutaneous Medicine
St John's Institute of Dermatology
Block 7
St Thomas' Hospital
Lambeth Palace Road
London SE1 7EH
UK

Jackie Middleton RGN DipHV
Health Visitor
Harrow & Hillingdon Healthcare NHS Trust
Harrow, Middlesex
UK

Keith R Middleton PhD BPharm MRPharmS
Principal Pharmacist
Northwick Park & St Mark's Hospital
Watford Road
Harrow, Middlesex HA1 3UJ
UK

David V Seal MD FRCPath FRCOphth DipBact MIBiol
Former Consultant Medical Microbiologist with the
Medical Research Council, National Health Service and
Public Health Laboratory Service and Senior Lecturer
with the University of Glasgow. Honorary Senior
Research Fellow with the City University, London, UK

Philip A Thomas MD PhD
Professor, Thomas Diagnostic & Research Centre and
Department of Ocular Microbiology
Institute of Ophthalmology
Joseph Eye Hospital
Melapudur Main Road
Tiruchirappalli
Tamil Nadu
India

PREFACE

This book has been written to further the understanding of both skin and wound infection and to consider the interactions that exist between the epidermis, dermis and subcutaneous tissue. Infections are described separately for each anatomical layer, rather than by organism, so that the reader can understand how different microbes may give similar clinical presentations. Some tropical infections are considered separately. We consider that this approach is beneficial here. We have included clinical descriptions and the relevant microbiological features, together with a synopsis of immunology and epidemiology. Tables have been constructed to highlight important practical points.

We are very grateful to all our colleagues, both in the UK and overseas, for their advice and assistance with this book. In particular, we would like to thank the following who have supplied clinical or laboratory photographs: Hugh Chadfield (deceased), John Chow (Hong Kong), Ray Clark, Paul Jacobs (deceased), Gavin Joynt (Hong Kong), David Kingston, Harold Lambert, Barbara Leppard (Tanzania), Donald Lyon (Hong Kong), Ian Mackie, Murray McGavin, M A Rajan (Kumbakonam), Keith Rodgers, G Senthamilselvi (Chennai), Hillas Smith, Rataporn Ungpakorn (Bangkok), Govinda Visvesvara (Atlanta) and Anthony du Vivier.

London
May 2000

1. PATHOGENESIS OF SKIN INFECTION AND THE LOCALIZED IMMUNE RESPONSE

Anatomical protection

The structure of the skin consists of a stratified cellular avascular layer – the stratum corneum and epidermis- and a fibrous, elastic and vascular layer – the dermis. This lies over the fibrous, fatty and vascular subcutaneous layer which is loosely joined to the fascial plane that separates it from muscle. The combination provides a barrier against infection which is considered below.

The epidermis is not uniform in thickness. The epidermal cells dip down into the dermis to form a network – the rete ridges – into which the papillary processes of the dermis protrude. Thus the surface area of the epidermal–dermal junction is much greater than that of the epidermis itself. The epidermis varies in thickness on different parts of the body, those sites subject to pressure being much thicker.

The superficial cells develop from the basal cells starting with prickle cells proceeding through granular cells to become non-nucleated keratinocytes (horn cells), constantly shed from the surface as microscopic scales (Fig. 1.1). The prickle cell layer undergoes thickening (acanthosis) when the skin is subjected

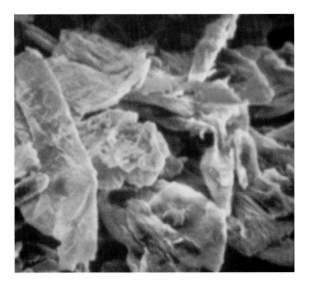

Figure 1.1: Electron micrograph of skin scales (horn cells).

to friction. It is also the site of intercellular and intracellular oedema in eczema. The insoluble protein – keratin – is formed in the outer layer, and the protective barrier is then complete.

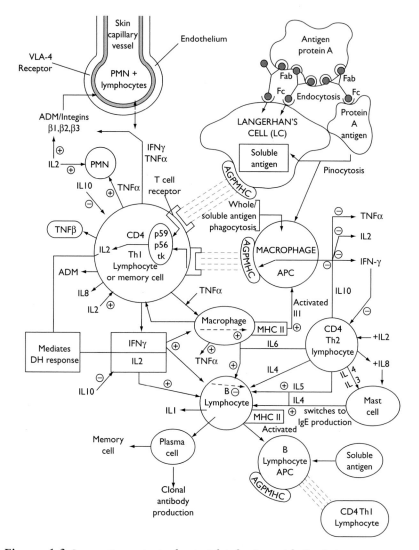

Figure 1.2: Immunity against a bacterial infection with *Staphylococcus aureus* protein A as the example antigen. PMN, polymorphonuclear cell; APC, antigen presenting cell; Th, T helper lymphocyte; CD, cluster determinant antigen; VLA, very late antigen (super IgG) receptor; ADM, adhesion molecules; tk, tyrosine kinase; MHC, major histocompatibility complex (II); AGPMHC, antigenic (oligo)peptide MHC group; cytokines including IL (interleukins), IFN (interferon) and TNF (tumour necrosis factor).

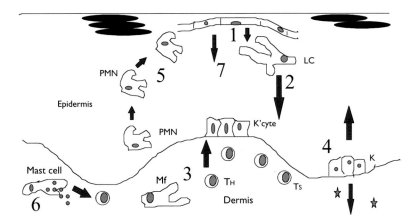

Figure 1.3: Immunity against a fungal infection. PMN, polymorphonuclear leucocytes; Mf, macrophages; TH, T helper cell; Ts, T suppressor cell; K, keratinocyte; LC, Langerhans' cell.

The horny layer protects the underlying cells against penetration by microbes and chemicals. It is resistant to common bacterial infections. In addition, there is a surface film over this layer derived from desquamated epidermal cells and sebaceous glands. Water penetrates hardly at all but fat-soluble substances will do so. Fat-soluble alkaloids penetrate easily, as do phenol and its derivatives, including salicylic acid. Fat-soluble vitamin D is synthesized in the surface film and absorbed through the epidermis.

The Langerhans' or dendritic cells are found in the epidermis. Their role is to process antigen and transfer it to T cells (Figs 1.2 and 1.3).

Scattered among the basal cells are the melanocytes, clear cells with small nuclei, which form the melanin pigment granules. These are conveyed by their dendritic processes to the epidermal cells, where they are deposited in their cytoplasm. Melanocytes are also present in the hair matrices.

The dermis varies in thickness and structure to provide a firm architecture with elasticity. It consists of the fibrous protein 'collagen'. This is embedded in a ground substance of mucopolysaccharides. Elastic fibres are present in small numbers together with fibroblasts (precursors of collagen and elastin), histiocytes, macrophages and mast cells. Melanophages are histiocytes which engulf melanin. The macrophages play a vital role in phagocytosing organisms.

The dermis has a rich blood supply. The deep arterial plexus supplies the skin appendages and the intermediate subpapillary plexus from which smaller vessels pass to the papillary bodies. Corresponding veins exist together with arteriovenous anastomoses which provide shunt systems to divert blood from superficial to deep vessels depending on the thermostatic requirements of the body.

The sensory nerves of the skin link up with the dorsal spinal roots and the central nervous system. There are free nerve endings beneath the epidermis for touch, pain and temperature and specialized end organs in areas of high tactile sensibility. The sweat glands, the musculature of the arterioles and the arrector muscles of the hair are innervated from the sympathetic ganglia of the autonomic nervous system. The sebaceous glands have no motor nerve innervation, being controlled by endocrine stimulus.

The hypoderm or fatty layer is the connective tissue layer between the dermis and the deep fascia adapted to the formation of aggregates of fat. Connective tissue strands run between the fat cells. The thickness and distribution vary according to age, sex, race, site, diet and nutrition of the individual. It provides for greater mobility of the overlying skin on the underlying structures. Both types of sweat gland are situated in the hypoderm, as is the pilosebaceous unit – a dermal papilla from which a hair grows in the follicle and a sebaceous gland secretes into it. In other areas the sebaceous glands open directly on to the surface. They secrete sebum, which is a complex mixture of lipids. Owing to lack of positive secretory pressure, they are vulnerable to infection. Their 'funnel' orifices accumulate surface bacteria and extraneous matter which can cause intense irritation.

Each nail is formed from its matrix in a fold of epidermis on the dorsum of the distal phalanx of a digit. The fold is lined by a soft keratin layer – the eponychium. Together with the cuticle, there is a protective barrier against entry of organisms into the paronychial fold. Nails grow at a rate of 0.5–1.2 mm each week.

Invasion of the skin or open wound by pathogenic microbes

Site of organism

The intact surface of the epithelium, attached to the dermis, provides a physical barrier of immense importance in preventing invasion by microbes. However, there are two potential routes of penetration either following an active process of adhesion between micro-organism and keratinocyte or through a break in the epithelial surface. Once breached, however, by physical or other trauma, even minor such as a mosquito bite, bacteria or fungal spores penetrate into the dermis and subcutis. A number of factors, reviewed below, will influence whether or not localized or systemic infection develops but initially it is the *site* of penetration that matters.

The effect of penetration to a particular site is best illustrated for infection by *Streptococcus pyogenes* (Fig. 1.4). Invasion by *S. pyogenes* at each layer gives rise to a different clinical condition separately reviewed in Chapters 3–5.

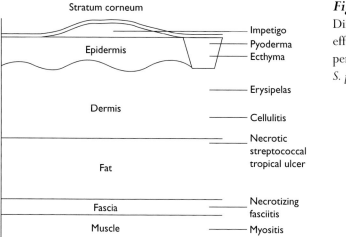

Figure 1.4:
Different
effects of
penetration by
S. pyogenes.

While there is evidence that certain M types of *S. pyogenes* can cause epidemics of impetigo (M types 2, 49, 53, 55, 56, 57 and 60), or are associated with impetigo and acute glomerulonephritis (M types 12 [commonly associated with pharyngeal infection as well] and 49), or pyoderma and acute glomerulonephritis (M type 55), or myocarditis with 'rheumatogenic' strains colonizing or infecting the throat (M type 5), the majority of isolates cannot be divided into subtypes which cause specific clinical conditions in skin and subcutaneous tissues. For example, both 'throat' and 'skin' strains can cause erysipelas, cellulitis and necrotizing fasciitis. It appears that the initial vascular and immune response within tissue at the site of invasion determines the host response, as well as the presence of other organisms such as *Staphylococcus aureus* that may cause a synergistic infection, with possible variations as given in Fig. 1.4. Similarly, no specific fungal subtypes are associated with skin infection. However, with viruses such 'subspecialization' does occur amongst the human papillomaviruses (HPV), where specific types are associated with different morphological variants of human warts.

Numbers of organisms

The number of organisms required to cause infection is influenced by the virulence factors produced, such as toxins and/or proteases, and their effect on the tissues – for example, alpha-lysin of *Staphylococcus aureus* 'paralyses' smooth muscle of arterioles leading to stasis and vasodilatation, and is lethal to polymorphonuclear cells, so inhibiting their phagocytosis. This toxic effect of *S. aureus* can cause inflammation without necrosis (Figs 1.5 and 1.6) (Seal and Kingston 1988) and varies in production between different strains.

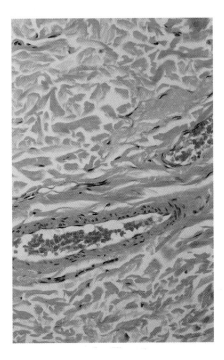

Figure 1.5: Histology (H & E stain) of normal rabbit skin injected with 0.9% saline (× 400).

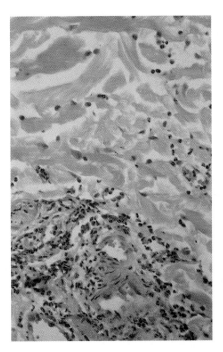

Figure 1.6: Inflammation (dilated vessels and polymorphonuclear cells) without necrosis given by alpha-lysin of *S. aureus* in rabbit skin (× 400).

For highly virulent bacteria such as *S. pyogenes*, which produces a variety of exotoxins (Belani *et al.*, 1991), as few as 10 cells may be sufficient to cause acute infection. Other bacteria such as Gram-negative rods like *Escherichia coli* have never established themselves as pathogens for the skin although they are pathogens at other sites, such as in the bladder, and they do cause polymicrobial infections in wounds. Whether small numbers of invading virulent bacteria for the skin such as *Pasteurella multocida* from a dog bite will cause infection or not will also be influenced by the host immune response (see below).

When there is an open wound, such as a diabetic foot ulcer, it is possible to study the effects of different numbers of bacteria (Sapico *et al.*, 1986). There is a minimum threshold required to cause infection by most bacteria, excluding *S. pyogenes*, and this is often at approximately 10^4. Below this number, active infection will not proceed and the organisms will be phagocytosed or remain to colonize the 'open' surface. When infection does occur, such as with *Pseudomonas aeruginosa*, there will be up to 10^6 or 10^7/ml (or g) bacteria present. The most important contributory factor to a minimum number of organisms causing infection is that of a foreign body. This point was proven very elegantly by the late Professor Elek when he injected subcutaneously the arms of medical students, in some of whom he had inserted black silk sutures, with varying numbers of *S. aureus*: 10^6 cells were required to cause infection on their own but only 10^4 cells were required in the presence of silk sutures, demonstrating the association of sutures (or, as later shown, foreign bodies such as plastic prostheses) with wound infection (Shulman and Nahmias, 1972). Virulence determinants of fungi are less well studied but *Candida albicans*, for instance, possesses an acid proteinase which is important both for tissue invasion and also for initiating the process of adhesion with host cells.

Polymicrobial and synergistic invasion

All too often, clinicians and microbiologists ascribe an infection to a single organism, reflecting the philosophy of the thirteenth century Occam's razor (no more things should be presumed to exist than are necessary). While this may be good advice for an infection such as tertiary syphilis, with various presenting features, it does not apply to most wound infections. Wound model studies in animals have shown that the infecting dose of a Gram-negative rod such as *E. coli* or an anaerobe such as *Bacteroides* spp. is approximately 10^6, but if these aerobic and anaerobic bacteria are combined as a joint infecting dose then the numbers required for each of them falls by 100-fold to 10^4 or even 10^3.

This reflects the clinical situation both for contaminated wounds, when the polymicrobial infection can result in synergistic microbial gangrene (Kingston and Seal, 1990), as well as for minor trauma such as a mosquito bite when a synergistic infection can develop rapidly from a combination of *Streptococcus pyogenes* and *Staphylococcus aureus* (Fig. 1.7). The common tropical disease 'tropical ulcer' is a

7

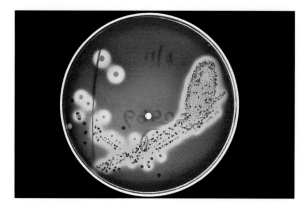

Figure 1.7: Primary blood agar culture plate of mosquito bite on foot with mixed isolation of *Streptococcus pyogenes* and *Staphylococcus aureus.*

further example of a synergistic infection comprising the anaerobe *Fusobacterium ulcerans*, a spirochaete and different aerobic bacteria (refer pp. 148–149).

A synergistic effect is believed responsible for initiating many cases of acute streptococcal necrotizing fasciitis (Seal and Kingston, 1988). In this situation, the alpha-lysin toxin produced by *S. aureus* allows vascular dilatation and is leucocidal so that a low inoculum of *S. pyogenes* can multiply and produce toxins to cause infection unless specific immunity is present (see below). Other combinations have been reviewed by Kingston and Seal (1990) and are discussed in Chapter 5. Not all combinations of organisms are synergistic, however, and they may be antagonistic. This can occur, for example, when the epithelium is colonized by bacteria and dermatophyte fungi, the latter producing penicillin inhibiting the former (Chapter 3) or giving rise to the possible development or selection of penicillin resistance.

Protection of skin by the colonizing microbial flora

The normal microbial flora within the epidermis consists of multiple different subtypes of coagulase-negative staphylococci (CNS), micrococci, corynebacteria of different species (diphtheroids) and small numbers of different types of alpha-haemolytic streptococci. Additional competing flora in hair follicles includes the anaerobic *Propionibacterium* spp. These bacteria act as 'competing' flora for pathogens which are inhibited in part by the production of extracellular products, namely bacteriocines, proteases and toxins. CNS in particular produce lipases which split fatty acids to triglycerides that can be toxic, resulting in chronic inflammation. When bacterial infection does occur, it usually involves minor (or major) trauma and is related to climate, being more frequent in hot and particularly humid areas such as tropical zones.

The cutaneous microbiology of normal human feet has been investigated in depth (Marshall *et al.*, 1987). There was a quantitative variation in numbers between different sites. The mean counts were as follows: toe web 1.04×10^7;

sole 4.1×10^5; and dorsal surface 1.2×10^3. Staphylococci predominated on the sole and dorsal surface while aerobic coryneforms predominated in the toe clefts. The skin pH was higher on the sole (6.25) than the dorsal surface (5.23). The prevalence of Gram-negative bacteria (GNB) varies with the conditions of the feet (Noble *et al.*, 1986). The authors found GNB in the foot flora of 8% normal students, 24% hospital out-patients with suspected tinea pedis, 41% industrial workers wearing protective clothing, and 58% coal miners. Prevalence was greatest in those exposed to wet conditions. In contrast, the dry diabetic neuropathic foot has been found devoid of Gram-negative bacteria and to be more likely to have staphylococci, streptococci and dermatophytes present (Seal *et al.*, 1988).

Successful attempts have been made in the past to colonize adults and babies with a known non-toxin-producing strain of *S. aureus* to prevent them becoming colonized with a virulent toxin-producing strain. It was found possible to colonize babies in a neonatal unit with such bacterial interference but this approach fell into disrepute when one baby developed sepsis with the 'colonizing' strain and died (Shinefield *et al.*, 1972). Preventing babies becoming colonized with virulent toxin-producing strains of *S. aureus* within a neonatal unit still depends on use of an antiseptic powder such as Ster-Zac (0.33% hexachlorophene), applied to the umbilicus and under the arms, or a bactericidal bathing soap such as Bacti-Stat (0.3% triclosan). It is our repeated experience, and that of others (Zafar *et al.*, 1995), that when this antiseptic therapy is withdrawn the neonates within a maternity unit very quickly develop spots with a common strain of *S. aureus* because of their lack of a normal colonizing skin flora.

Immunity against infection

Immunity against most microbes depends on specific and non-specific humoral antibodies, directed against both the organism cell wall and its toxins. Exceptions classically include *Mycobacterium tuberculosis*, which requires cell-mediated immunity (CMI) to protect against invasive infection, although this type of immunity also results in chronic inflammation. Inflammation of similar aetiology occurs with weak acid (5% acetic acid), non-alcohol-fast bacteria such as *Nocardia* spp., causing nocardiosis. In addition, it can occur with dissimilar bacteria such as *S. aureus*, which in certain circumstances leads to the host developing CMI to components of the bacterial cell wall, when it can cause chronic suppurative disease. Such inflammation can be destructive without controlling the infection. CMI is also required for inhibition of many fungal infections as well as certain viral diseases such as human papillomavirus infections.

Humoral immunity

The extensive microvasculature of the skin allows rapid vasodilatation and diffusion of humoral antibodies to invading sites of micro-organisms. This can involve either specific antibodies, such as IgG to alpha-lysin produced by *S. aureus*, which may or may not be effective in limiting the infection, as well as non-specific antibody such as IgG to the peptidoglycan of the bacterial cell wall which, together with the complement cascade, can 'puncture' the cell wall resulting in cell lysis and death. Deficiency in humoral immunity results in repeated skin infection, often with *S. aureus*, presenting in children (Monteil *et al.*, 1987; Seal and Lightman, 1987). This recurrent infection can be suppressed by repeated doses of 'normal' immunoglobulin. Deficiency states affecting humoral immunity seldom predispose to fungal, parasitic or viral infections of the skin, although specific antibodies are important in defence against certain cytopathic viruses, particularly in the early phases of infection. Deficiency in neutrophil function, such as the 'lazy leucocyte syndrome', may present similarly due to the failure of effective phagocytosis of the organism.

For humoral immunity to develop, particularly for organisms infecting skin, active CMI is required to process microbial antigens for presentation to B lymphocytes (see below). Following Langerhans' cell, macrophage and Th-1 lymphocyte stimulation, and processing of antigen, the oligopeptides of the bacterial antigen are presented to Th-2 and B lymphocytes (to produce antibody) under a 'feedback' mechanism of cytokine production as illustrated in Fig. 1.2.

Delayed-type hypersensitivity (DTH) due to cell-mediated immunity

Cell-mediated immunity (CMI) in the skin is dependent on Langerhans' cells (LC), which take up antigen by pinocytosis or endocytosis. An example for bacterial infection is given in Fig. 1.2 and for a fungal infection in Fig. 1.3.

Langerhans' cells are dedicated antigen-processing cells and, as such, express the major histocompatability (MHC) class II antigens without prior inducement by cytokines. Upon exposure to antigen, LCs and other antigen-presenting cells (APCs) undergo functional maturation and gain the ability to present the antigen to CD4 T helper cells attracted by cytokines. Antigens taken up into APCs are enzymatically degraded to oligopeptides with an unfolded secondary structure, which are expressed at their surface as antigenic peptides bound to MHC molecules.

Dermal macrophages can also function as APCs. Keratinocytes produce a number of cytokines such as IL(interleukin)-1 and granulocyte macrophage colony stimulating factor (GM-CSF). Interferon-γ produced by T lymphocytes induces the expression of MHC class II molecules on the surface of keratinocytes, although it is not known if these can function as APCs. Macrophages can also process particulate antigens, including whole bacteria such as staphylococci and free-living amoebae such as *Acanthamoeba*, but can more effectively process soluble antigens such as the protein A of *S. aureus*, internalized in endocytic vesicles. This is in contrast to Langerhans' cells, which only process soluble antigen.

T lymphocytes exert their local effector function by secreting cytokines in tissues which act directly on target cells (Cousins and Rouse, 1996). Interferon (IFN-γ) induces expression of MHC class II molecules on epithelial and endothelial cells and fibroblasts which can all, to a variable degree, act as APCs, processing and presenting immunogenic peptides complexed with MHC class II molecules. However, they differ in capacity to produce co-stimulatory signals and do not stimulate resting T cells, which require IL-2 to become activated.

Delayed-type hypersensitivity (DH) is induced by acid-fast bacteria, such as *M. tuberculosis*, and occasionally by *S. aureus*, by fungi such as dermatophytes, *Herpes simplex* viruses and helminths such as *Onchocerca volvulus*. They are able to induce a cell-mediated immune reaction, expressed by the T helper (Th)-1 lymphocyte cells and mediated by cytokines (Hendricks and Tang, 1996).

S. aureus repeatedly colonizes the lid margins, noses, axillae and perineum of both normals (approximately 10%) and atopics (approximately 50%) (Tuft *et al.*, 1992). It is likely that diffusable cell wall antigens from *S. aureus*, especially protein A but also ribitol teichoic acid, reach across the epithelium where these antigens are processed by dendritic Langerhans' cells. The LCs have receptors for the Fc portion of the antibody molecule, which assists endocytosis of antigen such as *S. aureus* protein A by binding of specific antibody. In the latter case, there can be cross-linking between specific (F_{ab}) and non-specific (F_c) sites both found on protein A.

The CD4 Th-1 lymphocyte is responsible for most DH reactions. The Th-1 subtype (as opposed to the Th-2 subtype), mediates DH by a cascade of cytokines produced by T cell clones. Th-1 cells produce IL-2 and interferon (IFN-γ), responsible in part for the induration response of the DH reaction in the skin. Th-1 and -2 cells regulate each other's actions on antibody production, i.e. IFN-γ produced by the Th-1 cell inhibits the stimulatory effect of IL-4, produced by the Th-2 cell, on antibody production by B lymphocytes. This may be the mechanism for the clinical observation that a strong DH response is associated with a weak antibody response and vice versa. This opposite situation often develops in chronic human infections due to certain dermatophytes such as *Trichophyton rubrum*, where Th-2 responses may dominate.

Activated CD4 Th-1 cells secrete IFN-γ at the site of antigen entry and induce MHC class II expression on 'non-professional' APCs, thereby activating them. The recognition of the MHC-peptide complex of the APC by a T cell receptor initiates an intracellular signal transduction pathway via the p56 and p59 tyrosine

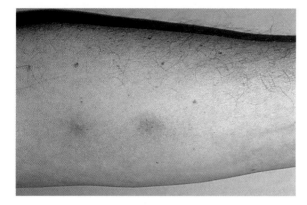

Figure 1.8: Delayed hypersensitivity (cell-mediated immune reaction) with induration at 48 hours to (left lesion) *S. aureus* protein A (significant reaction); (right lesion) thiomersal (significant reaction).

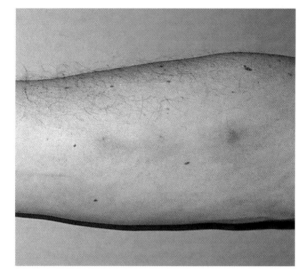

Figure 1.9: Delayed hypersensitivity (cell-mediated immune reaction) with induration at 48 hours to: (left lesion) killed coagulase-negative staphylococci (no reaction); (middle lesion) normal saline (no reaction); (right lesion) killed *S. aureus* (significant reaction).

kinases. The molecules that are then produced increase binding of Th cells to APCs and are called 'adhesion molecules' (ADM); for CD4 cells this includes the 55 kd monomeric transmembrane glycoprotein belonging to the Ig gene superfamily, and for CD8 T cytotoxic cells (CTC), two 34 kd alpha chain molecules.

The cellular response is regulated by expression of ADMs on inflammatory cells, suprabasal keratinocytes and vascular endothelium, which in turn is controlled by cytokines which can also act as chemotactic factors for polymorphonuclear cells (PMNs). These ADMs cause adhesion of PMNs and lymphocytes to the local vascular endothelium, when they bind to it and migrate to the site of activated lymphocytes in the skin.

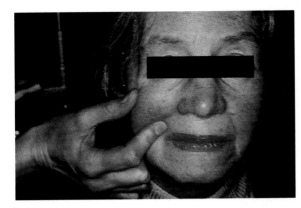

Figure 1.10:
Rosacea of face associated with chronic blepharitis.

Memory Th lymphocytes will also migrate to this site if the patient has undergone systemic enhancement of CMI to the particular antigen, in this example protein A of *S. aureus*. The expression of integrins (β1, β2, β3) attracts these activated Th-1 cells to the inflammatory site. The expression of β1 is up-regulated on the surface of activated memory cells which bind to the counter-receptor on vascular endothelium (VLA-4, a member of the Ig superfamily), and results in extravasation into the site of the processed antigen (in this example, protein A).

A clinical example of CMI at 48 hours is demonstrated in Figs 1.8 and 1.9 in which an individual with chronic blepharitis was injected in the left forearm with *S. aureus* protein A (2.5 ng) (White and Noble, 1980), and in the right forearm with killed *S. aureus* (10^7 cells), killed coagulase-negative staphylococci (10^7 cells) and saline as a control.

Rosacea (Fig. 1.10) is a unique condition in which there is both heavy skin colonization with *S. aureus*, noted particularly on the lid margins, and development of CMI to *S. aureus* (Seal *et al.*, 1995; Noble, 1997). This is associated with the typical histology in the skin of a perifollicular granuloma affecting the sebaceous gland. Treatment is discussed in Chapter 4 but it should be noted that rosacea patients with blepharitis improved considerably (and statistically) better than non-rosacea patients when treated with topical fusidic acid (Fucithalmic). It is believed that this occurred because of fusidic acid's cyclosporin-type effect, down-regulating Th-1 lymphocytes by inhibiting the tyrosine kinase pathway, as well as its antistaphylococcal activity (Seal *et al.*, 1995).

Contact dermatitis ('allergic' hypersensitivity)

This is an important manifestation of DH in the skin to an external antigen that has come into contact with its surface (Rietschel *et al.*, 1999). It often involves

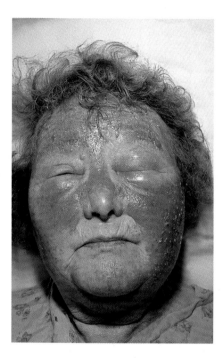

Figure 1.11: Acute contact dermatitis from Nivea cream.

skin creams (Fig. 1.11), lotions, eye drops or contact lens disinfecting fluids that contain a chemical compound acting as an allergen, or haptens including metal objects, such as buckles or wrist watches, that contain nickel and are held against the skin. The host gradually becomes 'sensitized' to the antigen from the development of activated Th-1 lymphocytes over time, varying from months to years. This results in the development of acute or subacute inflammation, from a minor eczematous response to severe induration, at the local site of antigen presentation, which subsides when the antigenic source is removed.

Thiomersal (thimerosal) is included as an antibacterial preservative in vaccines such as DPT (diphtheria, tetanus, pertussis) and tetanus toxoid and other products such as antiviral (*H. simplex*) creams (Rietschel *et al.*, 1999). This is not sensible as it is a well-known 'sensitizing' agent. Its use with vaccines, and their associated adjuvants, has resulted in causing DH to thiomersal in up to 7% of the Swedish population in whom sensitivity testing has been performed (Seal *et al.*, 1991). If any such 'sensitized' person then meets thiomersal as a component of a topical cream, drug or disinfecting fluid there will be acute or subacute inflammation at the site of application due to CMI (Fig. 1.8) until the offending product (antigen) has been removed. Since thiomersal *per se* is a weak bactericidal compound, and is rapidly broken down to toxic mercurial products, its use should be curtailed forthwith even though the toxic products are bactericidal

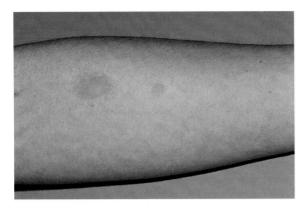

Figure 1.12: Wheal and flare at 15 minutes following subcutaneous injection of 2.5 ng *S. aureus* protein A.

(Seal *et al.*, 1991a; Seal and Amos, 1982). Other antimicrobial sensitisers include clioquinol (Vioform) and neomycin (Rietschel *et al.*, 1999). More rarely, therapeutic agents such as imidazole antifungal drugs and even corticosteroids can be 'sensitizers'.

While topical corticosteroids are often used to suppress inflammation of contact dermatitis, delayed hypersensitivity to them is being increasingly recognized by dermatologists. Boffa *et al.* (1996) found that 6% of their patients had a relevant DH reaction to corticosteroids, most commonly tixocortol-21-pivalate, hydrocortisone butyrate or budesonide (Wilkinson and English, 1991).

Immediate hypersensitivity (IgE) reaction

In sites such as the skin and conjunctiva, Th-2 lymphocytes play a key role in immediate hypersensitivity reactions. They produce IL-4 and IL-5 which stimulate B lymphocytes to switch to IgE production and to express IgE receptors (Fig. 1.2). Furthermore, IL-4 induces mast cell proliferation.

The typical presentation of the immediate hypersensitivity response in the skin is that of the 'wheal and flare' reaction occurring within 15 minutes of the allergen being in contact with the skin due to the release of histamine from mast cells. This can occur following natural exposure to the allergen or by skin testing with intradermal or subcutaneous injections. However, this type of reaction can also be elicited by purified protein A of the *S. aureus* cell wall (Fig. 1.12), following the subcutaneous injection of 2.5 ng. Protein A cross-binds the F_c receptors of IgE antibody fixed to mast cells, stimulating the release of histamine to give the 'wheal and flare' reaction.

Other presentations include that of acute papular dermatitis (Fig. 1.13), which is seen more typically with helminth and parasite infections. This type of

15

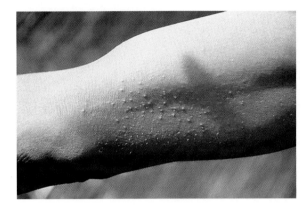

Figure 1.13: Acute papular onchodermatitis of *Onchocerca volvulus.* (Courtesy of Dr Murray McGavin.)

reaction occurs spontaneously, or when drug treatment is given, resulting in death of the worms and release of cellular antigens which can produce systemic reactions such as chills and fever. Diethylcarbamazine, a microfilaricide, is particularly associated with this reaction (Mazotti reaction).

The hyperimmunoglobulin E recurrent infection syndrome (Job's syndrome) was first described in 1966 for the presentation of recurrent 'cold' staphylococcal abscesses. The patients have eczema soon after birth and suffer from recurrent otitis, cellulitis and furunculosis. They have exceptionally high levels of IgE and a marked eosinophilia. Complement levels and PMN phagocytosis and killing are normal. Long-term antistaphylococcal antiseptic (chlorhexidine, hexachlorophene) and antibiotic therapy (Chapter 2) controls the recurrent infections for a reasonable period – relapse with pneumonia is a recognized complication.

Immune complex disease

This may cause skin sequelae from a systemic infection. This is reflected most seriously with necrotizing lesions in peripheral capillaries following systemic infection with *Neisseria meningitidis* (Fig. 1.14) or *Streptococcus pneumoniae* (Fig. 1.15), the latter causing bilateral peripheral symmetrical gangrene. It is thought that antigen–antibody complexes activate the complement cascade intravascularly, resulting in the disseminated intravascular coagulation (DIC) syndrome, which presents at the most extreme with peripheral symmetrical gangrene (Fig. 1.16). Early plasma exchange has been recommended to prevent progression of DIC and its sequelae. Restoring peripheral vascular perfusion is the main aim but often fails.

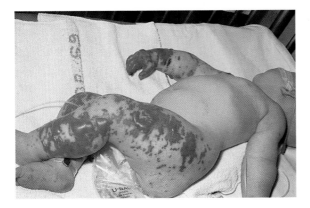

Figure 1.14: Late severe rash of meningococcal septicaemia.

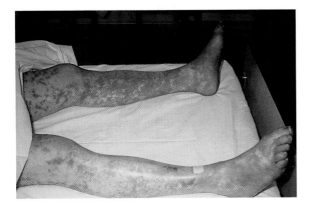

Figure 1.15: Early bilateral peripheral symmetrical gangrene due to *S. pneumoniae* septicaemia.

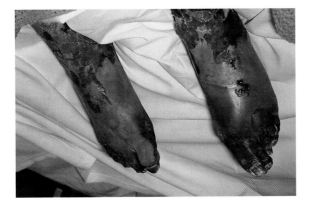

Figure 1.16: Late bilateral peripheral symmetrical gangrene due to *S. pneumoniae* septicaemia (cf. Fig. 1.15).

Other examples of immune complex-mediated skin disease during infections include papulonecrotic tuberculid and erythema nodosum or erythema multiforme. The latter are seen as manifestations of immune complex deposition in a variety of conditions from leprosy and coccidioidomycosis to orf and *Herpes simplex* infections.

Modification of the immune response

T cell function can be modified by drugs. Cytotoxic CD8 T cells are functionally inhibited by azathioprine. Cell-mediated immunity, or DH, can be modulated by drugs such as cyclosporin acting on Th-1 cells by suppressing the activity of the p56 and p59 tyrosine kinase cascade, blocking T cell activation. Fusidic acid, available as a topical skin preparation (Fucidin), as well as orally and parenterally, has a similar immunosuppressive action in addition to its antistaphylococcal effect. This may explain its beneficial effect in treating the blepharitis of rosacea, usually associated with both *S. aureus* colonization of the lids and systemically enhanced DH to its antigens (Seal *et al.*, 1995). However, topical use can lead to resistance developing in *S. aureus*.

Corticosteroids generally inhibit cytokine synthesis to suppress inflammation, including that resulting from infection (Rosenbaum, 1995). They reduce the activity of macrophages, but not necessarily their activation by cytokines. In addition, there is suppression of PMN activity. With corticosteroid treatment, there is progression of fungal, viral and protozoal infections, since functioning macrophages are required as 'scavenger' phagocytic cells to engulf and destroy these organisms. This has been well researched for *Acanthamoeba* in the cornea (van Klink *et al.*, 1996) and the results apply to the skin as well. While corticosteroids provide effective anti-inflammatory treatment in the short term, they are of no long-term benefit, and have no prophylactic role for managing infection. The use of corticosteroids for the late immunoinflammatory phenomena of onchocerciasis is considered specifically in Chapter 8.

2. ANTIMICROBIAL PHARMACOLOGY FOR THE SKIN AND WOUND

Antimicrobial effectiveness, tissue levels and drug interactions

The following section illustrates the efficacy of selected antimicrobial agents for pathogenic skin and wound organisms (Tables 2.1–2.6) and their adverse reactions with other drugs (Table 2.7). These data are tabulated below. For dosages of antibiotics for therapeutic use, refer to Appendix A. For laboratory methods, refer to Appendix B.

Mechanisms of action and effectiveness of selected antiviral drugs are given in Table 2.2. Mechanisms of action of the antibacterial and antifungal drugs are summarized in Table 2.5 and well described in detail in O'Grady F *et al.*, *Antibiotic and Chemotherapy* (1997).

Antimicrobial resistance is being recognized world-wide at an increasing rate. This can be due to mutation within individual bacteria or arise from transferable plasmids or transposons. Mutation tends to occur when surface infections, such as skin ulcers, are treated with a topical antibiotic and produces low-level resistance to a single antibiotic group in *S. aureus* and *Ps. aeruginosa* in particular. Plasmid transfer by conjugation can result in the rapid acquisition of high-level resistance to a number of different antibiotics simultaneously within and between bacterial species. In addition, progressive selection of resistant strains occurs with widespread use of an antibiotic such as ciprofloxacin, or other quinolones, with resistance now appearing in *S. aureus* and other important pathogens. This type of resistance has been very slow to develop in streptococci to penicillin but there are now penicillin-resistant pneumococci (*S. pneumoniae*), which can also be resistant to tetracycline and erythromycin. *S. pyogenes* (BHS Lancefield group A) has remained fully sensitive to penicillin, which is still the drug of choice to treat serious infection, but it may not be bactericidal in high dosage when clindamycin or vancomycin should be used in combination; this definitely applies for treatment of serious sepsis due to Lancefield group G BHS.

Table 2.2 lists the current drugs effective against HIV. The British HIV Association (BHIVA) guidelines for the treatment of HIV-infected adults with anti-retroviral therapy were first published three years ago (BHIVA, 1997). They have recently been revised and are now available on the BHIVA internet web site at 'www.aidsmap.com'. These guidelines have been written by physicians involved in the care of HIV-positive patients. Therapy now involves the use of three drugs, either two nucleoside analogue reverse transcriptase inhibitors (NRTIs) plus a protease inhibitor (PI), two NRTIs plus two PIs, two NRTIs plus a non-nucleoside analogue reverse transcriptase inhibitor (NNRTI) or three NRTIs.

Table 2.1 Antibiotic sensitivities and expected MICs for selected bacteria pathogenic for the skin and wound

	Penicillin	Ampl Amoxicillin	Flu/cloxacillin	Cefuroxime	Ceftazidime	Fusidic acid	Cipro-floxacin	Oxytetra-cycline	Chloram-phenicol	Vanco-mycin	Gentamicin/ Amikacin	Metroni-dazole
Staph. aureus[a,b]	R	R	S (0.1)	S (1–4)	(S) (2–6)	S (0.1)	S (1)	(S) (4)	S (4)	S (2)	S (0.25)	R
Coagulase-negative staphylococci[a,b]	R	R	S (0.1)	S (1–4)	(S) (2–6)	S (0.1)	S (1)	(S) (4)	S (4)	S (2)	S (0.25)	R
Streptococci[a,b]	S (0.03)	S (0.03)	S (0.1)	S (0.1)	S (0.25)	(S) (1–16)	(S) (4)	(S) (2)	S (4)	S (0.2)	R (16)	R
Corynebacteria and C. diphtheriae[a,b]	S (0.02–0.06)	S (0.02–0.06)	S (0.6)	S (0.5)	S	S	?S	?S	S (0.5–2)	S	S	R
P. acnes[b]	S (0.1)	S (0.1)	S (1)	S (0.1)	S (0.1)	S		S (0.1)	S (0.1)	S (1)	S (0.25)	R
Bacillus sp.[a]	R	R	R	R	R	S	S (0.25)	(S)	(S) (2.5–5)	S (0.2–4)	S (2)	R
N. gonorrhoeae/ meningitidis	S (0.1)	S (0.1)	R	S (0.06)	S (0.01)	S (0.05)	S (<0.1)	S (1)	S (2)	R	(S) (4)	R
H. influenzae[b]	(S) (1.0)	(S) (2–R)	R	S (0.5)	S (0.1)	R	S (<0.1)	(S) (8)	S (0.5)	R	S (0.5)	R
Coliforms	R	R	R	S (4)	S (0.1)	R	S (0.25)	(S) (8)	(S) (6)	R	S (0.5)	R
P. aeruginosa	R	R	R	R	S (4)	R	S (1)	R	R	R	S (2)	R
Anaerobic streptococci	S (1)	S (1)	(S)	S (1)	S (2)	R	R	(S) (1–12)	S (3–6)	S (0.5)	R	S (3–25)
Clostridia sp.[a,b]	S (0.3)	S (0.3)	S (1)	S (0.5)	S (1)	R	R	(S) (0.3/R)	S (4)	S (0.5)	R	S
Bacteroides sp.	(S) (0.1/R)	R	R	R	R	R	R	(S) (2/R)	(S) (8)	R	R	S

MICs: minimum inhibitory concentrations (mg/l).
[a] Sensitive to clindamycin.
[b] Sensitive to erythromycin and azithromycin.
S: sensitive.
(S): moderately sensitive.
R: resistant.

Table 2.2 Effects of selected antiviral drugs

Drug	HIV	CMV	HSV 1/2 HZV	HSV 1/2 IDU-R	HSV 1/2 VID-R	EBV	Adeno-virus	Measles Mumps
Inhibitors of viral DNA polymerase and nucleic acid analogues								
Ganciclovir (Cymevene)*	R	S	S	S	S	?	R	R
Foscarnet (Foscavir)	(S)	S	S	S	S	?	R	R
Cidofovir (Vistide)	R	S	S	?	?	(S)	S	R
Aciclovir (Zovirax)	R	R	S	S	?	(S)	R	R
Valaciclovir (Valtrex)	R	R	S	S	?	(S)	R	R
Penciclovir (Vectavir)	R	R	S	S	?	(S)	R	R
Famciclovir (Famvir)	R	R	S	S	?	(S)	R	R

Inhibitors of reverse transcriptase (nucleoside analogues)

Drug	HIV	CMV	HSV 1/2 HZV	HSV 1/2 IDU-R	HSV 1/2 VID-R	EBV	Adeno-virus	Measles Mumps
Zidovudine (azidothymidine, AZT) (Retrovir) Didanosine (ddI) (Videx) Zalcitabine (ddC) (Hivid) Stavudine (d4T) (Zerit) Lamivudine (3TC) (Epivir) Abacavir (Ziagen)	S/(R)	R	R	R	R	R	R	R

Inhibitors of reverse transcriptase (non-nucleoside analogues)

Drug	HIV	CMV	HSV 1/2 HZV	HSV 1/2 IDU-R	HSV 1/2 VID-R	EBV	Adeno-virus	Measles Mumps
Nevirapine (Viramune) Delavirdine (Rescriptor)** Efaviranz (Sustiva)	S	R	R	R	R	R	R	R

Protease inhibitors

Drug	HIV	CMV	HSV 1/2 HZV	HSV 1/2 IDU-R	HSV 1/2 VID-R	EBV	Adeno-virus	Measles Mumps
Saquinavir (Invirase) Indinavir (Crixivan) Ritonavir (Norvir) Nelfinavir (Viracept)	S	R	R	R	R	R	R	R

Valaciclovir is the oral pro-drug for aciclovir.
Famciclovir, the oral pro-drug for penciclovir, is effective against aciclovir-resistant HSV.
*Not an inhibitor of DNA polymerase.
**Not licensed.
S: sensitive;
(S): moderately sensitive.
R: resistant.
HIV: Human immuno-deficiency virus, CMV: Cytomegalovirus,
HSV: Herpes simplex virus, HZV: Herpes zoster virus,
EBV: Epstein-Barr virus.

Table 2.3 Antibiotic effects on selected fungi.

	Polyene antibiotics Amphotericin/ nystatin/ natamycin	Imidazole antibiotics Miconozole/ fluconazole etc.	Terbina- fine	5-Flucyto- sine
Candida albicans and yeasts	S	S	S/R	S
Aspergillus spp.	S	S/R	(S)	R
Malassezia spp.	(S)	S	S	?
Dermatophytes	(S)	S	S	R

Table 2.4 Antifungal agents used in dermatophyte infections.

Product	Available as
Benzoic acid compound	Whitfield's ointment
Undecenoates – various brands	Ointment, powder
Tolnaftate	Cream, powder, lotion
Imidazoles – clotrimazole, miconazole, econazole, sulconazole, ketoconazole, bifonazole	Cream, powder, lotion, spray, shampoo (ketoconazole)
Tioconazole nail solution[a], bifonazole urea[a]	Nail treatment
Itraconazole[a], fluconazole[a]	Oral preparations
Allylamines[a] – terbinafine, naftitine	Cream
Amorolfine[a]	Cream, nail lacquer
Ciclopiroxolamine	Cream
Griseofulvin	Oral preparations

[a]Expensive.

Table 2.5 Action of antibacterial and antifungal drugs relevant to the skin.

Class	Inhibitor of microbial function	Antimicrobial effect
Penicillins and cefalosporins	Cell wall production	Bactericidal
Fusidic acid	Protein synthesis	Bactericidal
4-hydroxyquinolones: ciprofloxacin, ofloxacin, sparfloxacin	DNA gyrase	Bactericidal
Tetracyclines: oxytetracycline, doxycycline	Protein synthesis	Bacteriostatic
Macrolides: erythromycin, azithromycin	Protein synthesis	Bacteriostatic/ Bactericidal
Aminoglycosides: gentamicin, amikacin, vancomycin	Protein synthesis	Bactericidal
Metronidazole	Metabolic function	Bactericidal
Aromatic diamidines: Propamidine, hexamidine, pentamidine	DNA synthesis	Staphylococcicidal/ Amoebistatic
Cationic antiseptics: chlorhexidine (bis-biguanide), PHMB (polyhexa-methylene biguanide)	Membrane function and leakage of cell electrolytes	Bactericidal/ Amoebicidal
Imidazoles: miconazole, fluconazole, ketoconazole	Cell membrane structure (14α demethylase)	Fungistatic
Allylamines: terbinafine, naftifine	Cell membrane structure (squalene epoxidase)	Fungicidal
Polyenes: amphotericin, natamycin, nystatin	Cell membrane structure	Fungicidal
Phenylmorpholine derivative: amorolfine	Ergosterol biosynthesis inhibitor	Fungicidal (dermatophytes only)

Table 2.6 Experimental concentrations of drugs (mg/l) within polymorphonuclear (PMN) cells and extracellular (EC) tissue. Data compiled from various sources including Lorian V (1996) Antibiotics in Laboratory Medicine; O'Grady et al. (1997) Antibiotics and Chemotherapy; Capecchi P et al. (1995) Pharmacokinetics and pharmacodynamics of neutrophil-associated ciprofloxacin in humans. *Clin Pharmacol Therapeut*, **57**, 446–453; and Pfizer Ltd (data on file for Azithromycin and Erythromycin).

	Ampi-cillin	Cephalo-thin	Cloxa-cillin	Fusidic acid	Peni-cillin	Tetra-cycline	Genta-micin	Rif-ampicin	Ciprof-loxacin	Erythro-mycin	Clinda-mycin	Azithro-mycin
PMN cells	8	<1	32.5	16	5	13	15	47	10.0	254	434	2260
Extracellular tissues	100	10	100	40	10	17.5	18	20	2.7	18	10	10
PMN (intra-cellular) :EC (extra-cellular) Ratio	0.08	<0.1	0.33	0.4	0.5	0.74	0.8	2.4	3.7	14	43	226

PMN = polymorphonuclear cell
EC = Extra-cellular concentration

Table 2.7 Drug interactions of systemic antibiotics used to treat skin and wound infections.

Systemic antibiotic	Interacting drug	Description of interaction
Antibacterial drugs		
Aminoglycosides	Cholinergics	Antagonizes the effect of cholinergics.
	Cytotoxics	Increases the risk of nephrotoxicity and ototoxicity from cisplatin.
	Diuretics – etacrynic acid and furosemide	Increases the risk of ototoxicity with high tone deafness and loss of balance. This combination is well recognized for toxicity to the neural epithelium of the inner ear but not the eye.
Cefalosporins	Alcohol	Cefamandole and cefoperazone can have an 'Antabuse' type of effect.
	Anticoagulants	Cefalosporins can enhance the effects of warfarin and nicoumalone.
	Probenecid	Increase serum concentration (deliberate) from reduced renal clearance.
Clindamycin	Muscle relaxants	Potentiates the effect of tubocurarine.
	Cholinergics	Antagonizes the effect of neostigmine.
Metronidazole	Alcohol	Gives an 'Antabuse' effect.
	Antacids	Decreases absorption.
	Anticoagulants	Enhance the effect of warfarin and nicoumalone by inhibiting metabolism.
	Antiepileptics	Inhibits the metabolism of phenytoin. Phenobarbital increases the metabolism of metronidazole.
	Cytotoxics	Inhibits the metabolism of 5-fluorocytosine (5-FC).
Macrolides	Any drug metabolized in liver	Inhibit hepatic metabolism of drugs.
Penicillins	Allopurinol	Ampicillin increases the occurrence of rashes by ×2 /×4.
	Anticoagulants	Potentiate their effect by decreasing vitamin K synthesis by bowel flora.
	Probenecid	Increase serum concentration (deliberate) from reduced renal clearance.
Quinolones	Any drug metabolized in liver	Inhibit hepatic metabolism of drugs such as warfarin and sulphonylurea (oral antidiabetic drugs) with risk of bleeding and hypoglycaemia; causes accumulation of theophylline and caffeine.
	NSAIDs (nonsteroidal anti-inflammatory drugs)	Increase risk of convulsions.
	Antacids, iron tablets	Decrease absorption of 4-hydroxyquinolones.

Table 2.7 *continued*

Systemic antibiotic	Interacting drug	Description of interaction
Rifampicin	Any drug metabolized in liver	Accelerates metabolism of most drugs.
Tetracyclines	Anticoagulants	Decrease plasma prothrombin activity. Decrease vitamin K production by gut bacteria, so increasing anticoagulant activity.
	Iron/antacids	Decrease absorption due to chelation
	Phenobarbital, phenytoin	Reduce plasma half-life by half for doxycycline.
Antifungal drugs		
Amphotericin	Aminoglycosides	Increases risk of ototoxicity and nephro-toxicity.
	Cyclosporin	Increases risk of nephrotoxicity.
5-fluorocytosine	Rifampicin	Increases metabolism, decreases efficacy.
	Anticoagulants	Increases anticoagulant effect.
	Sulphonylureas	Increases hypoglycaemic effect.
	Antiepileptics	Inhibits metabolism of phenytoin with increased risk of toxicity.
	Cyclosporin	Inhibits metabolism of cyclosporin with increased risk of toxicity.
Imidazoles (mico-nozole, fluconazole, etc.)	Antacids	Decreases absorption.
	Anticoagulants	Enhance the effect of warfarin and nicoumalone by inhibiting metabolism.
	Antiepileptics	Phenobarbital increases the metabolism of antifungal azoles.
	Cytotoxics	Ketoconazole/itraconazole/fluconazole inhibit the metabolism of cyclosporin.
	Antihistamines	Most azoles raise serum levels of terfenadine and astemizole.
Antiviral drugs		
Foscarnet	Pentamidine	Causes renal impairment and symptomatic hypocalcaemia.
	Gentamicin	Enhances renal toxicity of gentamicin.
Ganciclovir	Imipenem/cilastatin	Can cause 'Grand mal' epileptic seizures.
	Probenecid	Decreases renal elimination.
Zidovudine (AZT)	Pentamidine, ganciclovir, ampho-tericin, 5-FC	Enhances toxicity of nephrotoxic drugs.

3. INFECTION OF THE STRATUM CORNEUM AND EPIDERMIS

Bacterial infections

Impetigo

Impetigo is caused by *S. pyogenes* (BHS group A), *S. aureus* or by a mixed infection. Lesions begin as vesicles, rapidly becoming pustular, then develop thick yellow crusts (Fig. 3.1). When infection is due to *S. pyogenes* significant regional lymphadenopathy can occur. Impetigo is commonest in hot humid climates.

In the 1960s studies revealed that 50% of patients had one organism on culture, 75% of these due to *S. pyogenes* and 25% due to *S. aureus*. The remainder had mixed cultures of *S. pyogenes* and *S. aureus*, presenting with non-bullous pustular lesions. In many cases *S. pyogenes* could be recovered from clinically normal skin prior to the development of impetigo, and was considered the source of the infection. It was suspected, but not proven, that *S. aureus* was a secondary pathogen, rather than the primary cause of the infection, the source

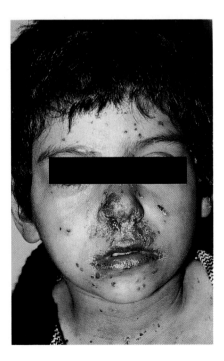

Figure 3.1: Impetigo due to *S. aureus*.

of which was thought to be nasal colonization. However, in recent years *S. aureus* has again become predominant, especially in most industrialized countries, as the cause of impetigo being found in approximately 85% of lesions and as the sole pathogen in 50% of cases (Darmstadt, 1997; Noble, 1997). An array of group I or II phage types of *S. aureus* are responsible. There is, however, an increasing incidence of streptococcal impetigo, due to *S. pyogenes* and group G beta-haemolytic streptococci, being reported from Japan (Adachi *et al.*, 1998) associated with atopic dermatitis; streptococcci were isolated alone in 28% of cases and with *S. aureus* in 72%.

Therapy should be given with topical antistaphylococcal (and antistreptococcal) antibiotics such as mupirocin or with an antiseptic cream such as chlorhexidine. Short-term systemic therapy with oral first-generation cefalosporins or Augmentin (amoxicillin/clavulanic acid) or erythromycin may be needed. Hygiene instruction should be reviewed for the family.

Bullous lesions are considered to be pathognomonic of infection due to *S. aureus*. They occur less frequently and in only 10% of patients from whom *S. aureus* is isolated. Patients present with both intact bullae and recently ruptured lesions (Fig. 3.2). A very thin golden 'varnish-like' crust forms which is difficult to elevate or remove. When these bullous lesions heal the skin can be depigmented, reflecting dermal involvement. Interestingly, scalp lesions of bullous impetigo never occur. This is one end of a spectrum of which staphyococcal scalded skin syndrome (SSSS) is the other. Like SSSS, the blisters are the result of epidermolytic toxins ETA and ETB (Chapter 4) which are serine proteases.

Exfoliative toxin (ET) production and coagulase serotypes have been examined recently in 283 isolates of *S. aureus* from impetigo with bullae, SSSS and non-toxic conditions using the polymerase chain reaction with primers for ETA and ETB (Kanazaki *et al.*, 1997). They found ET producers in 100% (6/6) of SSSS isolates and 69% (100/144) of impetigo isolates, compared to 3% (3/112) in atopic dermatitis and 0% (0/21) in furunculosis. Coagulase typing separated impetigo strains (type I or V) from furunculosis strains (type IV) – SSSS strains were all type I.

Its most severe form, 'pemphigus (impetigo) neonatorum', presents in newborn infants, in which it is highly infectious with a considerable mortality rate. Large bullae containing thin pus cover the body surface to be severe and fatal. There is little to separate this from the severe epidermal necrosis and blistering of exfoliative dermatitis of the staphlyococcal scalded skin syndrome (Fig. 4.10, Chapter 4); differential diagnosis is from congenital syphilis.

Multiple cases of *S. pyogenes* impetigo occur in families, particularly in hot humid regions, especially in children living closely together with poor hygiene and lack of fresh water. In subtropical areas, such as the southern USA, impetigo develops in July to September in contrast to the winter–spring seasonal incidence of streptococcal respiratory infections. Thus streptococcal skin infec-

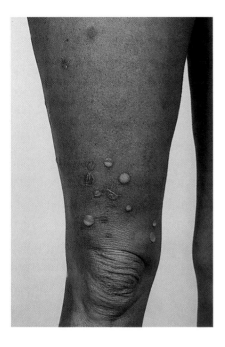

Figure 3.2: Bullous lesions (intact and ruptured) of impetigo due to *S. aureus*.

tion is spread from patients with active lesions to others in close contact without prior respiratory infection being required. This has led to the identification of 'impetigo' strains of *S. pyogenes* with T antigen complexes 3/13/B3264 and 8/25/Imp.19. These 'impetigo' strains may colonize the respiratory tract as a secondary event.

Association with minor trauma, especially mosquito bites (Fig. 1.7), is common. In addition, flies can carry *S. pyogenes* on their legs to transmit the organism between different individuals. Rates of infection are higher in hot humid than hot dry climates. This was well demonstrated in Colombia when the prevalence of impetigo was compared between a similar racial population living at sea level and at a height of 2000 metres. There may be various risk factors underlying this difference including climate and relative humidity, prevalence of biting insects, frequency of work-related trauma, personal hygiene and avail-ability of running water and type of crowded living quarters. Other factors include the presence of infestations, particularly scabies.

The association of acute glomerulonephritis with impetigo (or pyoderma) due to *S. pyogenes* was recognized in children 30 years ago (Poon-King *et al.*, 1973) and continues today but much less frequently in the southern USA. In contrast, rheumatic fever has never been described following *S. pyogenes* skin infection (only following throat infection), although this does not rule out the possibility.

The clinical features of impetigo associated with nephritis do not differ from those of uncomplicated streptococcal impetigo. The factor predisposing to the development of glomerulonephritis is the particular subtype of *S. pyogenes* involved – M type 49 and T type 25/Imp.19 are mainly implicated.

Specific gene correlates of 'skin' and 'throat' types of *S. pyogenes* have been investigated recently (Bessen *et al.*, 1996). The 'emm' gene structure was analysed for 105 isolates obtained from patients with well-defined impetigo, uncomplicated pharyngitis and acute rheumatic fever. Four 'emm' gene types were found to exist, defined by nucleotide sequence differences in regions encoding the peptidoglycan-spanning domain of M proteins. Strong correlations were made between disease patterns and the arrangements of these genes, providing a genetic basis for historical reference to 'skin', 'throat' and 'rheumato-genic' types.

Pyoderma

Pyoderma presents as single or multiple superficial pustular spots (Figs 3.3 and 3.4), often caused by *S. pyogenes*, together with respective lymphadenopathy which may form a purulent 'bubo'. Like impetigo, it is usually found in close contacts. There may be associated scabetic infection. Therapy with a penicillin or a cefalosporin is usually successful.

Pyoderma occurs in hot climates in similar circumstances to impetigo and may be associated with nephritogenic strains of *S. pyogenes*. Unlike impetigo strains, however, pyodermal strains of *S. pyogenes* do not normally colonize the throat, except during epidemics of nephritis, suggesting possible pathogenicity via this route.

When pyoderma is caused by *S. pyogenes* M type 55 ('Potter A'), acute glomerulonephritis may develop, especially in children under 14 years. In the past, this strain has caused large outbreaks of glomerulonephritis in Trinidad and Israel (Lasch *et al.*, 1971; Poon-King *et al.*, 1973). In contrast, *S. pyogenes* M type 52 ('Potter B') has caused outbreaks of pyoderma in Trinidad and Minnesota, USA, but without nephritis. Similarly, *S. pyogenes* M type 'Potter C' has been isolated from an outbreak of pyoderma in a kibbutz in Israel without sequelae (Seal *et al.*, 1991b), but an outbreak of pyoderma with it in South Africa was associated with acute glomerulonephritis. Interestingly, this latter strain ('Potter C') was first isolated from throat carriage of patients with rheumatic fever in Trinidad; its role there remains speculative but it may have been 'rheumatogenic' as other pyoderma strains may have been 'nephritogenic' when colonizing the throat.

An epidemic of acute post-streptococcal glomerulonephritis (APSGN) was reported among aboriginal children in Australia in 1995 (Streeton *et al.*, 1995). They screened children aged 2–14 to identify all cases and found it in 58 (10%)

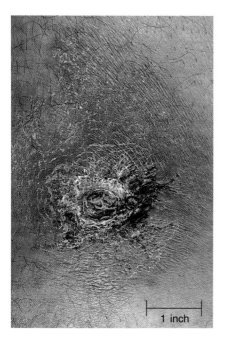

Figure 3.3: Pyoderma caused by *S. pyogenes*.

1 inch

of 583 children; a further 245 had microscopic haematuria. Some 34% of children had skin sores (pyoderma); *S. pyogenes* was isolated from 71% of skin swabs. The authors found that the prevalence of skin sores and *S. pyogenes* from skin swabs was greater in children with APSGN than those with microscopic haematuria than those with normal urine. A marked decline in APSGN occurred after the mass administration of penicillin.

In another recent study (Parra *et al.*, 1998), 153 patients from South America aged 2–23 with APSGN were studied. The site of initial infection was skin in 84 (55%), throat in 55 (36%) and unknown in 14 (9%). They tested serum for antibodies to streptococcal proteinase (erythrotoxin B) and its precursor, zymogen, which are putative nephritogenic antigens in these patients and controls with and without impetigo and pharyngitis. They found that anti-zymogen titres were consistently superior as markers of streptococcal infection in APSGN to either ASO or ADNase B titres.

Eczema and its relationship with *S. aureus*

Atopic subjects prone to eczema, but without active lesions, are heavily colonized (approximately 50% but up to 70%) by *S. aureus* on skin sites such as forehead, eyelids, cheek, axilla, groin, toe web and mucosae such as nose and

31

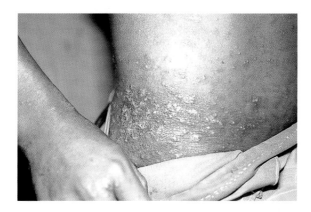

Figure 3.4:
Extensive scabies and pyoderma.

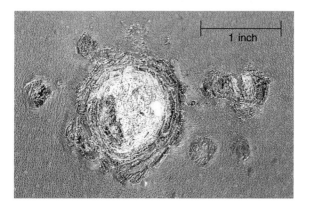

1 inch

Figure 3.5: Ecthyma due to *S. pyogenes*.

conjunctivae (Tuft *et al.*, 1992; Noble, 1997). In active atopic dermatitis these rates would approach 100%. Such skin colonization with *S. aureus* in atopes, who constitute 25% of the population, is often ignored or not understood by Infection Control personnel (Chapter 11).

The mechanisms that permit colonization of atopic skin, or prevent it in normal skin, may relate to susceptibility to particular fatty acids (linoleic and linolenic). Atopic subjects are considered to have a deficiency in their fatty acid metabolism (Noble, 1997). In addition, *S. aureus* adheres better to the keratinocytes of patients with atopic dermatitis than to those of normals, possibly due to the exposure of adhesins (Cole and Silverberg, 1986).

Ecthyma

Superficial ulceration (ecthyma) often occurs on the legs as multiple lesions (Fig. 3.5) due to *S. pyogenes* infection in hot climates with poor hygiene. The pathol-

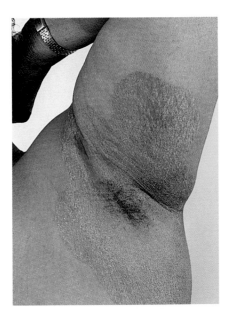

Figure 3.6: Erythrasma.

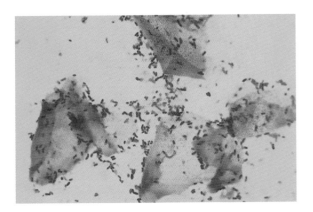

Figure 3.7: Gram stain of *Corynebacterium minutissimum* causing erythrasma ($\times$1000).

ogy involves both epidermis and dermis. It does not usually develop into deep ulcers but may do so. It is not associated with other streptococcal sequelae. Therapy with a penicillin or a cefalosporin is effective but post-infective scarring is common.

Erythrasma

Infection of the axilla, groin or interdigital spaces (Fig. 3.6) with irritation, inflammation and scaly lesions can be due to *Corynebacterium minutissimum* which is recognized as short Gram-positive rods on a skin scraping (Fig. 3.7). Lesions

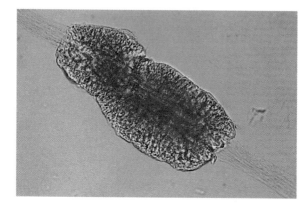

Figure 3.8: Trichomycosis axillaris of hair shaft due to *Corynebacterium tenuis* (×200).

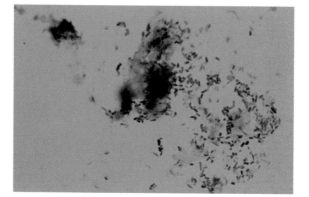

Figure 3.9: Gram stain of *Coryne-bacterium tenuis* (×1000).

do not have a prominent margin and the scales diffusely cover the surface. The organism possesses keratolytic properties. The clinical lesion is brown-red and shiny. It gives a striking pink fluorescence in ultraviolet (Wood's) light (365 nm). Treatment includes oral erythromycin 250 mg four times a day, azole creams (miconazole, clotrimazole), fusidic acid 2% (Fucidin cream or ointment) or neomycin cream. The infection is often indolent and may recur despite treatment.

Trichomycosis axillaris

This is due to *Corynebacterium tenuis*, which causes an infection of the external surface of the hair shaft with palpable nodules (Fig. 3.8). It is normally noticed as an accompanying feature of axillary hyperhidrosis but may present with variously coloured concretions on axillary or pubic hair. There is no pruritus and the patient is asymptomatic. The Gram-positive organism is illustrated in Fig. 3.9. Treatment involves shaving off infected hairs.

Otitis externa

Infection of the epithelium of the pinna, or external auditatory meatus, causing a weeping irritating inflammation, is due to Gram-negative bacteria such as *Pseudomonas aeruginosa*, Gram-positive bacteria including staphylococci, or fungi such as *Aspergillus niger* or *fumigatus*, *Scedosporium apiospermum* and *Candida* spp. In many cases the infection is secondary to another inflammatory process such as seborrhoeic dermatitis or allergic contact dermatitis, for example that due to neomycin or clioquinol in topical preparations applied to the ear. This results in cell-mediated immunity to the drug developing, with chronic inflammation. If the condition appears to be aggravated by therapy this should be withdrawn. Careful aural toilet is required with removal of debris and fungal material from the external auditory meatus. Cleansing can be performed with saline. A local astringent of aluminium acetate can be used as an 'ear drop'. If corticosteroids are introduced, they should *not* contain an antibiotic. An antibiotic should only be used selectively following culture for bacteria and fungi. Antifungals used successfully have included nystatin powder puffed into the ear for *Aspergillus* and *Candida* infections, as well as clotrimazole (Canestan), available as powder, solution and cream, and clioquinol (Vioform). Beware that allergic dermatitis can develop to clioquinol (Rietschel *et al.*, 1999).

Fungal infections

All fungi are heterotropic and must exist as saprophytes or parasites. Relatively few of the quarter of a million species recognized are pathogens of humans or animals. Those that are pathogenic in skin are either yeasts, such as *Candida albicans*, or dermatophytes. Subcutaneous mycoses are considered in Chapter 9. Sampling and identification are given in Appendix B, while therapeutic possibilities are listed in Chapter 2 and Appendix A.

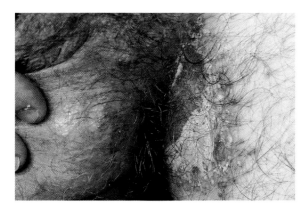

Figure 3.10:
Candida albicans
intertrigo of
perineum.

35

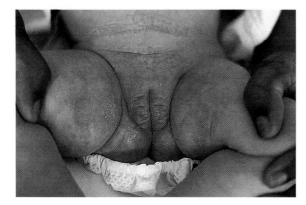

Figure 3.11: Nappy rash in baby due to *Candida albicans.*

Yeasts

Candida albicans is a budding yeast that forms a pseudomycelium when invading tissue. It stains Gram positive. It causes a bright red, irritating rash under warm, moist folds of skin such as the breasts, scrotum (Fig. 3.10) or prepuce (balanitis), under bandages (which can be due to cross-infection in hospital – Chapter 11) and in babies around the genitals and buttocks ('nappy' rash) (Fig. 3.11). A clinical hallmark of infection is the presence of satellite pustules distal to the edge of the rash. It can cause cross-infection in neonatal units (refer to Chapter 11). Occasionally, *C. albicans* will invade the tissue from these sites, particularly in immunocompromised individuals with long-term intravenous lines, to cause a candidaemia with vascular invasion of organs including the retina, to cause fulminant endophthalmitis. Refer to Chapter 2 and Appendix A for treatment.

Candida albicans can infect the nail in three ways. The commonest is onycholysis associated with paronychia. Complete destruction of the nail plate is seen in some patients with the rare immunodeficiency state of chronic mucocutaneous candidiasis (see below). In addition, uncommonly it can invade the distal and lateral nail plate, without causing total nail dystrophy, particularly in women with Raynaud's phenomenon or Cushing's syndrome. These cases respond well to oral antifungal imidazole drugs such as itraconazole. Finally, it may be isolated from under the nail plate in patients with onycholysis due to other causes, when it is present as a mixed colonization.

Persistent *C. albicans* infection of the mouth and sometimes the oesophagus, skin (intertriginous and other sites) and nails, refractory to conventional topical therapy, is a distinct syndrome – 'chronic mucocutaneous candidosis'. It may present in childhood associated with immunodeficiency or appear in adulthood associated with a thymoma or systemic lupus erythematosus, or it can be the initial presentation of HIV/AIDS. It is not possible precisely to identify the immune deficit responsible and a substantial minority have no apparent deficit at all. However, a variety of defects of cell-mediated immunity have been incriminated, together with defects in phagocytic killing by polymorphonuclear cells and macrophages. Predisposition in some individuals appears to be genetically determined as either an autosomal dominant or recessive trait which may be associated with endocrinopathy such as hypoparathyroidism or hypothyroidism. Treatment is difficult and requires a combined approach of systemic and topical antifungal drugs with maintenance therapy in between acute attacks.

Dermatophytes

The commonest fungal infections of skin are due to dermatophytes from three genera – *Trichophyton* spp., *Microsporum* spp. and *Epidermophyton floccosum*. In addition, there are the non-dermatophyte infections of skin and nails, such as the dermatomycoses caused by *Scytalidium* spp. and onychomycosis caused by other non-dermatophyte moulds. The tropical varieties are given in Chapter 9.

Invasion of the epidermis by dermatophytes begins with adherence between arthroconidia and keratinocytes of the stratum corneum, followed by penetration through and between cells and the development of a host response. Dermatophytes produce a variety of proteolytic enzymes with, as shown in *Trichophyton mentagrophytes*, both cell-free and membrane-bound keratinases. Clinically, there is heterogeneity in substrate preference. All dermatophyte species invade the stratum corneum but they vary in their capacity to invade the hair and nail. *Trichophyton rubrum* rarely invades hair but frequently invades nail. *Epidermophyton floccosum* never invades hair and only occasionally nail. Dermatophytes do not penetrate beyond the stratum corneum due to host defence from humoral and cell-mediated immunity. Humoral antibodies to dermatophytes are not protective. The development of sensitized T lymphocytes is essential for cell-mediated immunity (refer to Chapter 2).

The reason for persistent infections and the relationship to a failure of immunity is not well understood. There is an association between the presence of atopy and chronic dermatophytosis, with a high proportion of those with persistent disease having atopy with active disease (asthma or hay fever) and raised IgE levels. Patients with severe atopy are known to have a depression of cell-mediated immunity (Chapter 2) which is probably responsible. In addition, dermatophytes may produce immunomodulatory antigens.

When invading the epidermis, the dermatophytes cause intensely irritating lesions that weep from excoriation. They tend to invade moist skin sites such as toe webs (tinea pedis) (Fig. 3.12), perineal areas (tinea cruris) (Fig. 3.13), the face (tinea facei) (Fig. 3.14) and the scalp (tinea capitis) (Fig. 3.15), as well as the body (tinea corporis (Fig. 3.16) and the hands (tinea manuum) (Fig. 3.17). The clinical appearances are the result of direct damage to the keratinized tissue

37

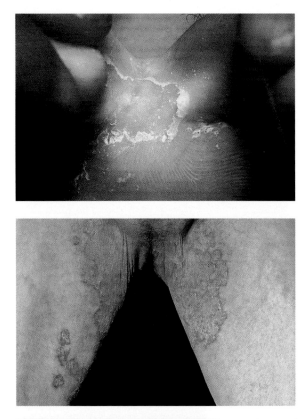

Figure 3.12: Tinea pedis due to *Trichophyton rubrum.*

Figure 3.13: Tinea cruris due to *Epidermophyton floccosum.*

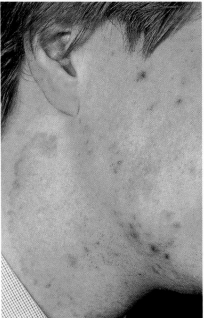

Figure 3.14: Tinea facei due to *Trichophyton rubrum.*

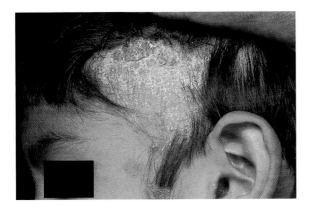

Figure 3.15: Tinea capitis due to *Trichophyton violaceum.*

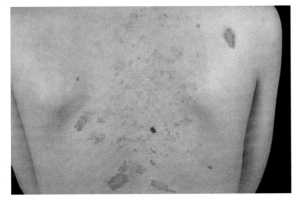
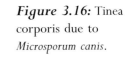

Figure 3.16: Tinea corporis due to *Microsporum canis.*

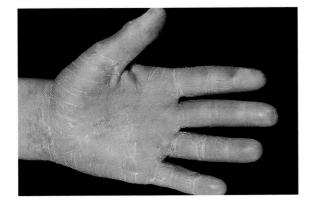

Figure 3.17: Tinea manuum due to *Trichophyton rubrum.*

39

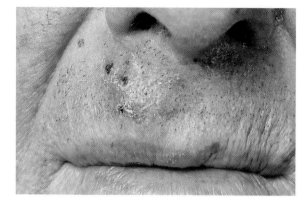

Figure 3.18: Tinea incognito (steroid treated) due to *Trichophyton rubrum*.

and of the inflammatory host response which varies widely. *Trichophyton rubrum* often causes a dry-type simple hyperkeratosis, while at the other extreme are the pustular highly inflammatory lesions or kerions seen most frequently in zoophilic infections such as those caused by *Trichophyton verrucosum*. The dermal infiltrate contains histiocytes and lymphocytes and is perivascular. However, there may be a pustular reaction with acute inflammatory changes in the epidermis mimicking 'contact hypersensitivity'. Other possibilities include lesions similar to erythema multiforme with subepidermal bullae and an infiltration by eosinophils.

In annular ringworm (tinea circinata), the rim of the lesion is marked by inflammatory changes with a perivascular infiltrate of lymphocytes. There is less inflammation in the central zone, probably because of elimination of the fungus from the stratum corneum, while fungal growth proceeds centrifugally. The epidermal turnover is normal within the ring but four times greater at its border. The exception to this is tinea imbricata, due to *Trichophyton concentricum*, in which central clearance is only partial with successive waves of fungal growth in skin previously cleared of infection, although overall expansion of the lesion is centrifugal.

Lesions can either resolve slowly on their own from the immunological reaction or persist for years if no treatment is given. If the patient is on corticosteroids, for a mistaken diagnosis or with systemic treatment, the lesion can be severe (tinea incognito – Figure 3.18). Typically, the raised margin is diminished, scaling is lost and inflammation is reduced. It keeps recurring, however, when the steroid treatment is stopped, resulting in a 'dermatitis' with papules, tiny pustules and nodules with a brownish discoloration, especially in groin infection. If steroid treatment is continued to suppress the inflammation, atrophy, telangectasia and striae occur. Antifungal treatment should be given to eradicate the infection – refer to Chapter 2 and Appendix A.

Dermatophyte infections can be more severe and extensive in diabetics and/or when the skin is enclosed, for example within a plaster cast (Fig. 3.19).

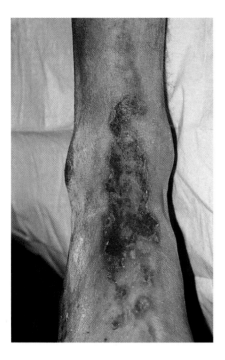

Figure 3.19: Ulcerated infection of dorsum and plantar surfaces of foot due to *Trichophyton mentagrophytes* var. *interdigitale* in a neuropathic diabetic whose leg had been placed in a plaster cast.

Tinea capitis, or ringworm of the scalp, presents with hair loss due to invasion of hair shafts by a dermatophyte fungus. Tinea barbae, affecting the beard area in males only, is essentially similar. Many species of dermatophyte are capable of invading the hair shaft but some species have a predilection to do so, for example *Microsporum audouinii*, *T. schoenleinii* and *T. violaceum*. In contrast, *E. floccosum*, *T. concentricum* and *T. mentagrophytes var. mentagrophytes* are exceptional in never causing tinea capitis. All dermatophytes invading the hair shaft can also

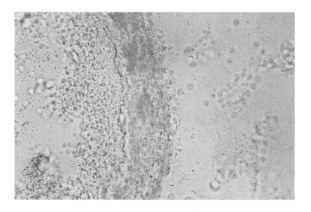

Figure 3.20:
Ectothrix of hair shaft (×200).

Table 3.1   Types of dermatophyte causing ringworm.

Name of lesion (synonym)	Site	Common causes
Tinea capitis	Scalp	Ectothrix: (large spore) *T. verrucosum, mentagrophytes,* (small spore) *M. audouinii, ferrugineum* and *canis* Endothrix: *T. tonsurans* and *violaceum* Favus: *T. schoenleinii*
Tinea barbae	Beard and moustache (male)	*T. verrucosum*
Tinea faciei (tinea faciale)	Chin and upper lip (female)	*T. mentagrophytes* var. *mentagrophytes, rubrum* and *concentricum; M. audouinii* and *canis*
Tinea corporis (tinea circinata)	Trunk and limbs	All dermatophytes
Tinea cruris (dhobie itch)	Perineum	*T. rubrum* and *mentagrophytes; E. floccosum*
Tinea manuum	Hand	*T. rubrum* and *mentagrophytes; E. floccosum*
Tinea pedis (athlete's foot)	Interdigital spaces of foot	*T. rubrum, mentagrophytes* var. *interdigitale* and *E. floccosum*
Tinea unguium	Nails	Associated with hand and foot infection: *T. rubrum, mentagrophytes* and *soudanense* and *E. floccosum* Associated with scalp infection: *T. tonsurans, violaceum* and *schoenleinii*
Tinea incognito (steroid-associated tinea)	Any part of body	All dermatophytes

invade the stratum corneum and many infect nails as well. The species of fungus causing scalp infections in a community varies geographically as well as over time.

Infection of hair shafts can involve the production of conidia (spores) on the external (ectothrix) (Fig. 3.20) or internal (endothrix) aspects of the hair shaft, or the fungi may die off within hair leaving air spaces, which occurs in favus. Very inflammatory lesions of the scalp are known as kerions. Tinea capitis varies widely in presentation depending on the level of host resistance and inflammatory response. It can vary in clinical expression from a few broken hairs with little scaling to a severe painful inflammatory mass covering most of the scalp. The cardinal features are partial hair loss with some inflammatory reaction. Hairs should be sampled as given in Appendix B.

Large-spored ectothrix infections, where chains of arthroconidia appear around the external surface of the hair shaft, are caused predominantly by *Trichophyton* species (Table 3.1). Small-spored ectothrix infections caused by *Microsporum* species (Table 3.1) present as circular patches of partial alopecia with numerous broken-off hairs. Inflammation is minimal but there is fine scaling with a sharp margin. Endothrix infections are caused by *T. tonsurans* or *violaceum*. They present as multiple patchy areas of baldness, often with little inflammation and thus minimal scaling. Often there are black dots of a swollen hair shaft when the affected hair breaks at the surface of the scalp. Favus infection, due to *T. schoenleinii*, is characterized by the formation of yellow crusts called scutula. Each scutulum develops round a hair which pierces it centrally. These crusts enlarge to become confluent. Early lesions are less dramatic with perifollicular redness and some matting of the hair. It can lead to extensive patchy hair loss with cicatricial alopecia. The best treatment at present is oral griseofulvin (Fulcin) 10–20 mg/kg once daily; contraindications include liver failure, lupus erythematosus, porphyria and pregnancy. Alternative treatments include terbinafine, itraconazole or fluconazole. Topical therapy alone is ineffective but shampooing with selenium sulphide or ketoconazole may limit spread within families and reduce carriage.

Tinea unguium or onychomycosis (due to dermatophytes) (Fig. 3.21) represents invasion of the nail plates by species of dermatophytes (Table 3.1). It occurs in all parts of the world and has been caused by various species, although *T. rubrum* is the commonest cause. Invasion of the nail plate occurs from the lateral nail fold or from the free edge. A network of channels and lacunae is formed, leading to opacity and eventual destruction of the nail plate. Oral therapy is required with terbinafine 250 mg daily for 6 weeks (fingernails) or 12 weeks

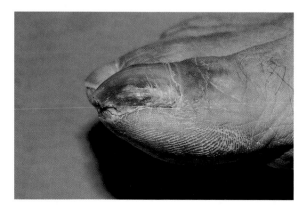

Figure 3.21:
Onychomycosis due to *T. interdigitale*.

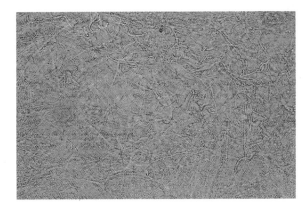

Figure 3.22:
Potassium hydroxide
preparation of skin
scraping showing
hyphae *(×200)*.

(toenails) or itraconazole 200 mg twice daily for 1 week repeated every month for 2–4 months. Fluconazole at 300 mg weekly is an alternative. Griseofulvin can be used but is less effective. Adjunctive topical therapy (Chapter 2 and Appendix A) can also be given – for instance amorolfine, as well as partial nail removal using 40% urea. Onychomycosis can also be caused by *Scytalidium* spp. (Chapter 9) and non-dermatophyte moulds.

Examination with Wood's light (ultraviolet wavelength at 365 nm) excites hair infected by certain dermatophytes (including all species of *Microsporum* genus) to produce a characteristic brilliant green fluorescence. The hair remains fluorescent after the fungus is no longer viable; the fluorescent substance can be extracted from the hair in hot water. Common sources of error with detecting fungus-infected hairs include a blue/purple fluorescence produced by ointments containing petrolatum; scales, serum and exudates; an insufficiently darkened room; light reflected from a white coat and the fact that not all fungi produce fluorescence. It is therefore most useful in areas of the world where infection by *Microsporum* spp. predominates.

Investigation should include skin scrapings (Fig. 3.22) and microscopy of hairs (Fig 3.20) and/or nail clippings. These should be sampled and examined as given in Appendix B. Hyphal fragments can be recognized when the sample is suspended in 5 to 30% potassium hydroxide. The sensitivity of various other techniques is given in Appendix B.

Dermatophytide ('id') reactions

These have been variously called microsporides, trichophytides or epidermophytides (according to genus). They represent a non-infective cutaneous eruption caused by an allergic response to a distant focus of dermatophyte infection. The suggested mechanism is one similar to that of erythema nodosum; on occasions only, erythema multiforme and annulare and urticaria may be manifestations of an allergic reaction to an active dermatophyte infection, but other causes should be excluded. Another common 'id' reaction is acute vesicular eczema. The requirements for the diagnosis are:

1. A proven inflammatory dermatophyte infection.
2. A distant eruption free of active fungus infection.
3. Spontaneous disappearance of the reactionary rash when the active lesion settles with or without treatment.

The dermatophytide can consist of a widespread eruption of small follicular papules, often symmetrical and severe on the trunk. The follicular papules may be topped by horny spines. The common cause is a scalp ringworm kerion due to *T. verrucosum*. It may also appear as a pompholyx-like lesion affecting the web spaces and palmar surfaces of the fingers.

Antibiotic production by dermatophyte fungi

Dermatophytes were first investigated for antibiotic production to explain why 86% of *S. aureus* isolates from the skin of hedgehogs were resistant to penicillin (Smith and Marples, 1965). An antibiotic substance resembling penicillin G was produced in the laboratory at a concentration of 7 U/ml by *T. mentagrophytes* var. *erinacei* isolated from the hedgehog. Penicillin production was also demonstrated in rabbit skin infected with this dermatophyte. It was considered that *S. aureus* caused secondary infection of the dermatophyte lesions in the animal and thereby developed resistance, representing a 'natural' source for the emergence of antibiotic-resistant mechanisms. This situation was later found in humans, when it was shown that patients infected with antibiotic-producing strains of dermatophytes more frequently carried cocci resistant to penicillin with a lower bacterial skin load (Youssef *et al.*, 1979). Hence, the bacterial flora causing secondary infection of a dermatophyte lesion will be influenced by the ability of the fungus to produce inhibitory substances.

Non-dermatophyte infections of the epidermis

Pityriasis versicolor

This is also known as tinea flava or dermatomycosis. It represents a mild chronic infection of the skin by *Malassezia* yeasts. It is characterized by scaly, discoloured areas on the upper trunk (Fig. 3.23), which may be depigmented to give rise to a differential diagnosis of vitiligo. There is complaint of a patchy and varying change of skin colour with mild irritation. If there is a cellular response, it

45

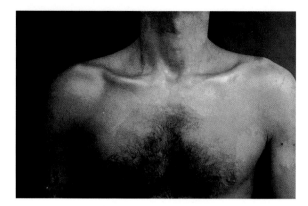

Figure 3.23:
Clinical lesion of
pityriasis versicolor
due to *Malassezia* spp.
(Courtesy of Prof. G
Senthamilselvi,
Chennai.)

consists of hyperkeratosis and a mild inflammatory infiltrate of cell-mediated type with memory T cells and macrophages. There can also be an accumulation of Langerhans' cells in the epidermis (Chapter 2). Skin scrapings should be performed with use of Parker's stain (Appendix B), when the presence of a characteristic coarse mycelium, fragmented to short filaments (2–5 μm wide × 25 μm long), and spherical yeasts (2–8 μm in diameter) confirm the diagnosis (Fig. 3.24). Laboratory culture with olive oil medium is not helpful as *Malassezia* spp. are members of the normal skin flora.

Other *Malassezia* spp. which are members of the normal flora have been associated with seborrhoeic dermatitis on the face and scalp. The pathogenesis of this condition still remains obscure, but the rash is thought to represent local failure of regulation of the inflammatory response. Seborrhoeic dermatitis may be particularly severe in HIV-positive individuals.

Black piedra

This consists of a fungal infection confined to hair shafts resulting in the formation of hard, dark superficial nodules 1 mm or more in diameter. It affects hairs on the scalp, beard, moustache or pubic areas. The mycelial fungus *Piedraia hortae* grows into the hair shaft, which may fracture easily. Treatment involves shaving the affected area to effect a cure. Whitfield's ointment (Appendix B) can be used to prevent recurrence.

White piedra

This consists of a fungal infection confined to hair shafts resulting in the formation of soft, white, grey or brown superficial nodules. It may affect the scalp, pubic

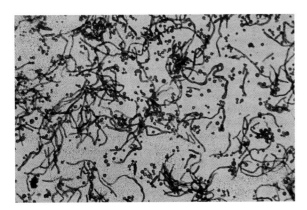

Figure 3.24:
Malassezia in skin scrapings (×200) (Parker's Quink stain).

area or axillae. It is caused by the *Trichosporon* spp. of yeasts including *T. beigelii*. It has a similar distribution to black piedra. The fungus grows around the hair shaft, which breaks off easily. Diagnosis is confirmed by examining the hair in Parker's stain when the gelatinous nodules around the hair formed by *Trichosporon* spp. take up the stain immediately. Treatment is best effected by shaving.

Viral infections

Poxvirus infections

One of the major medical advances of this century has been the global eradication of smallpox. However, the discontinuation of population-based vaccination with the vaccinia virus, derived from cowpox, has resulted in the majority of people now being susceptible to smallpox. Old laboratory stocks of the virus were destroyed, which was essential as the disease spread rapidly from person to person and was often fatal.

Vaccination

Vaccination was first practised in 1798 when Jenner inoculated a boy on the arm with exudate obtained from a cowpox lesion on the hand of a dairy-maid. When this boy was exposed to scarification with the variola (smallpox) virus 2 months later, no illness resulted and there was no local lesion demonstrating effective immunity. Present strains of vaccinia are avirulent mutants of obscure parentage. Vaccinia virus is a similar DNA virus to smallpox, of the same size and morphology on transmission electron microscopy (TEM), but can be distinguished by chick embryo inoculation.

47

Many techniques were described for vaccination but the simplest was a single scratch 5 mm long through one drop of the preparation (vaccine lymph) which was allowed to air dry in situ. In a non-immune person a papule developed at the site of the inoculation after 3–4 days, which became vesicular in 5–6 days and pustular in 8–10 days with surrounding inflammation. The pustule healed with a crust which was desquamated around the twenty-first day, leaving a depressed scar. Persons who had been recently vaccinated and possessed adequate immunity could give no reaction at all or an accelerated response of papule–vesicle–pustule. Primary vaccination of children was best performed in the second year of life but has not been performed routinely on children in the UK since 1971.

Problems with vaccination were legion. They included secondary cases (up to 55 per year in the UK), when approximately half were person-to-person spread from deliberate vaccination while, in the other half, infection arose by accidental use of the vaccine preparation – it was highly infective so that inadequate disinfection or sterilization of equipment, such as stainless steel bowls, could result in its unexpected application often with a venepuncture. Complications that were often fatal included generalized vaccinia, with a viraemia, eczema vaccinatum (resembling eczema herpeticum) and post-vaccinial encephalitis with an incidence of 1 in 8000 to 1 in 70 000 vaccinations. For these reasons, vaccination is no longer performed except for specified military personnel.

Cowpox

In the cow, the eruption appears on the animal's teats as small papules which later become vesicles and pustules without causing serious or generalized disease. Friction during hand-milking causes the infectious lesions to become raw. In man papular lesions thus begin in the interdigital clefts, on the back of the hands or on the forearms and face. The vesicular and pustular stages then follow, forming crusts which desquamate. The virus is a similar poxvirus to smallpox and vaccinia but can be distinguished by the type of lesions produced in a chick embryo. Cross-immunity to smallpox virus follows recovery from infection.

Orf

In the sheep there are pustules on the lips, mouth, cornea, legs and feet. Human infections occur as vesicular or bullous lesions on the hands of those who handle diseased animals. Secondary erythema multiforme is common. The causative DNA virus has the same size and morphology (brick-shape on TEM with an entwined pattern) as the vaccinia virus but does not grow in the chick embryo (refer to Appendix C).

48

Molluscum contagiosum

This poxvirus produces small, flesh-coloured warty papules on the trunk, buttocks, arms and face. This infection is seen most often in childhood, when it presents with discrete papules on the trunk or waist area. Papules often have central umbilication or necrosis. It is spread by direct contact or by contaminated fomites. The painless lesions are recognized by their central umbilications often filled with a keratin plug. Treatment is by curettage. The epithelial cells contain very large inclusion bodies, which eventually fill the whole cell, which contain the virus particles. The virus has a similar size and morphology to the vaccinia virus but does not grow in the chick embryo (refer to Appendix C).

Severe infections particularly affecting the face and eyelids are seen in HIV-positive patients and may be the presenting feature of AIDS, especially in children in Africa. Other systemic infections, such as histoplasmosis, may present with similar-looking lesions in AIDS patients.

Papillomaviruses

There are over 70 DNA types of human papillomavirus (HPV). Types 1–4 cause the common skin warts such as plantar (Figure 3.25), common and plane warts.

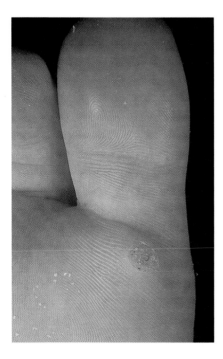

Figure 3.25: Plantar wart due to papillomavirus.

49

Genital warts are caused by a variety of types such as 6 and 11. Other associations include: type 6 meat handlers' warts, type 11 laryngeal papillomata, types 16 and 18 cervical dysplasia associated with carcinoma. Many of the other types are associated with anogenital or oral infection or infection in the rare condition epidermodysplasia verruciformis in which patients have an inherited susceptibility to extensive HPV infection.

The common warts are usually located on the hands or other exposed surfaces and are small hyperkeratotic papules which may amalgamate to form larger plaques. On the soles of the feet there is inward displacement of lesions so that plantar warts are often painful. Plane warts are smoother than the common warts and are often seen on the face. Diagnosis is considered further in Appendix B.

There is a clear association between certain cancers and certain HPV types, notably with cervical cancer. In these cases there is malignant transformation of squamous cells and the viral genome is integrated into cellular chromosomes. Warts associated with carcinoma are uncommon and are often located on mucosal or perimucosal surfaces such as the conjunctiva. However, some premalignant conditions such as bowenoid papulosis of the penis are associated with HPV. Extragenital warts in immunosuppressed subjects may also become malignant.

Herpesviruses

Refer to Chapter 4

Arachnida

Pediculosis (phthiariasis)

Infestation by the louse occurs on the hairs of the scalp (head lice or pediculosis capitis) or lice present in the clothing may affect the body (body lice or pediculosis corporis) – both caused by varieties of *Pediculus humanus* [Linnaeus] – or genital areas (*Phthirus pubis* [Linnaeus] (Fig. 3.26) the pubic or crab louse). *Phthirus pubis* can also involve the eyelids. There is considerable pruritus. Lice can be observed as motile 1–2 mm long grey-brown crawling ectoparasites or as 0.5 mm brown or white nits (eggs) attached to hair shafts; excreta apppear as tiny red dots on the skin amongst the hair. Effective treatment includes either permethrin 1% rinse (treatment of choice for head lice), pyrethroids and piperonyl butoxide or refer to Appendix A. Malathion and carbaryl are also satisfactory for head and pubic lice. Permethrin and phenothrin (pyrethroids) have good activity against the parasites except for the eggs. Old-fashioned treatment

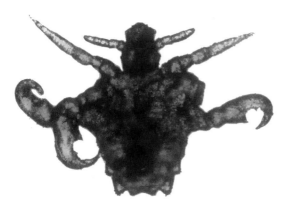

Figure 3.26: Pubic louse (*Phthirus pubis*) (×40).

included 6–10% sulphur ointment. Resistance is becoming a problem. The adults, eggs or nits can be removed by wet combing. Clothing or bed linen contaminated in the previous 48 hours should be washed before reuse.

Typhus

Epidemic or endemic typhus is caused by *Rickettsia prowazekii* and is transmitted between humans in the faeces of the human louse (*Pediculus humanus*). Transmission requires louse faeces to be rubbed into scarified skin which results from scratching. Direct transmission on a person-to-person basis does not occur under natural conditions. Man is, however, the reservoir host so epidemics are associated with wars, famines and unhygienic living conditions with 'epidemic' spread of lice within the population. Symptoms include headache and high fever, with a macular polymorphic exanthema which appears around the sixth day over the whole body excepting the face, palms of hands and soles of feet. Pneumonia, myocarditis, central nervous system signs and coma may ensue. Capillary endothelium is severely damaged – typhus macules contain perivascular haemorrhagic inflammation with leucocytes and macrophages. Chemotherapy with systemic tetracycline or chloramphenicol is effective but the mortality rate without treatment is 10–40%. In addition, there should be a systematic campaign of delousing the population with insecticides to remove the organism. No other rickettsiae are transmitted by human lice. Diagnosis can be confirmed by serology (refer to Appendix A)

Scrub typhus (tsutsugamushi fever) is caused by *Rickettsia tsutsugamushi*. Transmission is effected by the bite of the infected larvae of the mites *Trombicula akamushi* and *deliensis*. The larval mite remains on the host for 1–10 days and measures 0.6 mm when fully engorged. The larvae are infected from the adult female mites from which they were derived. The reservoir host is mainly rodents but latent infection can exist in humans. The infective bite results in a small ulcer

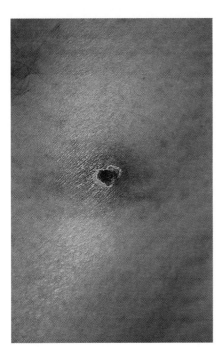

Figure 3.27: Scrub typhus eschar on buttock.

over which a reddish-black scab or eschar is formed (Fig. 3.27). Initially, multiplication of the rickettsiae is localized in this area but they invade systemically and after 5–8 days there is an exanthema with large macules. High fever, myocarditis and encephalitis develop with a mortality rate that may reach 50%. Chemotherapy with systemic tetracycline or chloramphenicol is effective. Insecticide spraying should be carried out to kill the mites and their larvae in clothes, tents, blankets, etc. Insect repellents may also be useful.

Scabies

Scabies is caused by infestation with the mite *Sarcoptes scabiei* (Fig. 3.28). After an incubation period of approximately 4 weeks, there is severe pruritus of the infected areas which is worse at night or after bathing. The diagnosis is confirmed by demonstrating the mite in unexcoriated papules or burrows. The female adult has a rounded body with four pairs of legs and is < 0.5 mm long. A hand lens is used to identify suspicious lesions. The classic linear burrows occur most frequently in the interdigital spaces and on the penis which are the best sites from which to collect scrapings. Penile or scrotal lesions are typical but the mites seldom infest the head except in the very young. Use a needle or scalpel blade to make a scraping along the length of the tunnel. The specimen is mounted in immersion oil under a glass coverslip and the mite observed under the high power 'dry' microscopy lens.

Effective treatment includes malathion lotion and permethrin 5% cream, applied to all areas of the body below the chin and washed off after 8 hours; application must be complete, including the interdigital spaces, and the hands must not be washed for 8 hours. Alternative therapy includes benzyl benzoate or oral ivermectin for Norwegian scabies. Other coexisting sexually transmitted diseases should be excluded. Clothing or bed linen contaminated in the previous 48 hours should be washed before reuse. Pruritus may persist for several weeks after adequate treatment and should be managed with calamine lotion. However, there should be a rapid decrease in the severity of symptoms within a few days of treatment. A single retreatment may be indicated if the pruritus persists. All members of the household should be treated.

A very severe form of scabies can occur, called Norwegian scabies, in elderly patients or those with HIV/AIDS (Figs 3.29 and 3.30). There is hyperkeratosis

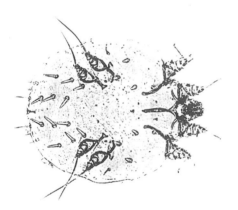

Figure 3.28: Mite of *Sarcoptes scabiei* (×40).

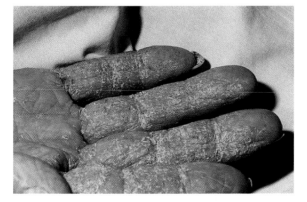

Figure 3.29: Norwegian scabies of hands.

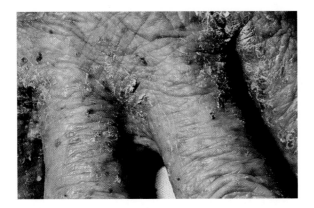

Figure 3.30: Close-up of Norwegian scabies of hands.

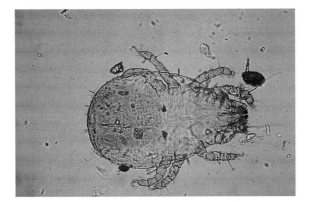

Figure 3.31: *Dermatophagoides pteronyssinus* (×100).

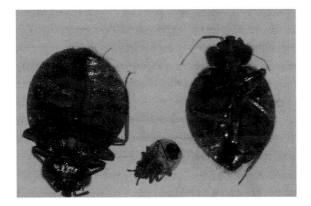

Figure 3.32: *Cimex lectularius* (bedbug) (×10).

of the epidermis, which is heavily colonized by the mite. There are widespread lesions covered in thick crusts surrounded by inflammation. These patients are highly infectious and should be managed in single-room containment. Staff should wear gloves and protective clothing or they can easily become infected by handling the patient. In this situation, the scabetic burrows will not be in typical sites and itching may be minimal. Staff first complain of severe generalized pruritus and may present with wheals or other demonstrations of allergy to the mite. It is usual to find that families of such staff members have also become infected from them, such is the contagious nature of scabies, so that family members of staff must also be treated when outbreaks occur.

Dermatophagoides pteronyssinus (the house dust mite)

This mite (<1 mm) (Fig. 3.31) feeds on shed human skin scales and causes allergic problems in atopic subjects, precipitating asthma in particular. Such patients need to frequently vacuum clean their bedding and household surroundings of shed skin scales (epidermal cells), which contain the mite and constitute part of household dust. The mite is thought to be the allergic component within it.

Demodex folliculorum

This mite of 0.1–0.4 mm colonizes the hair follicles and sebaceous glands in skin, particularly around the scalp, nose and eyelids. It is considered of no importance to man but may, under certain conditions, contribute to acne-like lesions.

Cimex lectularius ('the common human bedbug')

The family Cimicidae includes the bugs of man and animals. The adult bedbug is 5 mm long by 3 mm wide. The adult is reddish while the young are yellowish (Fig. 3.32). Bedbugs have been the companion of man since time immemorial, having been described by Aristotle. They do not colonize the epidermis but survive in cracks and crevices surrounding the bed and within seams of the mattress, leaving an unpleasant odour. The female deposits 200–500 eggs which hatch in 10 days and mature in another 37–128. It feeds at night, biting its victims lying on the mattress, particularly around the shoulders, and engorges itself with blood within 3–10 minutes. There can be a considerable inflammatory reaction, when each bite can reach 1 cm in diameter, due to an allergic reaction to the saliva. The bedbug can transmit experimentally the pathogens of leishmaniasis, leprosy, Chagas' disease, hepatitis B and others but there is doubt about whether it is an important vector.

Infectious agents associated with urticaria

The following have been associated with urticaria at some time: *Neisseria meningitidis*, *Shigella sonnei*, *Yersinia enterocolitica*, *Coxiella burnetii*, Coxsackie viruses A9, A16, B4, B5, echovirus, EBV, hepatitis B, mumps, *Mycoplasma pneumoniae*, *Giardia lamblia*, *Necator americanus*, *Plasmodium* spp., *Schistosoma* spp., *Trichomonas vaginalis*, *Wuchereria bancrofti*, bedbugs, fleas, mosquitoes, mites, *Trombicula irritans* (Chigger bites). In addition, chronic allergic reactions including urticaria and eczema can occur from skin contact with arthropod parts.

4. INFECTIONS OF THE DERMIS

Bacterial infections

Anthrax

Infection by *Bacillus anthracis* is still seen regularly in places with dry hot climates such as the Middle East. It commonly colonizes the skin of cattle and sheep and survives in hair and soil by forming resistant spores. Such spores can cause acute purulent infection, known as the 'malignant' pustule (Fig. 4.1), when inoculated into human skin at a site of trauma. This occurs in countries where the organism is endemic, as well as non-endemic areas when goods are imported carrying spores. It infects labourers or porters who handle contaminated goods such as bales of wool and leather.

The initial lesion of acute infection is often surrounded by a characteristic ring of vesicles (Seal *et al.*, 1998), when the lesion is oedematous. A scraping at that time can be simply stained with methylene blue to show large numbers of bacilli (Fig. 4.2) which would also be Gram-positive. This distinguishes the lesion from streptococcal infections. As the infection progresses it becomes acutely purulent; if septicaemia ensues it can be fatal. Treatment should be given with penicillin, to which the organism is very sensitive. Anthrax infection should be notified in non-endemic areas to the local Medical Officer of Health for epidemiological investigations (Chapter 10) to identify its source.

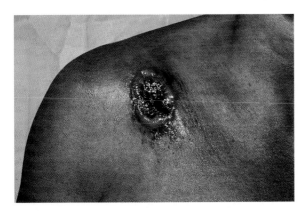

Figure 4.1: Acute 'malignant' pustule of anthrax infection.

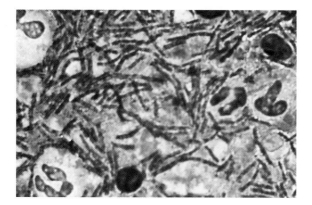

Figure 4.2:
Methylene blue stain
of anthrax bacilli in
purulent tissue
(×1000).

Erysipelothrix

Erysipeloid is cellulitis caused by the Gram-positive bacillus *Erysipelothrix rhusiopathiae*. It presents with severe pain and swelling of a finger or part of the hand after minor injury in workers who handle raw fish, pork or poultry. In contrast to streptococcal cellulitis, there is a well-marginated flat lesion with a violet colour. It heals spontaneously after a few weeks but responds sooner to penicillin or tetracycline.

It is seldom possible to recover *Erysipelothrix rhusiopathiae* from swabs. In order to culture the organism it is necessary to collect a biopsy from the advancing edge of the lesion. This should be incubated for 48 hours in 1% glucose broth, subculturing to blood agar.

Erysipelas

Erysipelas develops rapidly over 48 hours with acute inflammation and a firm raised red margin, as a result of *Streptococcus pyogenes* infection of the superficial layer of the dermis. The patient is generally febrile and has accompanying symptoms of malaise and chills. *S. aureus* does not cause skin infections with this appearance. It commonly arises on the face, possibly following infection from throat carriage of the organism, but can occur at any site (Figs 4.3 and 4.4). Blistering may develop at an early stage but this is not associated with necrosis. The well-defined lesion with a clear border, and little lymphadenopathy, distinguishes it from both cellulitis and necrotizing fasciitis (see below). Erysipelas should be treated with large doses of penicillin – for a severe infection this should be given as intravenous benzylpenicillin, while for less severe cases intramuscular penicillin or oral amoxicillin is suitable. A rapid response is usually obtained (Fig. 4.5)

58

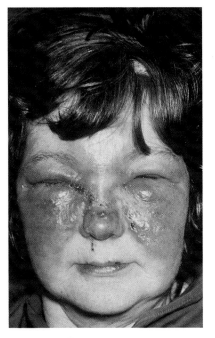

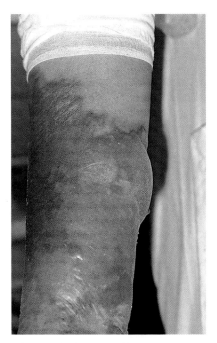

Figure 4.3: Acute blistering erysipelas of face due to *S. pyogenes.*

Figure 4.4: Acute blistering erysipelas of arm due to *S. pyogenes.*

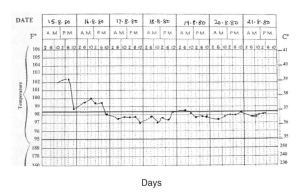

Days

Figure 4.5:
Temperature chart for expected response to penicillin in erysipelas.

It is seldom possible to recover *S. pyogenes* from swabs of the overlying skin but throat swabs may yield the responsible organism ('throat' strains) for facial lesions. In order to culture the organism from the skin, it is necessary to collect a biopsy from the advancing edge of the lesion. However, cultures are frequently negative. The diagnosis is best made on clinical grounds with serological evidence of acute infection, for example, raised antistreptolysin O (ASO) titre (but not high levels because of cholesterol neutralization of the streptolysin in the skin) and raised anti-deoxyribonucleaseB (ADNaseB) and anti-hyaluronidase (AHT) titres.

Cellulitis

Cellulitis develops less rapidly than erysipelas, with an ill-defined margin and marked lymphadenopathy. Blistering rarely occurs and, if it does, the possibility of necrotizing fasciitis developing should be considered. It is due to *S. pyogenes* infection of the dermis at a deeper level than that of erysipelas. While it can occur at any site, the foot and leg is commonest with the source being colonization of the toe web, when all five webs may be affected with or without concomitant infection with dermatophytes. Chiropody or an associated blister can act as portals of entry for the organism. Infection commonly occurs with 'throat' or 'skin' strains of *S. pyogenes* as well as by Lancefield groups C (Figs 4.6–4.8) or G beta-haemolytic streptococci. Cultures of overlying skin are usually unsuccessful – and unnecessary. Once again patients are generally unwell and may have an acute febrile episode prior to the development of the skin lesion. Serological investigation confirms the clinical diagnosis with raised ASO, ADNaseB and AHT titres. Occasionally, cellulitis may arise from infection by *S. aureus*.

Treatment should be given with a penicillin. If the cellulitis is severe, intravenous benzylpenicillin is required. It takes 5 days or more to gain a satisfactory response with a slow reduction of inflammation, in contradistinction to erysipelas (Fig. 4.9). If *S. aureus* is thought to be involved then an antistaphylococcal antibiotic such as flucloxacillin or fusidic acid (as Fucidin) is indicated.

Staphylococcus aureus 'scalded skin' syndrome

Patients present with a generalized exfoliative syndrome when there is splitting at a superficial level between cells comprising the epidermis due to the action of the epidermolytic toxin on desmosomes (Fig. 4.10). This is a biopsy feature that may help to distinguish this form of exfoliation from drug-induced scalded skin syndrome, when the split occurs at a lower level.

It occurs in infants and children under 5 years, presenting with extreme tenderness of the skin and widespread superficial blistering. Prior to onset of the rash, there will have been fever, malaise and irritability followed by pharyngitis, conjunctivitis and a generalized macular erythema. If it involves a neonate with bullous desquamation of large areas of the skin it is called Ritter's disease.

It is caused by infection with *S. aureus* strains that produce staphylococcal exfoliative (epidermolytic) toxin A (ETA) or toxin B (ETB) or both of them. It resembles bullous impetigo, where the same two exfoliative toxins are produced. Treatment includes antistaphylococcal antibiotics (flucloxacillin or fusidic acid) and supportive therapy.

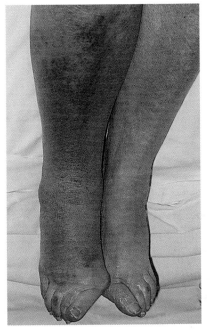

Figure 4.6: Cellulitis of leg due to group C beta-haemolytic streptococci from infected blister on toe.

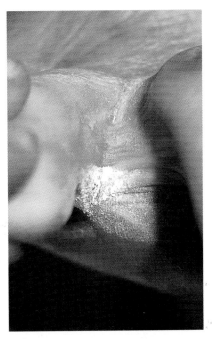

Figure 4.7: Close-up of toe web of the patient in Fig. 4.6 colonized with group C beta-haemolytic streptococci.

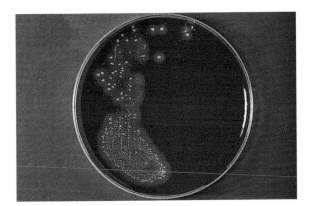

Figure 4.8: Pure culture of group C beta-haemolytic streptococci on blood agar from the toe web above.

61

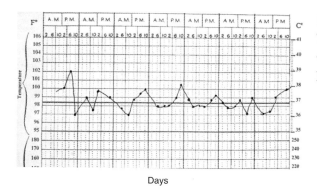

Figure 4.9:
Temperature chart for
expected response to
penicillin in cellulitis.

Days

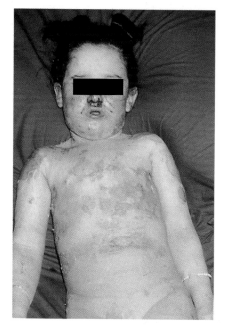

Figure 4.10: Staphylococcal
'scalded skin' syndrome in a child.

Toxic shock syndrome (TSS) in adults

Toxic shock syndrome (TSS) is an acute-onset multi-organ illness caused by *S. aureus* or *S. pyogenes*. Toxin-mediated disease (TMD) is a milder version of TSS that does not include 'shock' or hypotension (or multi-organ failure) in its presentation (Harvey Wood *et al.*, 1998). Toxin-mediated disease, rather than TSS, may occur in people who are partially immune to toxic shock toxin of *S. aureus* (TSST-1), or other toxins, or be caused by strains of bacteria that are only weak toxin-producers.

Staphylococcal TSS is generally divided into two types with different clinical associations; menstrual, when there has been bleeding within 2 days of onset; and non-menstrual, which affects males as well as females. Menstrual cases are primarily associated with the use of certain tampons in which the risk of TSS increases with increasing absorbency. Non-menstrual cases can occur with any type of *S. aureus* infection but notably with colonization of wounds, such as burns, in children (Chapter 7). *S. pyogenes* TSS has not been associated with tampon use but with penetrating and non-penetrating wounds.

Menstrual staphylococcal TSS is nearly always associated with toxic shock toxin-1 (TSST-1), whereas TSST-1 and enterotoxins B and C cause non-menstrual illness. Streptococcal TSS is mainly associated with pyrogenic exotoxin A.

The most widely used case definition was established by Todd *et al.* in 1987. It involves the establishment of three major criteria of high fever, rash and hypotension and three minor criteria as given in Table 4.1. However, the rash and accompanying diffuse dermal oedema are dwarfed by the severity of the systemic symptoms. This clinical case definition was designed for epidemiological purposes, to attempt to identify cases in the population, but does not include the important laboratory findings of:

*   isolation of *S. aureus* from a mucosal or sterile site and testing for TSST-1 production;
*   demonstration of lack of immunity to TSST-1.

Such findings should be included in future definitions. Various possibilities were considered at a recent European Conference on Toxic Shock (Arbuthnott and Furman, 1998).

The unique features of *S. aureus* TSS (Table 4.1) with erythroderma, mucosal erythema and shock are mediated by pure toxin. It can be demonstrated in the blood but bacteraemia is absent. *S. aureus* infection can be minor, and only consist of colonization rather than infection, which can present a bacteriological challenge to find it in the non-menstrual case except if burns are present; in the menstrual case, the organism has multiplied within the tampon producing toxin which is absorbed from the vaginal epithelium. For staphylococcal TSS, suitable antibiotics include flucloxacillin and first- or second-generation cefalosporins (such as cephazolin, cephradine or cefuroxime) but not third-generation drugs such as ceftazidime, which have a limited antistaphylococcal effect; combination therapy can be given with fusidic acid but the aminoglycosides should be avoided if there is any degree of renal failure. Intravenous therapy and supportive measures for the treatment of shock form a critical part of the management. It should be remembered that the antibiotics will prevent further multiplication of *S. aureus*, and production of its toxins, but will have no effect on toxins already circulating within the vascular system.

Table 4.1 Features of toxic shock syndrome (TSS) compared to toxin-mediated disease (TMD).

Expected criteria for TSS (Todd et al., 1987) and TMD	TSS	TMD
Major criteria		
fever: 38.7°C or >	+	+
rash: diffuse, macular	+	+
mucosal membranes: hyperaemia, oropharyngeal or conjunctival	+	+
desquamation: 1–2 weeks after onset	+	–
hypotension: 5th percentile by age	+	–
Minor criteria		
chest: tachypnoea (> 40 per minute)	+	+
chest tachycardia (> 160 per minute)	+	+
gut: vomiting and/or diarrhoea	+	+
renal function: diminished urine output or raised plasma creatinine	+	+
hepatic: serum bilirubin or liver enzymes (AST/ALT) elevated	(+)	(+)
CNS: confusion or irritability	+	+
haematologic: < 100 × 10^9/l platelets	(+)	–
haematologic: > 10.0 × 10^9/l neutrophils	(+)	(+)

S. pyogenes TSS is quite different, as the local clinical manifestations of the infective process, such as necrotizing fasciitis, are usually severe (Chapter 5). Erythroderma and mucosal erythema, distinct from the punctate erythema of scarlet fever (Chapter 7), are uncommon. Streptococcal TSS is also associated with less diarrhoea and vomiting. Patients are often reported as having bacteraemia (in > 50% of cases) when the toxin is released within the vascular system – a different situation entirely from staphylococcal TSS (Chapter 7). Rapid demise, in 30–100% of patients, is therefore greater with *S. pyogenes* TSS, for which large intravenous doses of benzylpenicillin are required with supportive intravenous therapy; plasmapheresis may be indicated. Surgical exploration of possible necrotizing fasciitis may be life-saving (Chapter 5).

Pyrogenic toxins, such as TSST-1 of *S. aureus* and exotoxin A of *S. pyogenes* (SPEA), are 'superantigens' (PTSAgs) that share many biological activities. They have enhanced cell-binding domains to CD4 Th cells, class II MHC receptors (Chapter 1) and liver cells resulting in excessive release of cytokines. They interact with specific Vβ regions of the T cell receptor resulting in significant production of TNFβ, which has similar biological activity to endotoxin. The precise molecular structures of TSST-1 and SPEA are considered by Schlivert (1998). These molecules interact with zinc, including enzymes containing this element, with variable biological effects. These PTSAgs enhance endotoxic shock by potentiating the effects of endotoxin up to five times, induce cytokine release and suppress B lymphocytes (Chapter 1), resulting in shock and multi-organ failure.

Not surprisingly, there is little antibody produced to an episode of TSS. Such antibody production, which provides protective immunity (Chapter 7), only develops in the presence of colonization with the organism (often nasal or mucosal but can involve absorption from burn wounds), when the toxin produced is absorbed as an antigen in the absence of TSS.

Toxic erythema

Patients present with a widespread reddening of the skin which may blister (Fig. 4.11) due to toxic agents. This may or may not be accompanied by fever. It can have a viral origin (*H. simplex*, varicella-zoster virus, measles, rubella, Coxsackie 'B' virus); a bacterial origin (*S. aureus*, *S. pyogenes*, *E. coli* septicaemia); or a fungal origin (pulmonary aspergillosis); be due to drugs (sulfonamides, penicillin, tetracycline, NSAIDs, anticonvulsants, allopurinol, chlorpromazine, dapsone, ethambutol, pyrimethamine with sulfadoxine (Fansidar), griseofulvin, isoniazid, pentamidine, quinine, streptomycin, tolbutamide, trimethoprim); immunizations (BCG, diphtheria toxoid, measles, poliomyelitis, tetanus toxoid); neoplasia (Hodgkin's disease, other lymphomas, leukaemia); or graft-versus-host reactions; and it can be idiopathic. Treatment is symptomatic.

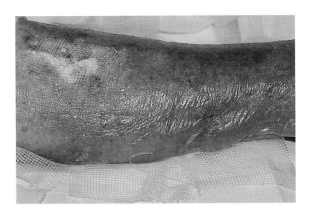

Figure 4.11: Toxic epidermal necrolysis (drug induced).

Specific erythemata associated with systemic infection

Erythema nodosum

Erythema nodosum is a tender nodular erythematous eruption appearing on the extensor surface of the legs in particular (Fig. 4.12). It is a type of cutaneous

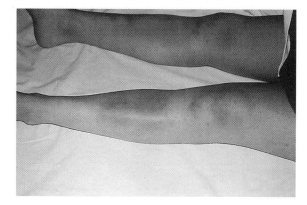

Figure 4.12:
Erythema nodosum
on legs.

vasculitis (vascular hypersensitivity) that produces bruising followed by resolution within a few weeks without ulceration, scarring or atrophy. Recurrences are rare except if precipitated by streptococci or sarcoidosis. It may follow an upper respiratory tract infection, often in a child or young adult. There is malaise and arthralgia, especially of the knees.

Infectious causes or sensitizing agents for erythema nodosum include *S. pyogenes*, meningococci, *Mycobacterium tuberculosis* and *leprae*, atypical mycobacteria, systemic fungal infecions (Chapter 9), cat-scratch disease, enteric bacterial infections, *Yersinia* infections, amoebiasis, giardiasis, *Rickettsiae*, *Treponema pallidum* and viruses including hepatitis B.

Non-infectious causes include drug reactions (oral contraceptives, antibiotics and sulfonamides), pregnancy, thyroid disorders, autoimmune diseases, sarcoidosis, lymphoma and leukaemia. Forty per cent of cases are idiopathic.

Erythema multiforme

Erythema multiforme affects young adults, tends to be recurrent and has no seasonal relationship. It involves the face and the distal parts of the limbs, as well as the mucosal surfaces of the lips, mouth and genitalia. There is malaise for 48 hours before the rash appears. The rash is polymorphic with maculoerythematous, papulovesicular, bullous and haemorrhagic varieties (Figs 4.13 and 4.14). Target lesions develop in which central darkening, or even frank blistering, appears (erythema iris). The rash, which does not itch, becomes dry and fissured followed by peeling and resolution. The mucosal lesions develop a moist ulcerative pseudomembranous appearance and are painful. There can be joint swelling, fever and albuminuria.

Infectious causes include *H. simplex* 1 and 2, Epstein–Barr virus, *S. aureus*, *S. pyogenes*, *M. tuberculosis*, *Yersinia* spp., *Mycoplasma pneumoniae*, *Histoplasma capsula-*

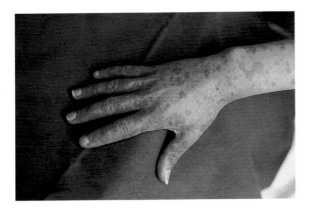

Figure 4.13:
Erythema multiforme
on hands.

tum. Non-infectious causes include drug reactions, radiotherapy for neoplasia, and pregnancy. Fifty per cent of cases are idiopathic, but HSV 1 and 2 infection should be considered in those cases where there is no obvious cause.

Stevens–Johnson syndrome and erythema multiforme major. This is a severe form of erythema multiforme. Particular problems develop with ulceration of the

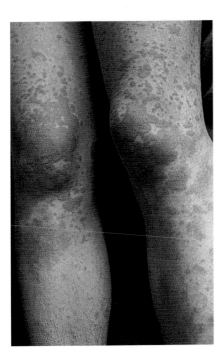

Figure 4.14: Erythema
multiforme on legs.

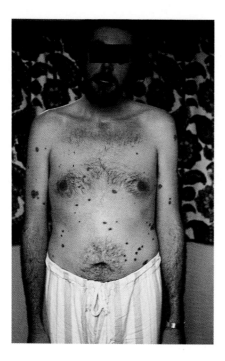

Figure 4.15: Stevens–Johnson syndrome secondary to mycoplasma infection.

conjunctival mucosa when 'rodding' to prevent adhesions has resulted in much worse scarring. It is common for blindness to develop as an end-result of the inflammatory process despite all attempts to prevent this severe complication. Therapy is not usually required for the infectious disease precipitating this syndrome but full supportive and anti-inflammatory therapy is needed with use of corticosteroids and immunosuppressive drugs.

It may follow the infections listed for erythema multiforme as well as mycoplasmas (Fig. 4.15). It also occurs as a consequence of drug therapy, particularly with sulfonamides, which should never be used unnecessarily. Not surprisingly, co-trimoxazole (sulfonamide/trimethoprim mixture) (Septrin or Bactrin) has also been implicated.

Erythema marginatum

This occurs in 10% of patients with acute rheumatism, mostly in children. The rash presents with red polycyclic flat rings. It is associated with rheumatic carditis that follows *S. pyogenes* throat infection.

Henoch–Schönlein (anaphylactoid) purpura

Purpura is caused by multiple spontaneous capillary haemorrhages into the skin and mucous membranes following abnormal bleeding tendencies or vasculitis. This type of purpura is characteristic, with symmetrical lesions found on elbows and buttocks and the extensor surfaces of the arms and lower legs and is due to a leukocyto-clastic vasculitis. Lesions are seldom found on the trunk and only occasionally on the face. The earliest lesions are urticarial and may even be itchy. Later the haemor-rhagic macules appear, changing colour from red to purple to brown. This sequence is easy to follow as the rash occurs in crops. It usually occurs in children under the age of 10. Joint involvement is common so that acute rheumatism may be suspected, but the fever is not high and the pain is not severe – in addition there is no relief from salicylate therapy. There may be an associated transient synovitis, usually of the knee. Glomerulonephritis with haematuria and intussusception may occur. In most patients symptomatic treatment alone is required.

There is often a history of an upper respiratory tract infection preceeding the onset by 10–20 days. The evidence incriminating *S. pyogenes* is not as good as for rheumatic carditis. The purpura represents the visible lesions of a widespread non-specific vasculitis thought to be due to a hypersensitivity reaction to micro-bial antigen. Leukocytoclastic purpura may also follow wound infections and allergy to drugs and foodstuffs; or no cause may be identified.

A generalized purpuric response may follow measles, rubella, chickenpox or mumps in children or be labelled 'idiopathic' if the precipitating antigen cannot be identified.

Lyme disease

Systemic infection with the spirochaete *Borrelia burgdorferi* arises from the bite of an *Ixodes* tick (Fig. 4.16) found on deer and other animals in wooded pasture-land.

Figure 4.16: Ixodes ticks – adult and progeny (×10).

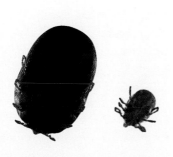

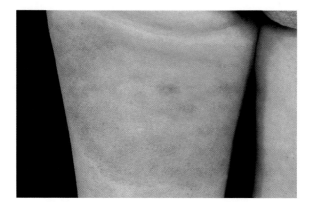

Figure 4.17:
Erythema chronicum
migrans of Lyme
disease.

Initial presentation includes fever, joint pains and the migrating rash of erythema chronicum migrans (Fig. 4.17). This rash begins 3–32 days after the tick bite with a median time of 7 days. The lesion may be located anywhere, but the thigh, groin and axilla are common sites. The median diameter is 15 cm with a range of 3–68 cm. The rash is hot but painless. Most lesions are flat with bright red outer borders and partial central clearing, but the changes can be very subtle. Multiple secondary lesions appear. If untreated, the main rash and secondary lesions usually fade within 28 days. There is occasional pigmentary change or residual scaling. If untreated there can be intermittent recurrences. Biopsy of the spreading lesion has demonstrated the organism.

The second stage follows weeks to months after the tick bite. There can be aseptic meningitis, neuritis, encephalitis, myositis and arthritis. The spirochaete invades the eye early in the infection causing a non-specific follicular conjunctivitis in 10% of patients with later keratitis and retinochoroiditis (Seal et al., 1998). Cranial nerve palsies can develop and, in endemic areas, it is responsible for approximately 25% of new-onset Bell's palsy. The third stage consists of frank arthritis and late neurological complications. Later atrophic skin lesions have been described and in some endemic areas morphea-like lesions have been ascribed to borreliosis. Lymphocytoma cutis may also be a feature of this infection.

The diagnosis is based on a history of exposure to woodland in an endemic area and positive serology using ELISA-based tests. The presence of *Ixodes* ticks (Fig. 4.16) alone is not predictive of human infection. It is the regional density of ticks and the percentage of them parasitized by *B. burgdorferi* spirochaetes that predict human risk. Measuring antibody may be useful at an early stage to show seroconversion or at a late stage to demonstrate an absence of antibody to refute the diagnosis. Approximately 8% of the UK population have antibodies to *B. burgdorferi*.

Oral antibiotic treatment of the rash shortens its duration and associated symptoms and prevents later illness in most patients. Therapy with oral doxycycline 100 mg twice daily or tetracycline 250 mg four times a day for 10 days to 3 weeks is recommended for men and non-pregnant women. The latter should be given amoxicillin 250 mg three times a day instead. This is effective in the early stages but late complications require high doses of intravenous penicillin (12 g or 20 million units/day) or ceftriaxone (2 g/day) for 14 days providing there is normal renal function.

Syphilis

Syphilis is due to *Treponema pallidum* and involves epidermal and dermal lesions in primary, secondary and tertiary stages. Diagnosis is clinical and confirmed by serologic testing using both the non-specific cardiolipin 'reagin' test such as the VDRL (Venereal Disease Research Laboratory) slide test, or the older Wasserman reaction, and specific tests such as TPHA (*Treponema pallidum* haemagglutination) or FTA (fluorescent treponemal antibody).

The primary stage lesion develops after 3 weeks and consists of the eroded indurated plaque or hard chancre, which arises at the site of contact (mouth, genital areas) with an open infectious lesion. It lasts for a few weeks but responds well to penicillin given as Bicillin (procaine penicillin 1.8 g, benzyl penicillin 360 mg) or as one intramuscular dose of 2.4 million units of benzathine penicillin. For penicillin allergy, use doxycycline 100 mg twice daily for 2 weeks instead. In this stage of syphilis, non-specific reagin tests are positive but specific tests may be negative.

T. pallidum disseminates throughout the body before the appearance of the chancre. Three weeks after the disappearance of the chancre this dissemination manifests as the secondary stage of syphilis. There is a generalized rash which is generally maculopapular, bilaterally symmetric and non-pruritic. There is an absence of bullous lesions. It is highly variable, however, and can be a diagnostic challenge. It may resemble pityriasis versicolor. It is associated with 'snail track' mouth ulcers and generalized lymphadenopathy in 75% of patients. There may be fever, sore throat and myalgias. If untreated, it will resolve, but 25% of patients will develop a mucocutaneous relapse within the first year of infection and be contagious for sexual transmission. Treatment is required with Bicillin or benzathine penicillin with weekly intramuscular injections for 3 weeks. Penicillin allergy is managed as given above. If not treated, progression advances to the tertiary stage in 50% of patients. In this secondary stage, both non-specific and specific serologic tests are positive.

Tertiary syphilis, if untreated, classically presents with various effects, mimicking many other conditions, including a stumbling gait (tabes dorsalis), aortitis,

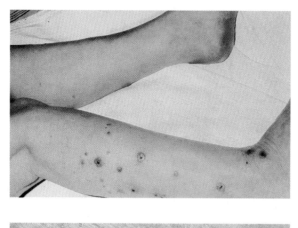

Figure 4.18: The great pox (or rupia) in a patient with tertiary syphilis (relapsing aortitis and positive TPHA test) after commencing penicillin.

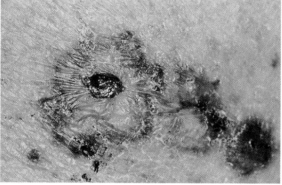

Figure 4.19: Close-up of patient in Fig. 4.18 (×4).

GPI (general paralysis of the insane), optic nerve atrophy, meningovascular lesions, gumma at any site or typical skin lesions (the great pox) (see above). The pathological disease is due to perivascular infiltration of lymphocytes around vessels causing chronic inflammation. Treatment is required with high-dose penicillin (900 mg or 1.5 megaunits intravenously 6-hourly or the equivalent) for a minimum of 14 days. In the tertiary stage, non-specific tests can be negative or weakly positive but specific tests remain positive.

During the apparent quiescent or latent phase of tertiary syphilis, when aortitis and other lesions may be developing, there can be a relapse with the great pox appearing. This rash, in contradistinction to smallpox, is also called 'Rupia', which is derived from the Greek word for dirty. Large pustular lesions ooze brown serosanguinous fluid (Figs 4.18 and 4.19) but respond rapidly to treatment with intravenous penicillin – without treatment large scars and new lesions coexist.

Tuberculosis

Tuberculosis of the skin (see below) is secondary to systemic infection with *Mycobacterium tuberculosis hominis* (spread via the pulmonary route) or *bovis* (spread from the infected cow via contaminated milk). *M. hominis* is the cause of most types of skin infection but, prior to milk pasteurization, scrofuloderma (see below) used to be common over tuberculous lymphatic glands in the neck infected with *M. bovis*. Such scrofuloderma was eradicated in Toronto, Canada, in 1920 by compulsory milk pasteurization, but this situation was not achieved in the UK for a further 20 years because of lobbies that favoured retention of raw milk for its nutritive and taste qualities (Hay and Seal, 1996b). The sale of raw milk is now condoned in the European Union, which may result in recurrence of this infection, since it is difficult to maintain a tuberculous-free herd. It is much safer to pasteurize milk.

A focus of active systemic tuberculosis should be sought especially in the population from the Indian subcontinent in whom extrapulmonary tuberculosis is much more common than in Caucasians. This can include cold abscesses at any site and bone involvement such as periostitis. This population is prone to trauma-associated tuberculosis, presenting with active infection at sites of injury that may include dermal involvement (Ferris *et al.*, 1987). This is due to the persistence of live tubercle bacilli in macrophages despite chemotherapy and previous healed lesions. Such macrophages are unable to achieve intracellular killing of live mycobacteria, which are then released from these cells at sites of trauma to cause reinfection.

Various theories have been proposed for this intracellular survival of mycobacteria, including the effects in the UK of the Indian vegetarian diet, when such patients have coexistent cobalamin deficiency and macrocytic anaemia (Chanarin and Stephenson, 1988). These authors recorded an incidence of tuberculosis in vegetarians of 133 per 1000 compared to 48 per 1000 in those on a mixed diet amongst the Indian population in West London. Such a big difference in incidence may support their hypothesis that dietary factors are of major importance in determining the susceptibility of Asiatic Indians to tuberculosis. Injury-associated tuberculosis is also seen occasionally in the Caucasian population and may follow surgical procedures such as total hip replacement as a late complication (McCullough, 1977).

Therapy includes systemic antituberculous drugs for at least 6 months (O'Grady *et al.*, 1997). There is no role for topical therapy and reliance should be made on systemic treatment alone.

Tuberculosis verrucosa cutis

Most cases are due to an exogenous reinfection in those with marked cutaneous hypersensitivity. The lesions start as indurated circumscribed warty plaques which

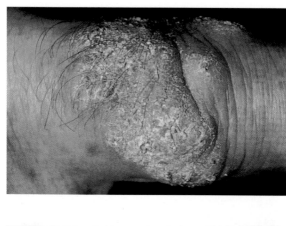

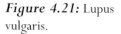

Figure 4.20:
Tuberculosis
verrucosa cutis
(warty tuberculosis)
due to *M. bovis*.

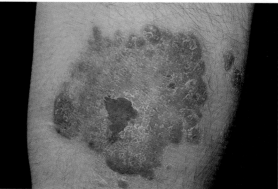

Figure 4.21: Lupus
vulgaris.

may be single or multiple and can coalesce to form large lesions. The most frequent sites involved are dorsal surfaces of hands (Fig. 4.20), feet, knees and buttocks. Tubercle bacilli are seldom found in the skin and the histology is of diffuse granulomata with overlying acanthosis and hyperkeratosis. The differential diagnosis is from atypical mycobacterial infection, such as *M. marinum* (Fig. 8.6). A history of occupational exposure is often helpful, as lesions are usually culture negative.

Lupus vulgaris

This occurs in those with adequate cell-mediated immunity (CMI) to the tubercle bacillus. It is prevalent on exposed parts, especially the face (Fig. 4.21) and the extremities. It is due to an endogenous source of tubercle bacilli from other active foci through haematogenous spread. The initial lesion is a small nodule with a pale brown-yellow (apple jelly) colour. The lesions enlarge considerably and can ulcerate. Acid-fast bacilli are almost never found in tissue sections but histology reveals tubercles composed of epithelioid cells and giant cells. Caseation necrosis is slight or absent. In late stages there is considerable scarring and secondary squamous carcinoma can occur in old lesions.

Scrofuloderma

Scrofuloderma involves the skin by direct extension from tuberculous lymph nodes, bones or joints. The nodules and 'gummata' appear over the lymph nodes of the neck, sternal region, knees or ankles. It begins with a deep purple induration of the skin that soon becomes fluctuant. The glands necrose to form chronic sinuses discharging purulent and caseous exudate. The differential diagnosis is from tertiary syphilis, systemic fungal infections (Chapter 9), actinomycosis and pyogenic lymphadenitis.

Papulonecrotic tuberculide

This is a diffuse cropping rash consisting of discrete papules, some of which develop central necrosis. It is due to dissemination of *M. tuberculosis* antigens and consequent vasculitis. The biopsies show periarteriolar inflammation with endarteritis and an infiltrate of giant cells and macrophages. Polymerase chain reaction (PCR) is frequently positive in this condition, which responds well to antituberculous chemotherapy.

Lichen scrofulosorum

This consists of very small lichenoid papules without itching or pain scattered over the trunk or extremities. Most are small, firm and flat (Figs 4.22 and 4.23). Most patients are young and have visceral tuberculosis. CMI to the tubercle bacillus is marked. Tubercle bacilli are not found in these lesions and cannot be cultured from them, although the histology shows dermal granulomata composed of epithelioid cells and Langerhans' giant cells.

Erythema induratum (Bazin's disease)

Erythema induratum (Fig. 4.24) develops in young women with glandular tuberculosis. CMI is marked. The rash usually occurs on the back of the lower calf. The lesions are soft recurrent nodules which are symmetrical and indolent. They persist for 3 months and may ulcerate with irregular shapes and deep undermined edges. The histology shows endothelial cell proliferation, thrombus formation and necrosis. Epithelioid cell tubercles and caseation necrosis support the diagnosis.

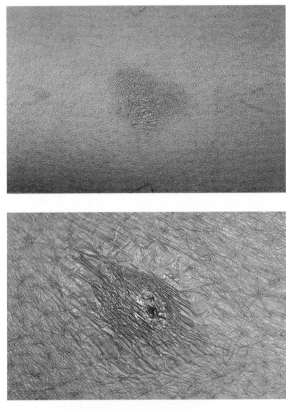

Figure 4.22: Lichen scrofulosorum on the leg in an Indian patient with a cold abscess of the thyroid gland due to active *Mycobacterium tuberculosis* infection (×2).

Figure 4.23: Close-up of lichen scrofulosorum (×4).

Figure 4.24: Erythema induratum.

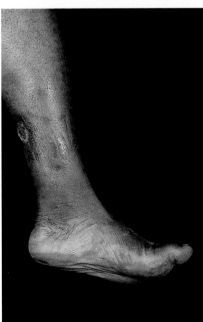

Erythema induratum is a form of nodular vasculitis of which tuberculosis is one cause; tuberculous cases respond well to antituberculous therapy, but this has no effect on non-tuberculous patients. It should be differentiated from erythema nodosum and syphilis. It responds better to corticosteroids than to antituberculous chemotherapy.

Non-tuberculous mycobacterial infection

Other mycobacteria may present with skin lesions (Chapter 8). Some, such as *Mycobacterium chelonae*, often cause injection abscesses. *Mycobacterium marinum* causes local indurated granulomata and ulcers and, in some cases, there is an accompanying chain of secondary lesions along the course of a lymphatic (sporotrichoid change). If possible, cultures and sensitivities should be obtained, as the response of these infections to chemotherapy is often unpredictable.

Leprosy

Leprosy is caused by *Mycobacterium leprae*, which has the following properties:

* it is a weakly acid-fast bacillus (AFB), which is an obligate intracellular organism that is non-cultivable in artificial media;
* it grows in Schwann cells and other nerve structures;
* it gives distinctive immunological reactivity.

The bacteriological (BI) and morphological (MI) indices provide information on the bacterial load and its viability, which is useful for following a response to chemotherapy. The BI is based on counting AFB in slit-skin smears based on a log scale from 1+ (1–10 bacilli per 100 microscope fields) to 6+ (> 1000 bacilli per field). The MI is based on the experience that viable bacilli stain in a uniform manner with even intact cell walls, and that fragmented, beaded or irregularly stained bacilli are dead.

M. leprae does not stain with the full Ziehl–Neelsen (acid/alcohol) stain used for *M. tuberculosis hominis*, as it is weakly acid but not alcohol fast. It requires to be stained by the modified Ziehl–Neelsen stain, using hot carbol fuschin for 20 minutes, but decolourizing with 5% acetic acid (vinegar) alone (Appendix B). A counterstain is used, such as malachite green, against which the red-staining bacilli can be seen (Fig. 4.25). It is often difficult to focus well on the bacilli because of the thick tissue section. The slit-skin smear technique is given in Appendix B.

Clinical forms of leprosy (Ridley–Jopling [1966] scale)

Lepromatous leprosy (LL) is characterized by a long period of incubation and latency. In the early stages the lesions are diffuse and erythematous with a weak

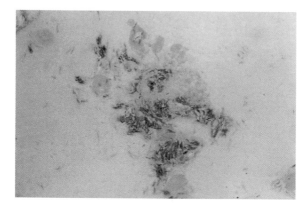

Figure 4.25:
Modified
Ziehl–Neelsen stain
of *M. leprae* in tissue
smear (×1000)
(weakly acid, non-
alcohol fast).

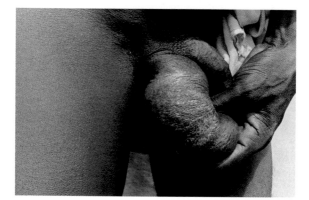

Figure 4.26:
Advanced
lepromatous leprosy
(LL) with diffuse
infiltrated lesions of
the scrotum and
penis. (Courtesy of
Dr MA Rajan,
Kumbakonam.)

brown pigmentation. They cover extensive areas of the body surface symmetrically. With progression the skin becomes more infiltrated and sometimes frank
symmetrical plaques and nodules appear (Fig. 4.26). These can become multiple to cover the trunk and arms. Neurological involvement begins with loss of
sensitivity followed by enlargement of nerve trunks with muscular atrophy and
deformities of hands and feet.

Lepromatous granulomata contain undifferentiated macrophages that may be
full of vacuoles – the foamy cells typical of LL. Stains for *M. leprae* reveal very
large numbers of bacilli present in the macrophages of active lepromatous lesions.

Borderline lepromatous lesions (BL) are similar to those of LL but the borders of the
plaques are more sharply defined (Fig. 4.27). Bilateral symmetry is not present and
the centre of the lesions has a normal appearance. Histology shows undifferentiated macrophages but without foamy cells and a much smaller number of bacilli.

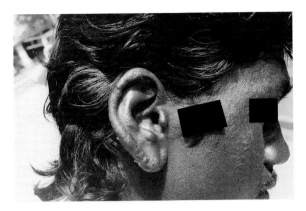

Figure 4.27:
Borderline
lepromatous leprosy
(BL) with ill-defined
lesion of ear.
(Courtesy of Dr MA
Rajan, Kumbakonam.)

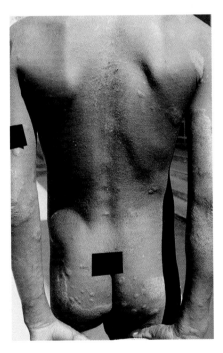

Figure 4.28: Borderline leprosy
(BB) with small to large ill-defined
raised erythematous lesions, with
nerve involvement. (Courtesy of
Dr MA Rajan, Kumbakonam.)

Borderline (BB) leprosy is very characteristic. There are numerous erythematous plaques
and nodules of varying size which can cover almost the entire surface of the body
(Fig. 4.28). Moderate anaesthesia is present. Histology shows a combination of undifferentiated macrophages and various numbers of epithelioid and giant cells. Large
numbers of weakly acid-fast bacilli are present. Lymphocytes are diffusely distributed.

Borderline tuberculoid (BT) leprosy is characterized by macules or plaques in
greater numbers than in tuberculoid leprosy (TT), but still with well-defined

79

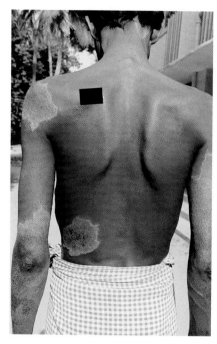

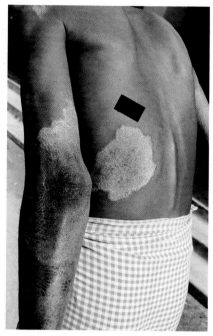

Figure 4.29: Borderline tuberculoid leprosy (BT) with multiple well-defined raised lesions with spreading margins. (Courtesy of Dr MA Rajan, Kumbakonam.)

Figure 4.30: Borderline tuberculoid leprosy (BT) (close-up). (Courtesy of Dr MA Rajan, Kumbakonam.)

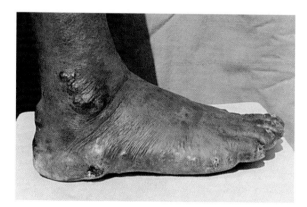

Figure 4.31: Ulcerative lesions of the lower limb in a patient with tuberculoid leprosy (TT). (Courtesy of Dr MA Rajan, Kumbakonam.)

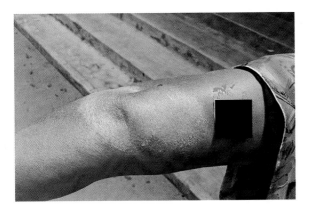

Figure 4.32:
Tuberculoid leprosy
(TT) with well-
defined lesion on the
arm. (Courtesy of Dr
MA Rajan,
Kumbakonam.)

borders and anaesthesia or hypoaesthesia (Figs 4.29 and 4.30). Inflammation of nerves is variable. Histologically, the lesions show some epithelioid differentiation and Langerhans' giant cells, similar to TT, but the granuloma is less organized and more diffuse. The main difference is the presence of small numbers of weakly acid-fast bacilli.

Tuberculoid leprosy (TT) affects both skin and nerves. Skin lesions are single or few and consist of infiltrated plaques with well-defined borders and a sunken centre. These lesions are anaesthetic, dry and are accompanied by dissociated anaesthesia at other sites. Thickening of nerve trunks is a prominent feature. Tuberculoid granulomata have well-defined characteristics but it may not be possible to demonstrate bacilli (Figs 4.31–4.32). They contain epithelioid cells surrounded by an abundant infiltrate of lymphocytes. The granuloma extends from the basal layer of the epidermis to the lower dermis. Nerves passing through these granulomata are obliterated.

Indeterminate leprosy consists of a single or few hypopigmented lesions which are anaesthetic. Small numbers of bacilli can be seen on biopsy within a superficial nerve. The inflammatory reaction is non-specific with a lymphohistiocytic infiltration around blood vessels.

Erythema nodosum leprosum is an exacerbation reaction of lepromatous leprosy (LL) during treatment, mimicking erythema nodosum clinically but differing histologically. The scars may ulcerate.

Immunopathology of leprosy
No exotoxins or endotoxins are produced by *M. leprae*. In lepromatous leprosy there are millions of bacilli per gram of tissue with a high level of antibodies produced but with absent CMI. The opposite situation occurs with tuberculoid leprosy, when

81

the CMI gives a strong reaction but without an antibody response. The phenomenon of CD4 Th-1 lymphocyte stimulation (for producing CMI) with CD4 Th-2 lymphocyte suppression (for reducing antibody production) and vice versa, mediated through the feedback cytokine system, has been reviewed in Chapter 1 and leprosy is no exception to the general mechanisms. However, why lepromatous leprosy should develop in one patient and tuberculoid in another is not understood, but is thought to involve the role of T suppressor cells in the particular individual. The expression of clinical disease and its type then depends on the immunological reaction to the organism mounted in the individual.

Therapy of leprosy

Dapsone was introduced in the 1940s and used successfully in many, but not all, patients for several decades until it became apparent that there was widespread resistance. In 1982 a WHO Study Group recommended that all patients with active leprosy should receive multiple drug treatment with different regimes according to their clinical-immunological state (the Ridley–Jopling scale). Multibacillary patients (LL, BL and BB) were given rifampicin 600 mg and clofazimine 300 mg as monthly supervised medication and dapsone 100 mg and clofazimine 50 mg as daily unsupervised medication. Patients were treated for 2 years and followed up for 5 years. Paucibacillary patients (TT and BT) were given rifampicin 600 mg monthly with daily unsupervised dapsone 100 mg. Therapy was given for 6 months and patients followed up for 2 years. These regimes have been implemented widely with good results; they are effective clinically and bacteriologically without undue toxicity but are still not available to many patients in the Third World.

Other infections

Embolic phenomena of septicaemia (bacteraemia) and SBE (subacute bacterial endocarditis)

Embolic phenomena of endocarditis with '*Streptococcus viridans*', and other alpha-haemolytic or non-haemolytic streptococci, include petechial (splinter) haemorrhages of the nails, tender nodules commonly found on the plantar surface of fingers or toes – Osler's nodes (Fig. 4.33) – and boat-shaped haemorrhages in the retina. While these are infected cutaneous emboli, they are not purulent unless acute infection is present with *S. pyogenes* or another pyogenic organism such as *S. aureus* or *Ps. aeruginosa* in an immunocompromised patient (Fig. 4.34). Similar lesions will be found in drug addicts injecting non-sterile products.

In addition, there will be a low-grade fever; evidence of systemic embolization, which can present with a cerebrovascular accident; cardiac symptoms and anaemia; an enlarged spleen; and in half the cases there is clubbing of the fingers. Red blood cells will also be found in the urine. Gram-negative septicaemias may

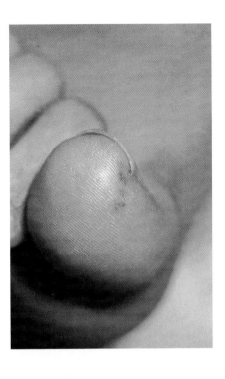

Figure 4.33: Pulp infarcts of the great toe due to septicaemia (Osler's nodes).

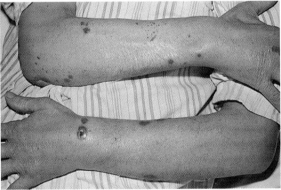

Figure 4.34: Septic emboli of the dermis in an immuno-compromised patient.

be accompanied by a specific skin lesion, ecthyma gangrenosum, which presents with a large indurated nodule or plaque with a central necrotic scab.

Typhoid and paratyphoid B fever

Typhoid and paratyphoid septicaemia produce characteristic 'rose' spots (Fig. 4.35) in the febrile phase, which may be missed. They soon disappear with chemotherapy.

83

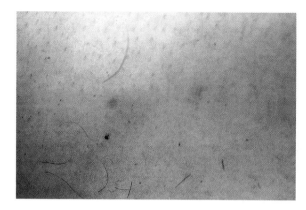

Figure 4.35: Rose spots of paratyphoid B fever.

Fungal infections

Systemic candidosis with *C. albicans*

In most cases the organism arises from the patient's own gut flora, particularly in those with leukaemia or immunosuppression. Drug addicts are at risk from use of contaminated products and equipment.

Typical lesions start as macules, becoming papular or nodular especially in hairy areas where they can become pustular. Some are haemorrhagic and may break down to form ecthyma-type lesions. This is associated with fever and muscle tenderness, when there may be widespread invasion of organs with candida.

Histology of a skin lesion shows both yeasts and hyphae in the dermis. This finding can provide a rapid diagnosis before broth-based blood cultures become positive after 3–4 days' incubation. It is much better to use a traditional agar pour-plate technique, incorporating heparinized blood from the patient with the Sabouraud agar. This technique yields growth after 18 hours at 37°C with yeast colonies in and on the agar surface.

Therapy requires intravenous amphotericin B or fluconazole (O'Grady *et al.*, 1997). Systemic invasion is usually widespread and only a minority of patients manifest skin lesions. The condition is often undiagnosed and fatal, when organ involvement with *C. albicans* is only found at necropsy.

Viral infections

Herpes infections

Herpesviruses contain DNA and have an icosahedral structure. They are classified on the basis of host range, duration of multiplication, cytopathology and the characteristics of latent infection. *Herpes simplex* viruses 1 and 2 (human herpes virus – HHV-1 and 2) and varicella-zoster virus (HHV-3) only infect humans, and can multiply within host cells in 24 hours to cause widespread destruction and maintain latent infection within neurones. Epstein–Barr virus (HHV-4) only infects humans, causes glandular fever and other lymphoid diseases and causes latency within lymphoid tissues. Cytomegalovirus (HHV-5) is also limited to humans but multiplies much more slowly and causes latent infection within secretory glands, lymphoreticular glands and other organs. HHV-6 was first isolated in 1986 and has a close relationship to HHV-5. It is implicated in two different syndromes: the first is exanthema subitum (or roseola infantum), a mild febrile illness of young children with a rash; the second is a lymphadenopathy in adults without other signs. HHV-7 has been isolated but is not yet associated with disease. HHV-8 has been isolated and associated with Kawasaki disease.

Herpes simplex *virus*

Herpes simplex virus (HSV) infection is endemic throughout the world. Different studies have found that around 90% of the tested populations have antibodies against HSV. The primary infection is most often asymptomatic but may be manifest in children as an acute localized vesicular rash with surrounding inflammation (Fig. 4.36). The lesion resolves over a few days without scarring. In young adults handling respiratory secretions, such as nurses handling tracheostomy wounds or young dentists, primary infection can present as a herpetic whitlow. There is a lesion on a finger which is very painful but heals without treatment; although swollen it should not be opened, as it contains necrotic material and not pus and incision will further spread the infection. Topical aciclovir can be given for severe cases but is most effective when used in the prodromal phase of recurrent lesions.

With recovery the virus becomes latent in the supplying neuronal ganglia for the affected sectors of skin. When this sector is stimulated, such as by excessive sunlight or another ultraviolet source, the virus travels along the nerve to cause repeated vesicular infection called a 'cold sore', which often occurs around the lips. The precise mechanism is an enigma and, while it is not impeded by serum antibodies, immunosuppression can result in reactivation (Fig. 4.37). *Herpes simplex* virus type 1 infects the face and neck region, while type 2 causes genital infection with recurrent ulcers on the glans penis and other sites. The rash may be preceded by prodromal symptoms such as itching or tingling in the same area. In HIV-positive patients *Herpes simplex* infection may present with a variety of different lesions from indolent ulcers to warty growths. *Herpes simplex* also causes a widespread infection with superficial ulcers and vesicles in patients with atopic dermatitis (eczema herpeticum).

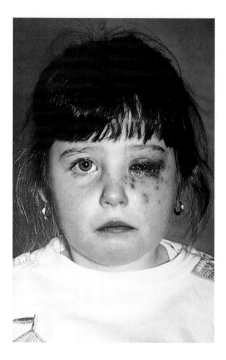

Figure 4.36: *Herpes simplex* as a primary infection.

Aciclovir is an acyclic nucleoside analogue of guanosine. It has potent antiviral activity against most herpes viruses. The selective activity for herpes virus replication is due to its selective phosphorylation by the herpes-encoded thymidine kinase within an infected cell to its monophosphate form. Cellular enzymes then convert aciclovir monophosphate to the di- and triphosphate. The latter is the active compound which is a selective substrate and inhibitor of herpes virus DNA polymerase (following incorporation into herpes virus DNA it lacks the 3'-hydroxy group necessary for further elongation, so terminating the viral DNA chain). It is also a competitive analogue inhibiting the incorporation of deoxynucleotide triphosphates into viral DNA. For other similar compounds refer to Table 2.2.

Penciclovir (for which the oral pro-drug is famciclovir) has been launched recently to treat *H. simplex* virus types 1 and 2 and *H. zoster*. It is converted *in vivo* to the triphosphate form by virus-induced thymidine kinase, as for aciclovir. It has been shown to be active against aciclovir-resistant *H. simplex*, which has an altered DNA polymerase.

Varicella-zoster virus (VZV)

This presents as chickenpox in childhood with 90% achieving satisfactory immunity before adulthood. A few remain susceptible, however, particularly

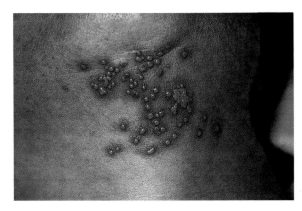

Figure 4.37:
Herpetic vesicles
under the chin of a
lymphoma patient on
chemotherapy.

young doctors and nurses, who catch the infection from unsuspected cases on the wards. Care is required on the maternity ward and if the diagnosis, supported by finding an absence of antibody or the acute phase IgM reaction, is in the first trimester of pregnancy then a termination may be considered. Chickenpox is safe in the third trimester but the baby can be born covered in a vesicular rash.

The illness begins with an incubation period of 14–21 days. Fever ensues with a vesicular rash which covers the entire body but is predominantly centripetal. The vesicular lesions, which develop at different stages, progress to become pustular and then heal with occasional scars. Cytology of the vesicular fluid shows multinucleate giant cells, while electron microscopy reveals icosahedral-shaped viruses.

In most patients there are no sequelae but the virus remains dormant in neuronal ganglia supplying respective areas of skin. These reactivate in later life to cause *Herpes zoster* or 'shingles'. There may or may not be a precipitating stimulatory event. There is a prodromal phase of increased sensitivity followed by a vesicular rash over that area of skin (dermatome) supplied by the nerve. This is followed by vesicles and pustules. There can be severe pain, not only at the time of the acute lesion but also after healing – the post-herpetic neuralgia syndrome. This commonly involves the Vth cranial nerve – trigeminal neuralgia – for which the patient may require relief by ablation of the ganglion with injection of alcohol. A severe side-effect of this procedure is trigeminal anaesthesia, when the lack of corneal sensation results in exposure (neuroparalytic) keratitis due to various microbes including *Candida albicans* (Fig. 4.30 in Seal *et al.*, 1998). Shingles can be recurrent. On occasions, particularly if the patient is immunosuppressed, localized shingles develops together with systemic chickenpox (Fig. 4.38). In HIV-positive patients, VZV may be severe, with long-lasting or haemorrhagic vesicles forming over wider areas of the skin (Fig. 4.43).

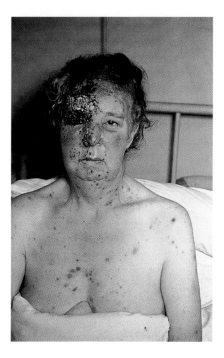

Figure 4.38: Herpes zoster ophthalmicus (shingles), involving the Vth cranial nerve, plus systemic chickenpox.

Aciclovir has been used intravenously in doses of 5 mg/kg 8-hourly for 5 days or at 10 mg/kg every 8 hrs for zoster in the immunocompromised. It is well tolerated and reduces the severity of the vesicular lesion but must be given in the prodromal phase to be really effective. It has been shown in some studies to reduce pain in the acute phase of the disease and to reduce the healing time of the rash. However, post-herpetic neuralgia has not been helped. Famciclovir (oral therapy as 250 mg tds for 7 days or 500 mg if immunocompromised) is a new alternative and is being marketed for its better effect in treating *Herpes zoster* infections.

Epstein–Barr virus (EBV)

Epstein–Barr virus causes the majority of cases of glandular fever in Europe in young adolescents, Burkitt's lymphoma in Africa and Papua New Guinea in children aged 4–12 and nasopharyngeal carcinoma in southern China in men aged 20–50. Most adults possess antibodies to it.

Glandular fever presents in teenagers with fever, malaise, pharyngitis, lymphadenopathy, mild hypersplenism and a transient macular rash. This rash is much enhanced if the patient is given ampicillin, due to the formation of antibodies to this antibiotic from EBV-transformed B lymphocytes which is a peculiar feature of this virus infection. There is a lymphocytosis when the B lymphocytes

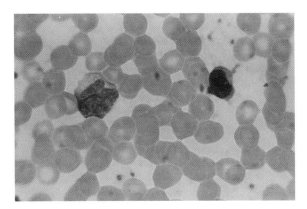

Figure 4.39:
Reactive lymphocyte
in a blood film of
EBV glandular fever
(×200).

are characteristically enlarged and reactive (Fig. 4.39). EBV transforms a proportion of them to blast cells that contain viral genome and divide indefinitely for the rest of the patient's life – hence the potential for oncogenicity.

The illness can take a protracted course with prolonged malaise lasting up to 6 months. Various systemic effects can develop, including encephalitis which may require attempted therapy with aciclovir (Bhatti *et al.*, 1990) that can be successful. Aciclovir has some antiviral activity against EBV but is not as effective as it is against *Herpes simplex*.

Specific and non-specific antibodies develop. Use has been made of non-specific antibodies for many years for diagnostic purposes with the Paul–Bunnell test. B cells transformed by EBV produce antibodies with a number of specificities – that for ampicillin has already been mentioned. Another is agglutinating antibody for horse or sheep red blood cells. This agglutinating ability can be removed by absorption with ox red cells but not with guinea-pig kidney tissue. This test was cumbersome and has been replaced with the slide agglutination test – the 'Monospot' test – using the same principle.

Burkitt's lymphoma presents mostly as a tumour of the jaw, less often of the orbit and other sites. EBV genome can be demonstrated in the tumour cells. There is much debate about the role of malaria as a cofactor. Malaria has a similar geographical distribution. It can cause immunosuppression, which may interfere with the control and destruction of tumour cell development by cytotoxic T lymphocytes.

Human immunodeficiency virus (HIV)

Early acute infection

Approximately 6–10 weeks after acquisition, when seroconversion is taking place, early acute infection can present with various systemic symptoms including fever,

89

headache and an exanthem (Figs 4.40–4.42). This rash, which does not itch, presents on most parts of the body and includes papular lesions and mouth ulcers. The rash is transitory within the spectrum of HIV disease and does not produce vesicles or pustules. The diagnosis may be confirmed either by identifying the P24 antigen or the virus load or by showing seroconversion with production of antibodies to HIV.

Complications of acquired immunodeficiency syndrome (AIDS)

Progression of HIV results in the acquired immunodeficiency syndrome (AIDS). Treatment is given with systemic therapy and involves a dual approach with an antiretroviral drug inhibiting production of reverse transcriptase required for virus replication, such as zidovudine (azidothymidine or AZT), and a protease inhibitor such as indinavir preventing virus particle function (Deeks *et al.*, 1997); at present combinations of three or four drugs are used. These drugs are listed in Table 2.2.

This combined approach is prolonging the lifespan of HIV-infected individuals and increasing their immune responsiveness so that the incidence of opportunistic infection is rapidly falling. There is a lack of HIV reproduction in lymphocytes, although the virus is not eradicated, and a CD4+ Th-lymphocyte count may rise above $200/mm^3$, at which level opportunistic infection is prevented by the immune response. Such chemotherapy has to be maintained for the lifespan of the individual.

Unfortunately, the drugs given above (Table 2.2) are expensive and only available to the 2% of cases worldwide presenting in Europe and the USA. The overall majority of infected individuals live in Africa, South America and the Far East, where opportunistic infection is the presenting symptom and the usual cause of death. Systemic infection with resistant strains of *M. tuberculosis* is an important problem. Another is the recurrence of severe *Herpes zoster* infection (Fig. 4.43), which becomes intractable, causing severe pain. Large doses of aciclovir or famciclovir should be given. In Thailand and the Far East, systemic infection by *Penicillum marneffei* is a particular problem, considered in Chapter 9. Chronic candidosis and other skin infections may occur.

Paramyxoviruses

The paramyxoviruses contain RNA and a surface coat with haemagglutinins which are used for testing antibody production. They produce characteristic exanthema.

Measles

Before measles vaccine became available, this was a widespread infection of childhood spread by the respiratory route. There is fever and a macular rash with

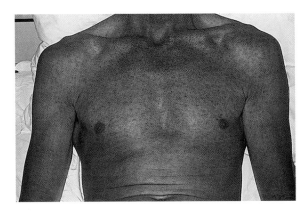

Figure 4.40:
Exanthem due to acute HIV infection showing appearance on chest.

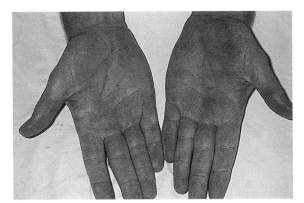

Figure 4.41: Close-up of exanthem on hands due to acute HIV infection.

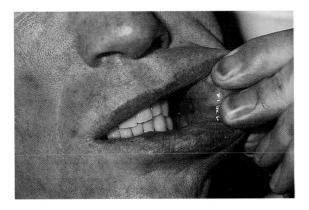

Figure 4.42: Close-up of exanthem on face and mouth ulcer due to acute HIV infection.

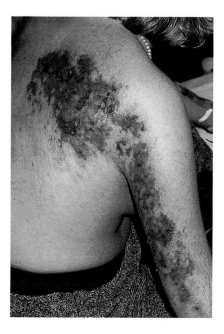

Figure 4.43: Severe *Herpes zoster* infection of the back and arm of a patient dying of AIDS due to HIV infection (prior to combination chemotherapy).

mouth ulceration (Koplik's spots). It causes severe symptoms in malnourished children, especially with vitamin A deficiency, when there is conjunctivitis and keratitis that can result in blindness; death occurs in 1 in 3000 cases. There can also be respiratory and neurological complications with encephalitis. Measles infection in the first trimester of pregnancy has a risk of inducing congenital malformation or spontaneous abortion. Subacute sclerosing panencephalitis is a rare devastating complication that has shown a striking decline since immunization was introduced. Immunization must be maintained.

Rubivirus

Rubella (German measles) is a common childhood disease with non-specific signs and symptoms including postauricular and suboccipital adenopathy, low-grade fever and a transient erythematous rash. It causes congenital deformation in the first trimester of pregnancy, for which reason there is a mass immunization programme which should be maintained. There are good antibody tests for this virus which allow successful screening of the antenatal population.

Parvoviruses

Parvoviruses can replicate only in the presence of another virus or of active DNA synthesis in rapidly dividing host cells. They are the smallest of all viruses with

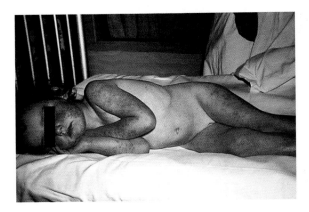

Figure 4.44: Rash of erythema infectiosum (fifth disease) due to parvovirus B19.

single-stranded DNA 5.5 kb long. They only code for three polypeptides (two of which are structural) and otherwise depend on the host cell. The pathogenic parvovirus B19 causes two types of infection.

Erythema infectiosum was also known as 'fifth' disease, on the basis that there were six recognized childhood exanthemata including measles, rubella, scarlet fever (due to *S. pyogenes*), exanthem subitum (or roseola infantum, due to HHV-6) and Duke's disease (a rash of obscure aetiology). It is also known as 'slapped cheek syndrome'. There is an incubation period of 13–18 days after which there is fever and malaise. A rash need not appear but, when it does, it presents as a maculopapular rash over the malar areas followed within the next 4 days by a rash on the trunk and limbs which may persist for 2–3 weeks (Fig. 4.44). Differential diagnosis from other febrile illnesses with rashes is not always easy and it can simulate rubella. Laboratory confirmation is given by detection of IgM antibody. Spread is by the respiratory route.

Adults can also acquire the infection with joint involvement, especially hand and fingers in women. Arthralgia can persist for a few weeks. There are no sequelae except in the case of pregnancy, when infection can result in foetal death.

Parvovirus infection (type B19) can cause aplastic anaemic crises in susceptible individuals by multiplying in red cell precursors (late normoblasts) with a lytic effect. Infection is not obvious with normal health but presents in those with chronic haemolytic anaemia due to sickle cell or thalassaemias.

Enteroviruses

Coxsackie and ECHO (enteric cytopathogenic human orphan) viruses are spread by both the respiratory and enteric routes. They owe their name to their initial identification from faecal pollution and only much later was cross-infection by

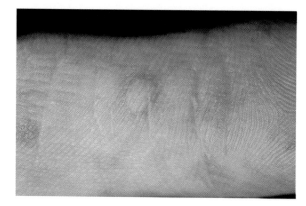

Figure 4.45: Papule on a finger of hand, foot and mouth disease (Coxsackie A virus).

the respiratory route proven. They cause systemic illness with non-specific signs and symptoms including fever and rashes. The most characteristic strains – Coxsackie A5, 10 and 16 viruses – cause hand foot and mouth disease (Fig. 4.45). From a few to a 100 lesions are found on the margins of the dorsum and palms of hands, soles of the feet as well as on the posterior oropharynx. They begin as erythematous macules or papules in the centre of which arises an oval vesicle which rapidly ulcerates. The infection lasts 7–10 days. Virus can be isolated from vesicle fluid, throat and stool cultures. Diagnosis can also be made by measuring rises in IgM antibody titres. The differential diagnosis is from *H. simplex* virus and other enteroviruses. Treatment is symptomatic.

5. INFECTIONS OF THE SUBCUTANEOUS TISSUE (HYPODERMIS) AND FASCIA

This chapter considers infections of the deeper tissues. Some of these infections are associated with penetrating trauma while others arise *de novo* in the tissues. Spread of infection internally is via the bloodstream from a distant focus. Such bacteraemias often settle out to cause infection at sites with internal bruising or vascular insufficiency. This may involve trauma, such as a fall from a horse, with *Clostridium perfringens* gangrene of a closed lesion.

Bites and stings

Dog bite

The classic dog bite involves laceration of tissues and inoculation of organisms indigenous to its mouth. These include in particular group G beta-haemolytic streptococci (Gaunt and Seal, 1987) and *Pasteurella multocida*. There is cellulitis around the wound which may or may not become purulent. Treatment should be given with oral amoxicillin, a cefalosporin or Augmentin.

Human bite

The human can also bite and lacerate the skin to produce a puncture wound. Possible infections include those found in serum and saliva such as hepatitis B virus, HIV and EBV. Bacterial infections are uncommon but infection due to *S. pyogenes* is quite possible, as it is carried in the saliva and throat, as can be *S. aureus* and *S. pneumoniae*. Chemotherapy depends on the circumstances of both the culprit and the recipient, but if there is a possibility of inoculation with hepatitis B virus then the recipient, if hepatitis B negative, should be offered a combination of active and passive immunization. Likewise, if the person responsible for the bite is known to be HIV positive the victim should be offered screening after appropriate counselling.

Saliva is considered a low risk material for HIV. Its contamination of a human bite wound, from an HIV positive individual, is not considered a high-enough risk in itself to warrant post-exposure prophylaxis (PEP) unless there has been blood-staining within the mouth, such as that following dentistry. If PEP is warranted, combination therapy should be given for 4 weeks with

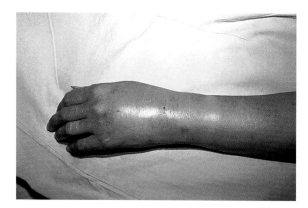

Figure 5.1: Severe inflammation of the dorsum of hand, wrist and forearm following a monkey bite.

zidovudine (200mg tds or 250mg bd) plus lamivudine (150mg bd) plus indinavir (800mg tds). Further advice is given by the UK Department of Health, 'Guidelines on Post-Exposure Prophylaxis for Health Care Workers Occupationally Exposed to HIV', June 1997.

Monkey bite

This is the most serious bite of all. Monkeys carry herpes B virus systemically and in their saliva. Infection is associated with a high mortality rate. Aciclovir should be given as prophylaxis as soon as possible. Severe inflammation, without identification of the organism, is shown in Fig. 5.1.

Snake bites

Snake bites cause problems from toxic venom injected into the skin (Fig. 5.2). This may be absorbed to cause DIC (disseminated intravascular coagulation) with

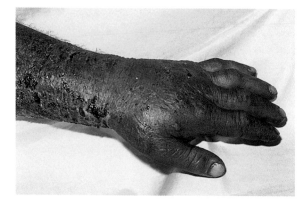

Figure 5.2: Necrosis (toxic necrolysis) due to a snake bite on the wrist.

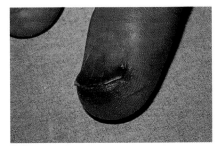

Figure 5.3: 'Seal' finger.

shock and acute respiratory distress syndrome (Chapter 1) or cause local toxic necrolysis. If the type of snake is known then it may be possible to inject antivenom serum, otherwise full supportive therapy is required.

In the UK the only indigenous venomous snake is the adder (*Vipera berus*), the bite of which can cause local and systemic effects. Local effects include pain, swelling, bruising and lymphadenopathy. Systemic effects include syncope, angioedema, colic with diarrhoea, ECG abnormalities, DIC and adult respiratory distress syndrome. Indications for antivenom include either local extension of swelling 4 hours after the bite or severe systemic effects. Treatment is given with one vial (10 ml) of European viper venom antiserum (available from Farillon) by intravenous injection over 15 minutes. The same dose is given to adults and children and can be repeated after 2 hours if symptoms persist. Adrenaline (epinephrine) injections must be available in case of anaphylactic reactions to the antivenom. For information on snake identification and other available antivenoms, contact the following numbers: London, 020 7635 9191; Liverpool, 0151-708 9393; Oxford, 01865-220968.

'Seal' bite

The bite of a seal, or contact when, for example, performing a post-mortem, can cause an infection known as 'seal' finger (Fig. 5.3). This infection is well known in Canada and Norway and is caused by an unidentified organism. Treatment should be given with tetracycline – penicillin and sulfonamides are ineffective.

Insect stings

These cause local pain and swelling but seldom severe direct toxicity unless many stings are inflicted simultaneously. Treatment can be given with an oral antihistamine. The main problem is that of anaphylaxis due to massive histamine release from previous exposure to the antigen from former stings. There can be collapse

Table 5.1 Spreading infections of the dermis and hypodermis mostly but not always synergistic (adapted from Kingston and Seal, 1990).

Clinical entity	Rate of spread	Principal microbial cause	Clinical subtypes	Animal model
Necrotizing fasciitis	Hours	BHS +/– S. aureus Mixed aerobes/anaerobes Mixed aerobes/anaerobes	Streptococcal or 'hospital' gangrene Non-streptococcal necrotizing fasciitis Fournier's gangrene	Seal and Kingston, 1988 — —
		Mouth anaerobes	Cancrum oris (noma)	Macdonald et al., 1956, Hampp and Mergenhagen, 1963
Anaerobic cellulitis	Hours or days	Mixed clostridia Mixed aerobes/anaerobes	Clostridial cellulitis Non-clostridial anaerobic cellulitis	— Onderdonk et al., 1979, Brook, 1988
Spreading ulcers				
Decubitus	Days or weeks	Mixed aerobes/anaerobes	—	—
Tropical	Days or weeks	BHS +/– S. aureus– Mixed aerobes/anaerobes	— Tropical phagedenic ulcer	— —
Diabetic foot	Days or weeks	Mixed aerobes/anaerobes	—	—
Meleney's progressive postoperative 'synergistic' gangrene	Weeks	? Entamoeba histolytica ?? synergistic or fastidious bacteria of unknown type	—	Brewer and Meleney, 1926[a]
Cutaneous amoebiasis	Weeks (occasionally rapid)	Entamoeba histolytica and bacteria	—	Mirelman, 1987

[a] It is not considered that Brewer and Meleney's (1926) animal model adequately reproduced the disease.

of the stung person within minutes. Immediate treatment is needed with intramuscular adrenaline (epinephrine). EpiPen is the best self-administered preparation, when 300 μg (0.3 mg) of adrenaline at 1 mg/ml (1 in 1000) is administered intramuscularly by the autoinjector; 1.7 ml of solution remains in the autoinjector for further use. The same dose of 300 μg is given to adults and children (over 30 kg) and can be repeated after 15 minutes if necessary. For children under 30 kg, EpiPen junior is available and delivers 150 μg (0.15 mg).

Ulcers and gangrene

Bacterial

With the exception of myositis, the following infections are considered by their rate of spread and are reviewed in Table 5.1.

Necrotizing fasciitis

Necrotizing fasciitis due to S. pyogenes (and synergistically with S. aureus). Necrotizing fasciitis is a clinical diagnosis of acute gangrene of the tissues immediately above the fascial plane involving the subcutaneous tissue, hypodermis and dermis. Its appearance begins with a patchy erythema of the skin that is swollen and very tender. The edge is not raised and demarcated as in erysipelas. Lymphangitis is absent in contrast to cellulitis, when it is prominent. The patient is febrile, later becoming toxaemic with confusion and disorientation. After 24 hours dusky purple areas develop with blistering and bullae, within islands of normal-looking skin, while the erythema and tissue oedema spread further (Fig. 5.4). Rapid necrosis of subcutaneous tissue occurs with deep undermining of

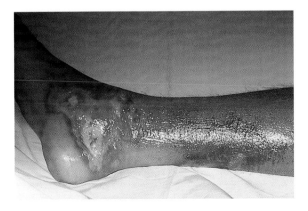

Figure 5.4: Acute *S. pyogenes* necrotizing fasciitis of the leg in a diabetic showing the lesion in its different stages of spread.

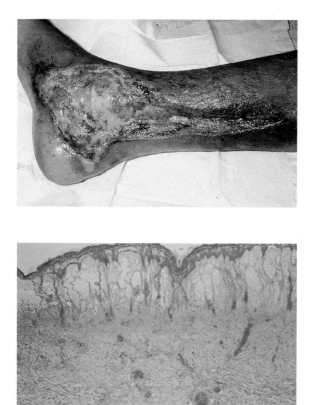

Figure 5.5: Acute debridement of *S. pyogenes* necrotizing fasciitis.

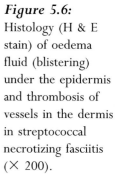

Figure 5.6: Histology (H & E stain) of oedema fluid (blistering) under the epidermis and thrombosis of vessels in the dermis in streptococcal necrotizing fasciitis (× 200).

ulcerated areas but superficial to the fascial plane. Unless controlled by surgery, with deep incisional drainage or debridement (Fig. 5.5) of the infected necrosing area, there is rapid progression over several days up a limb or across the abdomen with a fatal result from septicaemia or toxaemia. The edge of the spreading lesion should be marked with a pen and its advance followed hourly. There should be no delay in debridement with attention to necrosis underlying the blistering ulcerated lesions. Fatality often takes place within the first 24 hours either due to uncontrolled or inadequately managed *S. pyogenes* septicaemia, associated with toxic shock syndrome (TSS) and organ failure, or due to disseminated intravascular coagulation (DIC) from liberated exotoxin-A with a fatal embolus in a brain or heart vessel.

The nidus of the infection, often associated with minor trauma, is due to *S. pyogenes* and in 25% of cases there is an identified combined infection with *S. aureus*. Occasionally, necrotizing fasciitis is due to *S. aureus* alone – five childhood cases involving the mammary region have been reported recently

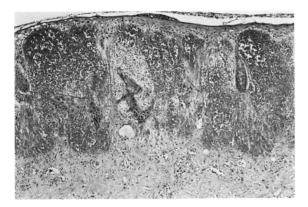

Figure 5.7: Histology (H & E stain) of haemorrhage into the dermis in the streptococcal necrotizing fasciitis shown in Fig. 5.4 (× 200).

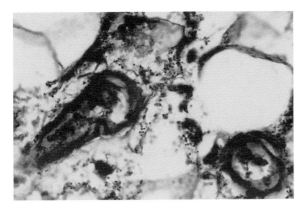

Figure 5.8: Gram stain of streptococci around thrombosed vessels in the dermis in the necrotizing fasciitis shown in Fig. 5.4 (× 200).

in France (Bodemer *et al.*, 1997) and two cases in Israel following needle puncture wounds (Regev *et al.*, 1998). It is thought that the alpha-lysin toxin produced by *S. aureus*, which paralyses the smooth muscle of arterioles and is leucocidal, not only initiates thrombosis of the subcutaneous vessels, but predisposes towards multiplication of *S. pyogenes* by impeding host defences, so allowing it to spread through tissue in the direction of the lymphatics (Seal and Kingston, 1988). *S. aureus* is left behind at the site of trauma. This explains the patchy clinical appearance, due to the irregular subcutaneous thrombosis, which in itself is diagnostic. Recognition and early therapy are all-important in this medical and surgical emergency (Sellers *et al.*, 1996). When the diagnosis is missed there is a 100% fatality rate while, when the condition is recognized, this rate can be reduced to 25% (Sellers *et al.*, 1996; Li *et al.*, 1997a).

Histology of tissue, using haematoxylin and eosin staining of paraffin-embedded sections, shows extensive thrombosis of vessels which results in necrosis of

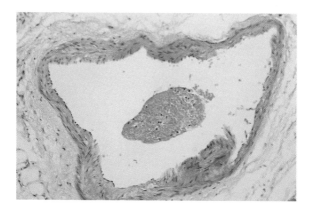

Figure 5.9: Ante-mortem thrombus in a coronary vessel of a patient who died of necrotizing fasciitis, septicaemia and DIC due to *S. pyogenes* (× 200).

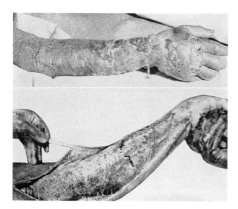

Figure 5.10: Successful debridement of necrotizing fasciitis in China without antibiotics. (Reproduced from Meleney FL, *Archives of Surgery*, 1924, **9**, 317–64.)

the epidermis and dermis (Barker *et al.*, 1987). This presents clinically as blistering, with accumulation of fluid under the epidermis (Fig. 5.6), which then separates the dermal layer. This is accompanied by the purple discoloration which is due to haemorrhage into the dermis (Fig. 5.7) followed by ulceration. Gram staining shows many streptococci in the tissue around the vessels (Fig. 5.8). These effects result in the variable clinical features of blistering and discoloration alongside normal and gangrenous skin with no clear distinguishing margin between them. In addition, there will be evidence of DIC in some patients. Figure 5.9 shows ante-mortem thrombus in a coronary vessel of an elderly patient who died of DIC after presenting 24 hours earlier with necrotizing fasciitis beginning around one ankle; *S. pyogenes* was isolated from tissue and blood cultures. A similar strain of *S. pyogenes* to that infecting the patient was isolated from throat carriage in the family. The necrotizing effect can be considered protective in that the greater the degree of thrombosis in tisssue, the less likely

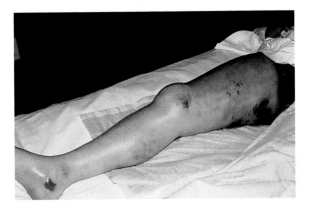

Figure 5.11: Acute *S. pyogenes* necrotizing fasciitis involving the entire leg.

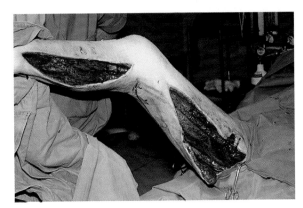

Figure 5.12: Incisional drainage of the calf and thigh, as practised by Meleney, together with antibiotics which resulted in control of the infection without amputation.

there is to be a fatal septicaemia with DIC, although both have been witnessed together, as here.

Therapy should include very large doses of intravenous benzylpenicillin, with 14.4 g or 24 megaunits per day, or a cefalosporin if the patient is allergic to penicillin, or erythromycin or clindamycin if allergic to both. The use of heparinization should be considered as part of the therapeutic strategy but may be contraindicated if early surgery is to proceed. Heparin has been used successfully to control the DIC and to prevent further thrombosis in vessels of the subcutaneous tissue and hence to stop the spreading gangrenous process (Hammar and Wanger, 1977). In addition, antibiotics will not penetrate through the tissue in the presence of widespread thrombosis, which is another reason to heparinize the patient – the danger is possible massive bleeding into the tissue, which must be carefully observed.

Meleney (1924) first demonstrated in Beijing, China, in the preantibiotic era, that incisional wound drainage or debridement of necrotizing fasciitis (thought to

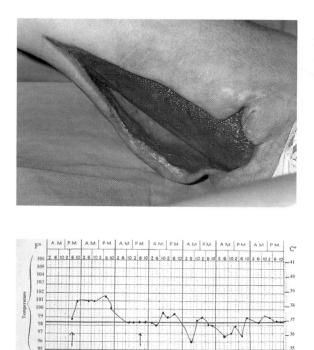

Figure 5.13:
Satisfactory drainage
while granulation
tissue forms in the
patient in Fig. 5.12.

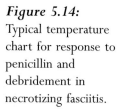

Days

Figure 5.14:
Typical temperature
chart for response to
penicillin and
debridement in
necrotizing fasciitis.

be due to *S. pyogenes*) could successfully prevent further spread of the infection and promote healing (Fig. 5.10). He wrote a fundamental treatise on the surgical management of this condition which is still fully relevant and applicable today. Indeed, surgical drainage or debridement similar to his techniques is required today, with the role of antibiotics being to control septicaemia and prevent recurrence (Figs 5.11–5.14). Antibiotics alone in the absence of surgery will not work because the infection spreads with further thrombosis. If surgery cannot be used then a combination of antibiotics and heparin should be considered. Amputation is occasionally required, particularly if fingers are involved (Fig. 5.15), but it can usually be avoided because the infective thrombotic process is above the fascial plane and not below it, in contrast to myositis particularly by *Cl. perfringens*.

Necrotizing fasciitis due to other beta-haemolytic streptococci (BHS). This occurs in the elderly. It has been associated with colonization of toe webs by BHS Lancefield group C or G isolates and has followed chiropody or blisters on toes. It presents similarly to the *S. pyogenes* disease (Fig. 5.16) but

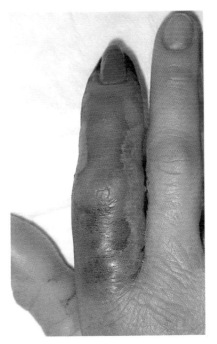

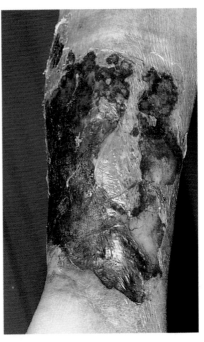

Figure 5.15: Acute *S. pyogenes* necrotizing fasciitis of the finger, following a minor burn, requiring amputation.

Figure 5.16: Acute necrotizing fasciitis of the calf due to BHS Lancefield group C treated with penicillin.

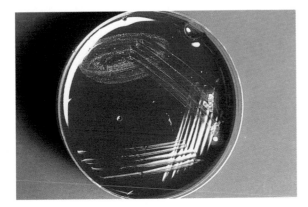

Figure 5.17: Single colony of BHS Lancefield group C cultured from the necrotic tissue shown in Fig. 5.16 in the presence of penicillin, by inhibiting the antibiotic with dilution or 'spreading out' on agar.

the degree of subcutaneous thrombosis is less and there is better penetration of penicillin into the tissues which requires inactivation to culture the organism (Fig. 5.17).

Necrotizing fasciitis due to *Vibrio vulnificans*. Refer to Chapter 8.

Necrotizing fasciitis due to mixed aerobic/anaerobic bacterial infection. The similar clinical syndrome of necrotizing fasciitis can develop due to a mixture of aerobic and anaerobic bacteria albeit in particular circumstances. In some areas, such as the USA, a mixed aerobic–anaerobic bacterial flora has accounted for 68% of specimens, with anaerobic bacteria only accounting for 22% of specimens (Brook *et al.*, 1995); a similar situation has also been reported from a detailed bacteriological study in India, with 50% of cases due to aerobic bacteria alone and 50% due to aerobic/anaerobic combinations with up to 9 isolates of bacteria present from the necrotic tissue (Singh *et al.*, 1996). A trend towards polymicrobial infection has also been reported from Singapore when the majority of patients had some form of underlying disease (Li *et al.*, 1997a). Polymicrobial infection is identified following abdominal injury, due to gunshot wounds or trauma, and good use of anaerobic culture techniques (Brook 1995, 1996; Singh *et al.*, 1996). This mixture can involve Gram-negative coliform bacteria, *S. pyogenes* and *S. aureus* and various anaerobes including peptostreptococci, *Bacteroides* spp. and *Clostridia* spp. This type of necrotizing fasciitis may arise after surgery or a compound fracture. It can also be due to a neoplasm of the gastrointestinal tract perforating and penetrating into surrounding tissue or to severe immunosuppression. It is also more likely to occur in diabetic patients, Fournier's gangrene and cancrum oris (Table 5.1).

Incidence of necrotizing fasciitis. There is a clear need, both in the public interest and for health surveillance, to ascertain the risk of necrotizing fasciitis. Such knowledge contributes to planning for emergency treatment with appropriate surgery and antibiotics. The requirement for cohort studies to ascertain correct figures of incidence is discussed in Chapter 10.

Low (1995) and Kaul *et al* (1997) recently presented Canadian incidence figures from the Ontario study of invasive group A beta-haemolytic streptococcal (GAS) disease, when the incidence figure given for necrotizing fasciitis was 1/200 000 population with 25% mortality. Extrapolation to the UK population of 60 million would suggest 300 cases per year and 75 deaths.

Evidence from the Swedish reporting system for GAS was given with 21 cases of necrotizing fasciitis including 7 deaths in 1994 (Holm, 1995). Extrapolation to the UK would mean 105 cases per year and 35 deaths. Because any routine reporting system, as opposed to a study, depends on clinical identification premortem followed by successful laboratory isolation of GAS from routine cultures (often swabs rather than tissue), when patients have already received antibiotics, the real number of expected GAS cases will be at least three times those recorded, that is 315 with 105 deaths – a similar figure to Canada.

These figures contrast with those from the Public Health Laboratory Service (PHLS) in England and Wales, which recorded 49 proven cases of GAS necrotizing fasciitis in 1994. Comparison with the results above suggests that the PHLS figure is an underestimate by sixfold. The English reporting system was similar to that in Sweden (that is, expected to miss two-thirds of cases) but was also open to error by twofold because only 25% of hospitals have a PHLS laboratory. This suggests that the real English figure for GAS necrotizing fasciitis was approximately 294 cases during the year.

In addition, neither the English, Canadian or Swedish figures included cases due to either beta-haemolytic streptococcus Lancefield groups C or G or anaerobic or mixed aerobic/anaerobic synergistic mixtures which present with a similar clinical syndrome (Brook 1995, 1996; Singh *et al.*, 1996). These cases must be considered in the overall incidence figures of necrotizing fasciitis. In some, but not all, hospitals these types are less common than GAS disease. They are expected to be seen once per year in most large UK hospitals with approximately 75 cases of each per year in the UK.

Unfortunately, the incidence figure for necrotizing fasciitis as a clinical entity has still to be estimated in the UK because the diagnosis has not yet been made a reportable disease (Seal, 1995, 1996). If the Canadian study figure is accepted as real, and the English (PHLS) figure as an underestimate by six times, then 300 cases of necrotizing fasciitis per year can be expected in the UK due to GAS, 75 due to BHS group C/G and 75 due to synergistic aerobic/anaerobic bacteria. The condition has not disappeared, as predicted by some, but continues to be reported in the lay press. Medical awareness must be maintained at all times. In other areas, such as Hong Kong and Southeast Asia, it is important to know the incidence of necrotizing fasciitis due to *Vibrio vulnificus* (Chapter 8).

Acute gangrene due to Ps. aeruginosa

This only occurs in immunosuppressed individuals and is a particular problem in the treatment of leukaemias with whole-body irradiation (Fig. 5.18). Large intravenous doses of several antipseudomonal antibiotics including either ciprofloxacin, ceftazidime, gentamicin or tobramycin, and piperacillin, azlocillin or Timentin (ticarcillin/clavulanic acid) should be given; laboratory sensitivity tests are required.

Anaerobic cellulitis

This develops more slowly than necrotizing fasciitis over several days but usually has the same aetiology. Quite why a similar mixture of aerobic and anaerobic bacteria should produce this syndrome rather than necrotizing fasciitis relates more to host susceptibility and the site of the lesion than to the types of bacteria. Exceptional to this are mixed clostridia or *Cl. perfringens*, in which case severe anaerobic infection develops, especially if muscle is involved in a penetrating injury, when gas

107

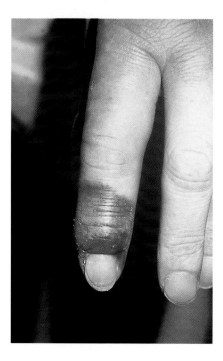

Figure 5.18: Acute gangrene of the index finger with *Ps. aeruginosa* septicaemia in a patient with acute myeloid leukaemia.

gangrene occurs and necessitates amputation. In the latter case there is usually trauma and mud splashing, as in the case of war wounds, but severe bruising with a fall can act as a nidus for clostridial gas gangrene, presumably due to a bacteraemia with the organism seeding into the anaerobic environment of injured muscle.

Description of the clinical presentation and bacteriology for anaerobic infections of war wounds in the preantibiotic era cannot better that of MacLennan (1943). Prophylaxis of such wounds should include large doses of a cefalosporin to inhibit clostrida and peptostreptococci which is also effective against beta-haemolytic streptococci and *S. aureus*. Metronidazole is required to inhibit *Bacteroides* spp. An effective alternative combination, but single drug to administer, is Augmentin (amoxicillin + clavulanic acid).

Spreading ulcers

Decubitus or pressure sores. Unrelieved pressure on the skin, in circumstances in which the patient cannot move, results in its necrosis from lack of perfusion. While this does occur to patients entering hospital with strokes or movement disabilities, it should not happen if they are managed with due understanding. Prevention of such 'pressure sores' is fully described in the literature – the patient must either be turned frequently and regularly or be placed on an air ripple bed

108

which frequently changes the pressure points on the skin. This is especially important near bony projections. Patients who are wheelchair-bound, such as those with multiple sclerosis, can develop several pressure sores at once and then be confined to bed for months while waiting for them to heal (Fig. 6.5).

When the epidermis/dermis is broken, the 'ulcer' quickly becomes infected. If this is situated near the sacrum then faecal flora predominates and the ulcer develops a foul smell. Continued pressure and bacterial infection contribute to failure of these ulcers to heal. Twenty-five such pressure sores were investigated by Sapico *et al.* (1986) in their classic study of the quantitative bacteriology in different stages of healing. They found that when grossly necrotic tissue was present, there was a density of $10^{6.4}$ bacteria per gram tissue for both aerobes and anaerobes; in the absence of nectrotic tissue but in the presence of undermining of the ulcer edge, there were $10^{2.7}$ aerobic and 10^{-1} anaerobic bacteria per gram tissue; without necrosis and undermining the ulcer yielded little growth. Foul smell was usually associated with the presence of anaerobes.

Management with caustic antiseptics such as Eusol will also delay healing particularly when applied for weeks, instead of days, at a time. This is exacerbated by gauze packs which tear out early formation of granulation tissue when removed. The beneficial effect of sugar paste for inhibiting bacterial growth and contributing to wound healing in this situation is considered in Chapter 6. Appendix F provides an algorithm for 'Which dressing?, a pharmacopoeia of possibilities' together with a listing and description of appropriate hydrocolloid, alginate and other dressings.

Tropical ulcers. These are considered in Chapter 8.

Diabetic foot. This is a unique situation. There is often a neuropathy present with decreased sensation together with a vasculopathy with decreased perfusion. There is also an impaired ability to produce an early vascular response as part of the host immune response to invading bacteria when the skin is broken. In addition, phagocytosis of bacteria is much less effective than in the non-diabetic, giving rise to frequent staphylococcal and streptococcal infections. It is for this reason that diabetic patients with ulcers on their feet have been given long-term prophylactic oral (first-generation) cefalosporins, such as cefradine, which have been claimed to reduce the number of patients presenting with progressive serious infection requiring amputation.

A small ulcer develops on the foot often following minor trauma. This becomes colonized with anaerobic bacteria in particular but may also be contaminated by toe web organisms such as BHS and *S. aureus* (Seal *et al.*, 1988). It is not uncommon for all three major species of anaerobes to be isolated from the ulcer – clostridia, bacteroides and peptostreptococci. These ulcers are peculiarly resistant to all attempts to promote healing and are often present for

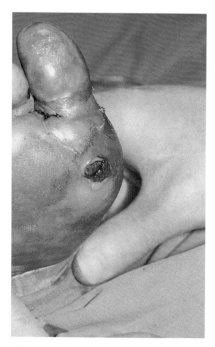 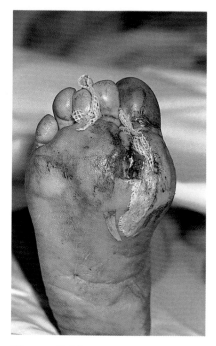

Figure 5.19: Anaerobic streptococcus (peptostreptococcus) infection of a plantar foot ulcer in a diabetic.

Figure 5.20: Debridement of ulcer of the patient in Fig. 5.19; the procedure failed, requiring amputation 3 days later.

months or years, gradually eroding the tissue surrounding them. Acute necrotizing infection is the usual end-stage result possibly due to increasing vascular insufficiency further decreasing host defences. The necrotizing infection spreads along the tissue plane of the plantar surface of the foot (Fig. 5.19) from the ulcer towards the lower leg. Despite very large intravenous doses of antibiotics including metronidazole (for anaerobes) and cefalosporins or Augmentin (for aerobic bacteria), it is usually necessary to amputate the foot or even the lower leg. This is necessary because the spreading necrotizing infectious process is not controlled by antibiotics alone, and debridement surgery as practised for necrotizing fasciitis is not possible within the confines of the foot (Fig. 5.20). There is also the background problem of vascular insufficiency.

Meleney's progressive postoperative 'synergistic' gangrene (ulcer). Whether synergy plays an important role or not in this syndrome is not clear. The disease presents as progressive postoperative gangrene at an abdominal or thoracic

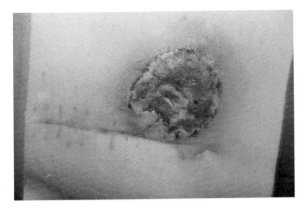

Figure 5.21:
Meleney's progressive postoperative 'synergistic' gangrene of the abdomen of questionable aetiology. (Courtesy of Abbott Laboratories.)

wound site, frequently when wire retention sutures are used. A few days following surgery, a tender, red, swollen and indurated area develops near the wound. This slowly becomes a shaggy ulcer with undermined purple oedematous gangrenous margins (Meleney's ulcer) (Fig. 5.21). There is relentless spread without treatment to become an enormous size with severe pain but little toxicity. Multiple fistulae can be present. Therapy has depended on further surgery with limited success. Claims have been made of successful treatment with hyperbaric oxygen.

Davson *et al.* (1988) carried out a retrospective and comparative review of 127 case reports of Meleney's progressive postoperative 'synergistic' gangrene and of 62 examples of postoperative amoebic (*Entamoeba histolytica*) skin gangrene for cases published between 1924 and 1985. This review found that these two entities were clinically indistinguishable. There were also no distinguishing bacteriological results using the older methods given in each paper. The histological features were entirely non-specific, precluding a definitive diagnosis. They concluded that if Meleney's progressive postoperative 'synergistic' gangrene cannot be diagnosed pathologically then its existence becomes debatable and offered the alternative aetiology of cutaneous amoebiasis due to *Entamoeba histolytica*. This might respond to hyperbaric oxygen, as this amoeba needs low oxygen levels for growth.

There are certain reservations however. Cutaneous amoebiasis is rare even following amoebic abscesses (Guerrant, 1986). If *Entamoeba histolytica* is the cause of Meleney's progressive postoperative 'synergistic' gangrene, then it should be more common in countries where infection by *Entamoeba histolytica* is more common – this has not been shown. Such cases warrant study with modern bacteriological methods including prolonged incubation for fastidious and anerobic bacteria as well as sensitive techniques to identify *Entamoeba histolytica*. Finally, the amoebic–bacterial relationship needs exploring as there is evidence

111

for an effect of bacteria on the growth rate and possible pathogenicity of the amoeba (Mirelman, 1987).

Brewer and Meleney (1926), who originally described the condition following operation for acute perforative appendicitis, also produced a putative animal model to support their hypothesis of synergistic bacterial gangrene. This model involved injecting the animal subcutaneously with various mixtures of bacteria isolated from their patients, including microaerophilic streptococcus and *S. aureus*, with observation of a gangrenous process over the following days. This does not explain the clinical condition since it develops over weeks and not days. Thus Brewer and Meleney's model is *not* considered adequate to reproduce the disease (Kingston and Seal, 1990). It is quite remarkable how textbooks of surgery have reproduced Brewer and Meleney's unproven hypothesis for 70 years! The unanswered conundrum, however, is whether their patients at the time of their appendicitis in the early 1920s also carried *Entamoeba histolytica* in their gastointestinal tract which proceeded to infect the wound and surrounding skin; this is quite feasible.

Myositis

Acute rhabdomyolysis (pyomyositis) is usually due to *S. pyogenes* in temperate climates and *S. aureus* in tropical climates (Nather *et al.*, 1987). The infection is rare. It is possible that it only occurs after there has been a viral myositis, often due to enteroviruses, followed by a *S. pyogenes* (or *S. aureus*) bacteraemia (Porter *et al.*, 1981). Most reported cases have been fatal but two survivors are recorded (Nather *et al.*, 1987). The patient presents with acute toxaemia and swelling of muscle groups (Figs 5.22 and 5.23). The situation needs to be recognized as a medical emergency. Large doses of intravenous penicillin together with supportive therapy for streptococcal TSS, due to exotoxin A, as well as heparinization for an expected DIC, and supportive intravenous therapy possibly including plasma exchange should be given. Pyogenic muscle requires radical excision and drainage to help control the infection (Nather *et al.*, 1987); it may not be necessary to amputate. Because of the very high mortality rate all therapeutic modalities are needed.

Fungal

Zygomycotic gangrenous cellulitis can cause severe destruction of tissue in an immunocompromised patient who is often a grafted organ recipient; it may also affect otherwise healthy individuals. Fungi that can cause this type of necrosis include *Rhizopus*, *Absidia* (Amin *et al.*, 1998), *Rhizomucor* and *Saksenaea* species. Patients have usually had prior tissue injury, including burn wounds, at the original site of infection. Half these patients are diabetic, who are more prone to this type of gangrene for the reasons given above. The infection is often misdiag-

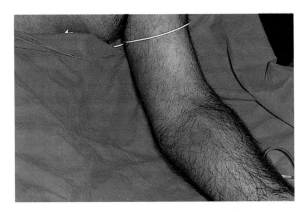

Figure 5.22:
Swollen arm and rash of fatal acute pyomyositis due to *S. pyogenes*.

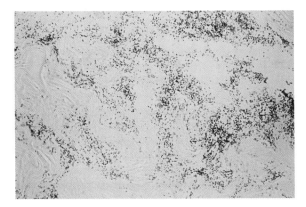

Figure 5.23: Gram stain of muscle from patient in Fig. 5.22 showing massive overwhelming infection with *S. pyogenes* (× 1000).

nosed, progresses rapidly and is fatal. It should be considered in the differential diagnosis of progressive necrotizing lesions. Identification requires histology and culture of tissue. Therapy involves extensive debridement and intravenous amphotericin; hyperbaric oxygen may be useful as well (Bentur *et al.*, 1998).

Viral

Recurrent *Herpes simplex* infection can result in severe necrosis of the epidermis and dermis but does not involve the hypodermis as in necrotizing fasciitis; it may, however, begin to look similar (Fig. 5.24). This is most unusual and can occur in an otherwise healthy individual. Deep necrotic herpetic lesions can occur in AIDS patients.

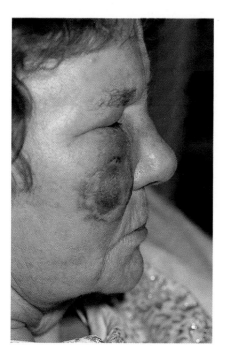

Figure 5.24: Herpes simplex
necrosis of cheek.

Successful therapy with famciclovir has been reported recently following failed therapy with aciclovir – it may become the antiviral drug of choice for necrotizing herpetic lesions because it has good bioavailability and is effective against aciclovir-resistant *H. simplex*.

Protozoal

Cutaneous amoebiasis due to Entamoeba histolytica

This usually starts with swelling and induration which rapidly breaks down to leave an irregular undermined ulcer. This lesion is not diagnostic in itself but is either a deeply invading ulcer or an ulcerated granuloma (amoeboma). It usually involves the abdomen with a wound infection following bowel surgery or may develop around the anal margin. The onset is often delayed but it can spread rapidly and cause fatality. There is severe pain and inexorable progression. There is a triple zonation of colour and a serpiginous outline (which mimics Meleney's progressive postoperative 'synergistic' gangrene). Treatment is given with metronidazole. The adult dose is 800 mg orally three times daily for 5 days.

Examination of fresh material from the lesion usually reveals amoebae. Material should be collected from the edge of the ulcer avoiding necrotic tissue and examined immediately. The presence of motile trophozoites containing red cells is diagnostic. Diagnosis by haematoxylin and eosin stain on fixed tissue is very unreliable. Repeated investigation of faeces for motile trophozoites and cysts should also be made as this is the usual source.

Cutaneous amoebiasis due to Acanthamoeba

This has so far only been identified in immunocompromised individuals. In such patients, any chronic discharging sinus or wound should be investigated by

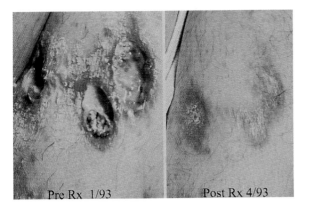

Pre Rx 1/93   Post Rx 4/93

Figure 5.25: Discharging sinuses and abdominal wound infection due to *Acanthamoeba rhysodes* in an immuno-compromised individual. (Courtesy of Dr G Visvesvara, CDC Atlanta.)

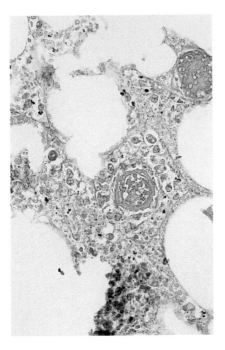

Figure 5.26: H & E section of trophozoites of *A. healyi* causing infection of the dermis and hypodermis (×100). (Courtesy of Dr G Visvesvara, CDC Atlanta.)

115

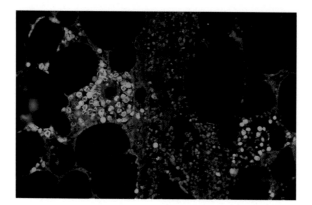

Figure 5.27:
Immunofluorescence of trophozoites of *A. healyi* shown in Fig. 5.26 (×40). (Courtesy of Dr G Visvesvara, CDC Atlanta.)

microscopy and specific culture for the free-living protozoa (Appendix B). *Acanthamoeba* is one of many free-living amoebae (Page, 1988), but the only one to have been clearly identified as pathogenic to both man and monkey, albeit in particular circumstances.

Slater *et al.* (1994) described the first case of disseminated infection due to *Acanthamoeba* spp. The patient had undergone a renal transplant and was on immunosuppressive therapy. The infection was characterized by granulomatous infiltrates in the brain and skin (Fig. 5.25) from which *A. rhysodes* was isolated. There was chronic discharge of necrotic purulent tissue from five different ulcers, ranging in size from 2 to 5 cm, that was uncontrolled by antibiotics. The concomitant immunosuppression including the use of prednisone will have inhibited both cell-mediated immunity and ingestion of the amoeba by macrophages, which are the most important cells for preventing tissue invasion.

Figures 5.26 and 5.27 are taken from a patient with multiple cutaneous ulcers (Visvesvara, unpublished). One formalin-fixed, paraffin-embedded section was stained by haematoxylin and eosin (H & E), while the other was treated with different rabbit anti-sera raised to a panel of acanthamoebae. This amoeba was identified as *A. healyi* on the basis of the highest intensity of fluorescence gained with the sera (Visvesvara, unpublished).

Successful systemic therapy has been given with 4 weeks of intravenous pentamidine isethionate (Slater *et al.*, 1994). In addition, topical therapy was given with chlorhexidine gluconate (concentration not stated, ? 0.2%) and 2% ketoconazole cream. The result was a dramatic improvement in skin lesions. Therapy was complicated by signs of nephrotoxicity so oral itraconazole therapy was given instead until all the skin lesions had healed, which took 8 months. The imidazoles are partially effective against *Acanthamoeba* spp. and this is assisted by the good absorption and tissue penetration of itraconazole.

6. WOUND HEALING AND THE USE OF SUGAR PASTE

Origins of use

Honey and sugar (sucrose) have been used to treat wounds for hundreds of years. Documents dating back to 1700 BC describe the treatment of battlefield wounds in ancient Egypt. The most reliable regimen employed utilized a mixture of honey with greases such as lard or resins which was packed into the wounds and held in place with muslin. Sculteus in 1679 described the use of finely powdered sugar for cleansing wounds and Zorin in 1714 reported on the value of sugar in promoting the healing of wounds and ulcers (Selwyn and Durodie, 1985).

Honey has good *in vitro* antimicrobial properties (Jeddar *et al.*, 1985; Cooper *et al.*, 1999) but it is not widely used to treat wounds. This is partly because its major components are glucose and fructose, which can be absorbed from a wound surface and may cause metabolic problems, particularly in diabetics. In addition, honey is difficult to standardize and sometimes contains resistant contaminating micro-organisms, particularly *Clostridium* spp.

Sugar is a disaccharide of glucose and fructose and is not metabolized if absorbed from a wound, and so is safe to use in diabetics. In 1976, Herszage and Montenegro of Argentina began to use ordinary granular sugar to treat the wounds of patients with postsurgical necrotic cellulitis. Further successes followed and in 1980 Herszage *et al.* reported on the use of ordinary granular sugar in 120 infected wounds and recorded a cure rate of 99.2%. The time taken for the wounds to heal varied between 9 days and 17 weeks, but it was observed that odour and secretion began to diminish within 24 hours of treatment commencing and disappeared totally after 72–96 hours. Knutson *et al.* (1981) reported on 5 years' experience of the use of sugar and povidone-iodine to enhance wound healing. They had treated 605 patients with a wide variety of wounds and noted rapid healing and debridement of eschar, a reduced requirement for skin grafting and reduced hospital costs, and concluded that the combination of sugar and povidone-iodine outperformed all other products for wound care and was the combination they most depended upon for wound, burn or ulcer treatment. In 1985 and 1988, Trouillet *et al.* described the use of sugar in the treatment of 19 patients with mediastinitis following cardiac surgery. Wounds were packed every 3–4 hours with ordinary commercially available granular sugar. The authors noted near complete debridement followed by the rapid formation of granulation tissue and eradication of bacterial infection after an average of 7.6 days of treatment. Topham (1992) from Zanzibar reported on the successful use of sugar pastes (with either povidone-iodine or chlorbutol) to treat pressure sores, burns and wounds, and observed that they offered workers with minimal resources a cheap, chemically pure and effective aid to wound healing.

Sugar was first used as a dressing in Northwick Park Hospital in 1982 (Middleton and Seal, 1985), when it was placed into infected radical vulvectomy wounds that had not responded to more conventional treatment. However, such wounds are difficult to pack with ordinary sugar which has the additional disadvantage that it is often contaminated with *Bacillus* spp., which is a contaminant derived from the packaging. Paste formulations, which allow the easy application of sugar to most wound types, were developed at Northwick Park in the mid-1980s and they overcame these problems. They have been used continuously since that time within the hospital with great success for treating infected and malodorous wounds (Gordon *et al.*, 1985; Seal and Middleton, 1991). They are now used at other centres throughout the UK.

The pastes are prepared in the hospital pharmacy by first mixing the hydrogen peroxide with the polyethylene glycol (PEG 400), which is then combined with the previously mixed sugars in a heavy-duty blender and mixed until homogeneous. The pastes are chemically and physically stable for at least 6 months at room temperature if kept in a tightly closed container and for 12 months if kept at 2–8°C. Their formulae are given in Table 6.1.

Caster and icing sugars were selected for the formulations as they help produce a smooth paste that is not prone to forming a solid 'cake' on storage. PEG 400 was chosen as the binder for the pastes as it does not interact with the other components and is readily available and relatively non-toxic. It can be absorbed from mucous membranes and high blood levels can be nephrotoxic (Wilson and Thomas, 1984). Although no toxic side-effects have been noted in our patients, many of whom are elderly and frail, sugar paste should be used

Table 6.1 Formulae of sugar pastes.

	Thin	Thick
Caster sugar[a]	1200 g	1200 g
Icing sugar (additive free)[b]	1800 g	1800 g
Polyethylene glycol (PEG) 400	1416 ml	686 ml
Hydrogen peroxide 30%	23.1 ml	19 ml

The final concentration of hydrogen peroxide is 0.15% v/w.
[a]Caster sugar is finely ground granular sucrose (cane or beet).
[b]Icing sugar is powdered sucrose (cane or beet). Ordinary icing (powdered) sugar usually contains calcium phosphate or sodium aluminium silicate which is added to prevent 'caking' on storage.

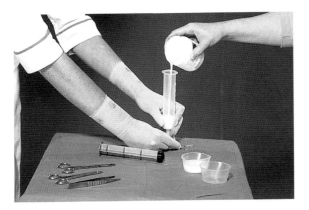

Figure 6.1: Thin sugar paste being poured into a syringe barrel ready for use.

with care in patients with impaired renal function as absorbed PEG is excreted renally (Archer *et al.*, 1987).

Thin sugar paste

Thin sugar paste has a similar consistency to that of thin honey and can be instilled via a syringe and fine plastic tube into abscess cavities with small openings (Fig. 6.1). Traditionally, such cavities are packed with ribbon gauze soaked in chemicals such as Eusol (Edinburgh University solution of lime containing not < 2500 ppm available chlorine) or povidone-iodine, which is often painful and of dubious efficacy.

Clinical examples of the use of thin sugar paste

Case 1. A 27-year-old patient with hypogammaglobulinaemia had two large abscesses, one in each buttock, and a smaller abscess in the right shoulder, all of which were infected with a variety of micro-organisms including *Mycoplasma* spp. The cavities had small openings and had previously been packed with ribbon gauze soaked in Eusol or povidone-iodine solution. Packing took place every 2 days and was so painful that general anaesthesia was required. The ribbon gauze became hard as it dried out within the cavities and was painful and difficult to remove. Antibiotics had been ineffective at controlling the infection which delayed healing of these abscesses. After 3 days of painless packing of the abscesses with thin sugar paste, instilled via a large-bore Argyll catheter (Fig. 6.2), the patient was able to walk, having previously been bed-bound. After 6 weeks, the buttock abscesses had healed completely.

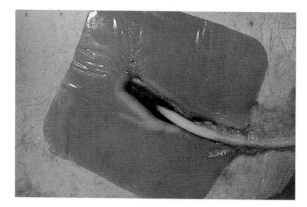

Figure 6.2:
Successful treatment of a large buttock abscess with thin sugar paste through a large-bore catheter.

Case 2. A 15-year-old patient with hypogammaglobulinaemia had multiple abscesses in the neck which had failed to respond to antibiotic therapy over the previous 6 months (Fig. 6.3). They exuded a copious yellow purulent discharge. Thin sugar paste was instilled into these abscesses and exuded out of the communicating branches. After 6 weeks, the various communicating abscesses had healed and the patient was discharged.

Thick sugar paste

Thick sugar paste has a consistency similar to that of modelling clay. It can be moulded in the gloved hand to the correct shape for packing into cavities with large openings such as pressure sores (Fig. 6.4).

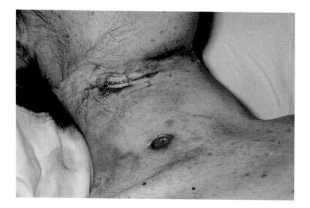

Figure 6.3: Multiple inter-communicating abscesses in the neck into which thin sugar paste was instilled by syringe and kwill.

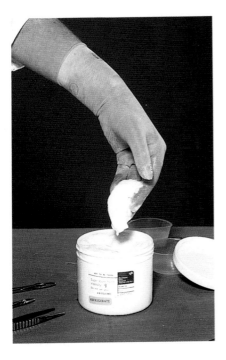

Figure 6.4: Gloved hand preparing to apply thick sugar paste.

Clinical examples of the use of thick sugar paste

Case 3. A 55-year-old male patient with multiple sclerosis had three large pressure sores in the sacral area. The wounds had enlarged over 1 year despite 'conventional' treatments (Fig. 6.5). He had been unable to cope at home and was bed-bound in hospital. The wounds (pressure sores) were packed twice daily with thick sugar paste (Figs 6.6 and 6.7). After 1 month, granulation tissue had formed (Fig. 6.8) and it continued to do so. After 3 months the wounds had virtually healed (Fig. 6.9). The patient was able to return home with healed wounds (Fig. 6.10) and live independently with use of his wheelchair.

Case 4. A 57-year-old man had undergone successful cardiac bypass surgery in a tertiary referral hospital but the wound became infected with methicillin-resistant *S. aureus* (MRSA). After 3 months of treatment with various wound dressings including Eusol, povidone-iodine and Debrisan, the wound was still infected with MRSA and had failed to heal (Fig. 6.11). The wound caused the patient much distress because, each time he breathed, it opened up and gave a gurgling sound, which was repeated on expiration. The wound was packed deeply twice daily with thick sugar paste (Fig. 6.12). Two weeks later the wound had healed sufficiently for

121

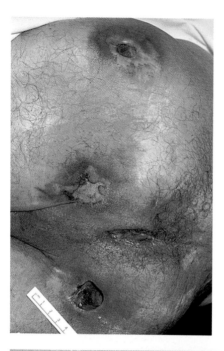

Figure 6.5: One-year-old non-healing bedsores in a multiple sclerosis patient.

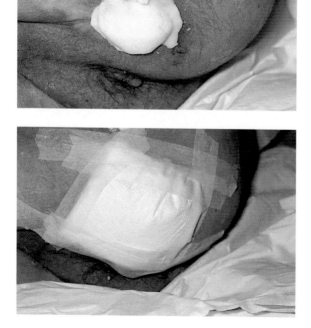

Figure 6.6: Thick sugar paste in wound.

Figure 6.7: Bandage to hold sugar paste in place (if the wound is in a suitable position, silastic foam is used instead of gauze).

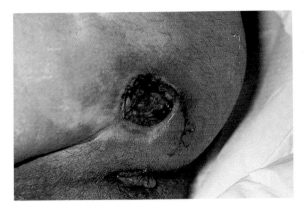

Figure 6.8: Early healing with sugar paste showing satisfactory formation of granulation tissue.

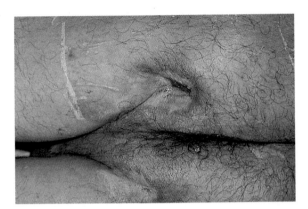

Figure 6.9: Late healing – sugar paste therapy now stopped and replaced with silastic foam.

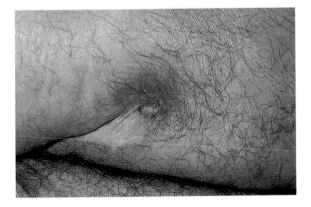

Figure 6.10: Finally healed bedsore returning wheelchair mobility to the patient.

123

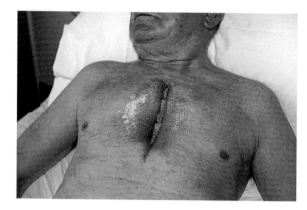

Figure 6.11: Non-healing thoracotomy wound after 3 months infected with MRSA.

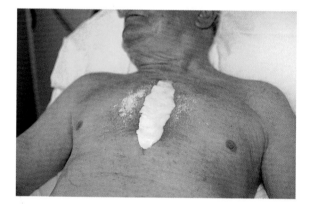

Figure 6.12: Treatment of patient in Fig. 6.11 with thick sugar paste.

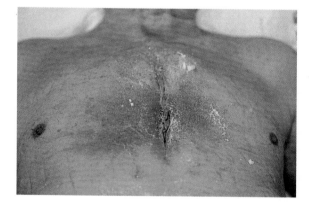

Figure 6.13: Wound of patient in Fig. 6.11 healing well after 2 weeks of sugar paste therapy.

the gurgling sounds to have disappeared (Fig. 6.13) and MRSA was no longer able to be isolated. Sugar paste treatment was continued and within 6 weeks the wound had healed completely. This reflects the successful treatment of postoperative mediastinitis by Trouillet *et al.* (1988) when raw granulated sugar was poured into the open wounds.

Method of use

Sugar paste is effective in treating many infected and/or malodorous wounds. When applied to a wound, sugar paste will normally dissolve within 4 hours. As it dissolves in the wound it also acts as an irrigant and further rinsing is not usually necessary. To maximize the antibacterial effects, twice-daily packing is suggested. Once packed the wound can be covered with another dressing to absorb the exudate, the choice of dressing being dependent on the location of the wound. Normally, treatment with sugar paste can be stopped when the infection has resolved: typically this takes 5–7 days. After this, we suggest that a dressing requiring fewer changes, such as a hydrogel or hydrocolloid, should be used until the wound is healed. For details of sugar paste application to the wound, refer to Appendix E.

Mode of antibacterial action of sugar pastes

Micro-organisms require water to grow and reproduce and such water requirements can be defined in terms of water activity (a_w) of the substrate rather than water concentration (Chirife *et al.*, 1983a). The water activity of a solution is

Table 6.2 Minimum a_w values and equivalent sugar concentrations for growth of various bacteria pathogenic to humans. Values were obtained by various workers and summarized by Chirife *et al.* (1983a).

Bacteria	Minimum a_w	Equivalent sugar conc. (g/100 g water)
Klebsiella spp.	0.96	66.7
	0.94	92.3
Salmonella oranienburg	0.96–0.94	66.7–92.3
Pseudomonas spp.	0.95	78.6
"	0.97	51.5
Cl. perfringens	0.97	51.5
E. coli	0.95	78.5
S. aureus	0.864	185.7
"	0.88	167.4

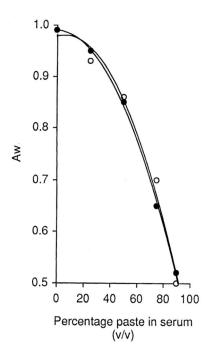

Figure 6.14: Effect on a_w of adding hydrogen-peroxide-free sucrose and xylose paste to serum. (Reproduced with permission from Ambrose *et al.*, *Antimicrob Ag Chemother,* 1991, **35**, 1799–803.) ●–●, xylose paste; O–O, sucrose paste.

Percentage paste in serum (v/v)

expressed as $a_w = p/po$ where p is the water vapour pressure of the solution and po is the vapour pressure of pure water at the same temperature. Addition of a solute (such as sucrose) to an aqueous solution in which a micro-organism is growing will have the effect of lowering the a_w with a concomitant effect upon cell growth. Every micro-organism has a limiting a_w below which it will not grow (Table 6.2) , for example, for streptococci, *Klebsiella* spp., *E. coli*, *Cl. perfringens* and *Pseudomonas* spp., the value is 0.95. *S. aureus* is most resistant and can proliferate with an a_w as low as 0.86 (Chirife *et al.*, 1983a).

The effect on a_w of adding serum to thin sugar paste (without hydrogen peroxide) is illustrated in Fig. 6.14. This graph indicates that an a_w of 0.86 is achieved with a mixture of approximately equal parts sugar paste and serum, which suggests that the pastes should have good antimicrobial activity.

In vitro antimicrobial activity

Antibacterial activity of sugar paste agars

Thin sugar paste (peroxide-free) was added to Columbia agar to give 10, 20, 30, 40 or 50% (vol/vol) sugar paste in agar. All the agar–sugar paste mixes were then autoclaved at 121°C for 15 minutes, and when cool, sterile horse blood

Table 6.3 Effects of various amounts of thin sugar paste (without hydrogen peroxide) incorporated in blood agar on the growth of micro-organisms.

Organism	Bacterial growth on blood agar plates containing the following % of sugar paste				
	10	20	30	40	50
Staphylococcus aureus	+	+	+	–	–
Streptococcus faecalis	+	+	–	–	–
Escherichia coli	+	+	–	–	–
Streptococcus equisimilis	+	–	–	–	–
Staphylococcus epidermidis	+	+	–	–	–
Klebsiella spp.	+	+	–	–	–

[+] = growth present; [–] = growth absent.

was added to a final concentration of 7%. Approximately 20 ml sugar paste agar was then dispensed into each Petri dish and allowed to set. Blood agar plates were used as controls.

Organisms under test were inoculated into nutrient broth and incubated for 5 hours at 37°C. Cultures were then diluted 1 in 10 000 with peptone water, and one standard loopful of each was inoculated on to the sugar paste–blood agar plates and control plates. At the same time, a viable count was performed on the broth cultures. All plates were incubated for 24 hours at 37°C. The results shown in Table 6.3 indicate that *S. equisimilis* was most easily inhibited, whereas *S. aureus* was the most resistant.

Bactericidal effects of sugar pastes

Thick and thin sugar pastes, with and without hydrogen peroxide, were incubated with potentially pathogenic organisms to determine the *in vitro* bactericidal/fungicidal effects. Fresh cultures of *S. aureus*, *S. faecalis*, *E. coli* and *Candida albicans* were suspended in 0.1% peptone water and the concentrations adjusted to approximately 10^{10}/ml. One millilitre of each was then added to approximately 100 g of the paste under test in a sterile container and mixed thoroughly. Samples were removed at intervals (Table 6.4) for serial dilution and subsequent viable counting (Ambrose *et al.*, 1991).

A similar experiment was conducted as a control with PEG 400 and *S. aureus* (that is, no sugar or hydrogen peroxide was present) (Fig. 6.15). A 95% reduction in viable numbers was noted within 2 hours. Chirife *et al.* (1983b) also

Table 6.4 Microbial challenge tests of thick and thin sucrose pastes with and without hydrogen peroxide.

Sucrose pastes and organism	Initial	Log_{10} bacteria/ml of sucrose paste at the following times of sampling (h):					
		0	6	24	48	168	672
Thick paste							
Without peroxide							
S. aureus	1×10^8	3×10^7	2×10^5	7×10^1	3×10^3	<10	<10
S. faecalis	1×10^9	2.3×10^7	7.3×10^4	7×10^3	8×10^1	2×10^1	<10
E. coli	1×10^8	7×10^4	<10	<10	<10	<10	<10
C. albicans	3×10^8	3.5×10^6	<10	4×10^1	<10	<10	<10
With peroxide							
S. aureus	1×10^8	$>10^8$	<10	<10	<10	<10	<10
S. faecalis	1×10^9	1.3×10^6	<10	<10	<10	<10	<10
E. coli	1×10^8	$<10^3$	<10	<10	<10	<10	<10
C. albicans	3×10^8	3×10^5	<10	<10	<10	<10	<10
Thin paste							
Without peroxide							
S. aureus	5.2×10^8	ND^a	1.2×10^5	9.6×10^3	5.8×10^2	<10	<10
S. faecalis	4.4×10^{10}	ND	1.5×10^4	7.8×10^4	1.0×10^4	4.3×10^2	<10
E. coli	5.5×10^8	ND	<10	<10	<10	<10	<10
C. albicans	5.5×10^6	ND	1.3×10^3	<10	<10	<10	<10
With peroxide							
S. aureus	1×10^8	1×10^7	<10	<10	<10	<10	<10
S. faecalis	1×10^9	6.6×10^7	<10	<10	<10	<10	<10
E. coli	1×10^8	$<10^3$	<10	<10	<10	<10	<10
C. albicans	3×10^8	$<10^3$	<10	<10	<10	<10	<10

[a] ND, not determined.

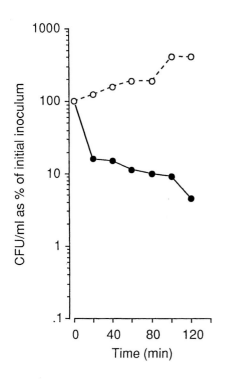

Figure 6.15: Effects of PEG 400 on the colony-forming ability of *S. aureus*. (Reproduced with permission from Ambrose *et al.*, *Antimicrob Ag Chemother*, 1991, **35**, 1799–803.)
●–●, PEG 400; ○–○, broth control.

noted the bactericidal effects of PEG 400 and suggested that concentrated solutions may have value as a topical antibacterial agent.

Viable count determinations

These studies were carried out on *S. aureus* and *Proteus mirabilis* because they are commonly found in infected wounds. In addition, *S. aureus* was demonstrated to grow in 30% sucrose in blood agar (see above) and thus presented the most severe challenge to the antimicrobial efficacy of the pastes.

Thin sugar paste, with and without hydrogen peroxide, was used alone and also diluted with an appropriate amount of human serum to give 25, 50 and 75% paste in serum. The final volume of paste and serum was 50 ml, and nutrient broth was used as the control. All were kept in stoppered conical flasks which were wrapped to exclude light. A 4-hour broth culture of either *S. aureus* or *P. mirabilis* was diluted tenfold with peptone water and 0.5 ml of the resultant cell suspension was added to the paste–serum mixes and control flasks. All flasks were incubated at 37°C for 130 minutes. Samples were taken at approximately 30-minute intervals and serially diluted with peptone water for estimation of viable numbers. Cysteine-lactose-electrolyte-deficient (CLED) agar was used for culturing *P. mirabilis* and nutrient agar was used for culturing *S. aureus*. All plates were incubated at 37°C for 24 hours and the colonies counted (Figs 6.16 and 6.17).

These data (Figs 6.16 and 6.17) indicated that *P. mirabilis* was very susceptible to the antibacterial activity of the pastes, which continued when they were diluted to 50%. The additional bactericidal effect of hydrogen peroxide is partly eliminated by the addition of serum because of the well-described inactivation of peroxide by organic matter. As predicted, *S. aureus* was more resistant to the bactericidal effects of the pastes. Serum alone was found to be bacteriostatic.

The effects of sugar paste on wounds in vivo

Because of the difficulty of conducting a controlled trial of sugar paste in human wounds, an animal study has been conducted (Archer *et al.*, 1990) using a method similar to that reported by Winter (1962) and Winter and Scales (1963). Full-thickness wounds, 25 mm square and 9 mm deep, were made in the backs of pigs and around each was placed a colostomy stoma ring. Wounds were then either covered with a semipermeable plastic film (Opsite), packed with thick sugar paste or packed with cotton gauze soaked in various antiseptic solutions and then covered with Opsite. The entire area was then covered with a stockinette body bandage to keep the treatments in place. Wounds were inspected after 48 and 96 hours and the wounds containing sugar paste were repacked. The other wounds containing gauze packing were not disturbed but the antiseptic under test was replenished by injecting 2 ml directly into the packing.

After 7 days the experiment was terminated and the wounds biopsied. Tissue was dissected to a depth of 12–15 mm and normal skin was removed from around the wound and subjected to microscopic examination. The results are shown in Table 6.5. Representative transverse sections ($\times$ 1 magnification) of some of the wound treatments are shown in Figs 6.18–6.23.

These data indicate that the antiseptics tested, namely Irgasan (triclosan) (and its diluent), chlorhexidine and povidone-iodine, all inhibited the healing process to some degree. Interestingly, in this animal model, Eusol did not appear to inhibit wound healing seriously, which is perhaps surprising in view of the data of others, who have found that this once widely-used product can cause severe damage to living tissue (Brennan and Leaper, 1985). The reason that little impairment of healing was noted here may be that the Eusol was applied at intervals of 48 hours (it is normally applied every 12 hours – it was originally used as a continuous irrigant) and the active ingredient is chlorine, which is volatile and would soon be vaporized once added to the warm open wound. Chlorine would also diffuse through the Opsite film.

At the termination of the experiment, many of the gauze-packed wounds had evidence of new granulation tissue growing into the cotton fibres of the packing (Figs 6.23 and 6.24). This reflects what happens in patients when their wounds

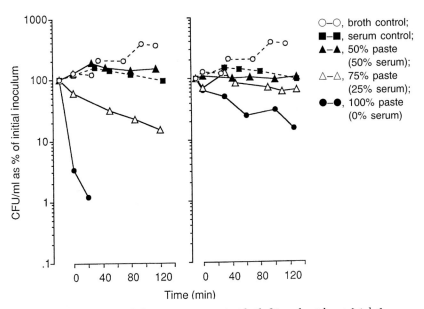

Figure 6.16: Effects of thin sugar paste (with [left] and without [right] hydrogen peroxide) diluted with serum on the colony-forming ability of *S. aureus*. (Reproduced with permission from Ambrose *et al.*, *Antimicrob Ag Chemother*, 1991, **35**, 1799–803.)

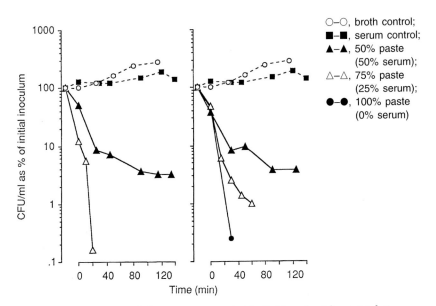

Figure 6.17: Effects of thin sugar paste (with [left] and without [right] hydrogen peroxide) diluted with serum on the colony-forming ability of *P. mirabilis*. (Reproduced with permission from Ambrose *et al.*, *Antimicrob Ag Chemother*, 1991, **35**, 1799–803.)

131

Table 6.5 Comparison of morphology of wound treatments.

Wound treatment	Average % infilling	Epidermal regeneration	Collagen maturation	New vessel formation	Gauze present
Opsite	90	+++	+++	+++	–
Sugar paste	87	+++	+++	+++	–
Irgasan (triclosan) diluent	63	++	++	++	+
Irgasan (triclosan) 0.2%	63	++/+	++	++	+
Chlorhexidine gluconate 0.2%	25	+/-	+/-	+/-	+
Povidone-iodine 0.8%	83	++	++	+++	+
Eusol half-strength	90	++	++	+++	+

– to +++ represents increasing presence.

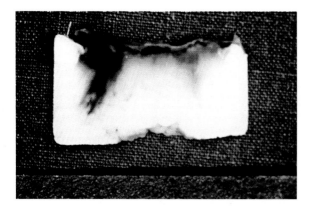

Figure 6.18:
Transverse section of pig wound model showing satisfactory formation of granulation tissue under Opsite plastic film.

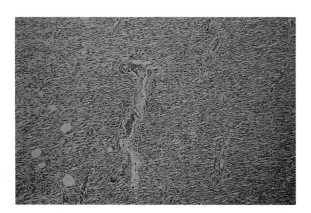

Figure 6.19:
Histology (H & E) section of granulation tissue from the same wound as in Fig. 6.18, showing well organized fibroblasts with new vessel formation ($\times$ 400).

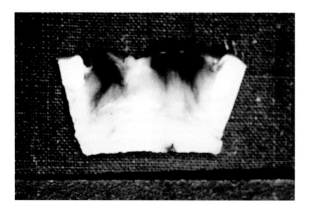

Figure 6.20:
Transverse section of pig wound model showing satisfactory formation of granulation tissue under sugar paste.

133

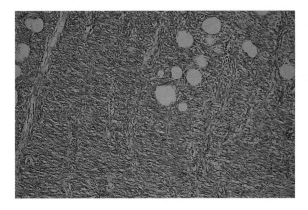

Figure 6.21:
Histology section of granulation tissue from the same wound as in Fig. 6.20, showing well organized fibroblasts with new vessel formation (× 400).

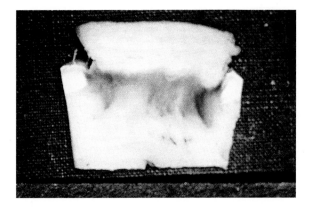

Figure 6.22:
Transverse section of pig wound model showing less satisfactory formation of granulation tissue under cotton gauze packing soaked with Eusol.

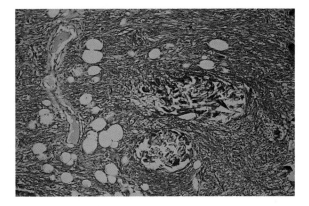

Figure 6.23:
Histology section of granulation tissue from the same wound as in Fig. 6.22, showing poorly organized fibroblasts around gauze fibres with less satisfactory new vessel formation (× 400).

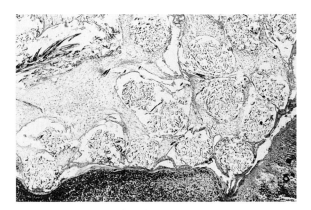

Figure 6.24:
Histology section of new tissue growing into the gauze dressing of the pig model above (× 400).

are packed with gauze and similar products; new tissue that has grown into the packing material is torn away when the packing is removed, thus further delaying the healing process. Packing of wounds with gauze is not recommended now that dressings are available that do not become incorporated into new tissue formation (Appendix E).

Unlike the antiseptics included in this study, sugar paste did not impair the wound-healing process and wounds healed at a similar rate to the Opsite-treated wounds. The antiseptic treatments can be counter-productive and possibly harmful. There is now a general policy of avoiding the regular treatment of wounds with antiseptics and our data support that notion. Sugar paste has been used on many patients with infected and malodorous wounds with excellent results (Middleton and Seal, 1985; Seal and Middleton, 1991). Our experience suggests that sugar paste may be the treatment of choice for many wounds that were traditionally treated with antiseptics.

Effects of sugar paste and antiseptics on the viability of polymorphonuclear leucocytes

Polymorphonuclear leucocytes (PMNs), also known as leucocytes, granulocytes and neutrophils, comprise 59% of all white blood cells and are present in large numbers in wounds. They migrate to sites of inflammation and tissue damage and have an important role in phagocytosing and destroying invading micro-organisms. The healing process is likely to be inhibited if any chemical or dressing added to a wound has an adverse effect on PMNs.

PMNs were isolated from fresh human blood and suspended in minimal essential media (MEM). The concentration of leucocytes was adjusted to approximately

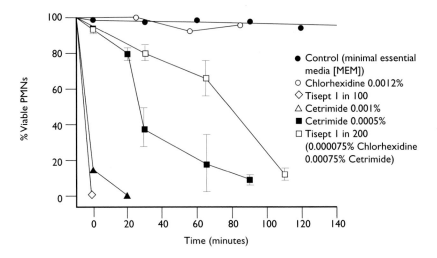

Figure 6.25: Effects of diluted chlorhexidine gluconate 0.015%/cetrimide 0.15% (e.g. Steripod chlorhexidine/cetrimide, Trisept/Travasept 100) and components on the viability of PMNs.

2×10^{6}/ml and various antiseptics were added. Samples were removed at intervals and the viability of the leucocytes was determined by the trypan blue dye exclusion test method.

A mixture of chlorhexidine gluconate 0.015% and cetrimide 0.15% (e.g. Steripod chlorhexidine/cetrimide, Trisept/Travasept 100) is widely used

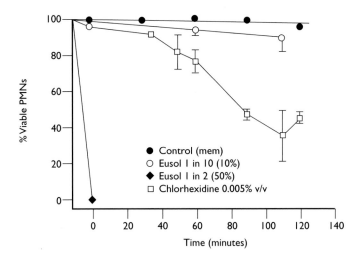

Figure 6.26: Effects of Eusol (diluted) and chlorhexidine on the viability of PMNs.

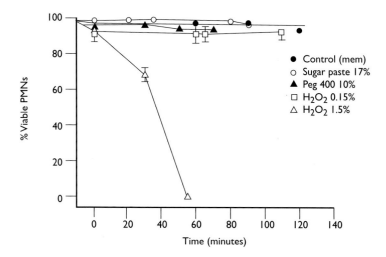

Figure 6.27: Effect of sugar paste (thin) and its components on the viability of PMNs.

undiluted as a wound irrigant. Figure 6.25 illustrates the effects of these diluted products and their components on PMNs and it is apparent that the mixture, even diluted, is rapidly lethal to these cells. Similarly, Eusol diluted 1:2 with minimal essential media was rapidly lethal (Fig. 6.26) but Eusol diluted 1:10 had little effect of the viability of PMNs.

The effects of thin sugar paste and its components on the viability of PMNs are shown in Fig. 6.27. The highest concentration of sugar paste that could be used in this experiment was 17%; higher amounts inhibited the motility of the PMNs . The components of the paste and the paste itself had little effect on the viability of PMNs over the 2-hour test period. The concentration of H_2O_2 in the sugar paste is 0.15%. If increased to 1.5%, this concentration becomes very toxic to PMNs, and yet this concentration has been applied directly to wounds.

These data suggest that some of the commonly used antiseptics are rapidly lethal to leucocytes and may inhibit the wound healing process. In addition, povidone-iodine is known to be 10 times more toxic to PMNs than to bacteria (Broek *et al.*, 1980). In contrast, sugar paste and its components had little detrimental effect on PMN viability and may be preferable to antiseptics for treating infected wounds.

Wound healing

Wound healing is facilitated, with the formation of granulation tissue and inward growth of epithelium, if the wound is kept moist (Winter and Scales, 1963;

Ferguson and Leigh, 1998). Healing is delayed by a variety of factors including certain chronic illnesses, poor nutrition, ischaemia, lack of PMNs and infection (Anonymous, 1991). The rate of clinical infection, from published trials of dressings, is lower under occlusion than when non-occlusive dressings are used (Hutchinson and Lawrence, 1991; Lawrence 1996). However, it must be realized that bacteria and yeasts multiply well under conditions of occlusion, which can result in infection and cross-infection particularly in neonates (Marples *et al.*, 1985). In such special situations, non-occlusive dressings should be used to attach catheters etc. to the skin.

In infected wounds, hypoxia impedes the destruction of bacteria by leucocytes while bacterial proteases have an adverse effect on the tissue repair processes. Sugar, in various formats including our sugar paste, has been used by many groups of workers who have shown it to be an effective treatment for the management of infected and malodorous wounds. Unlike the common practice of packing wounds with gauze soaked in chemicals such as povidone-iodine or Eusol, sugar paste does not disrupt the architecture of the healing wound, it appears not to damage leucocytes and yet is a very effective *in vivo* antimicrobial agent. Many clinicians continue to pack wounds with gauze and toxic, and often expensive, chemicals in the belief that this is the only correct way to treat infected wounds. There is now a growing amount of evidence to suggest that sugar is effective and non-toxic. It has the additional benefits of being readily available and inexpensive.

7. Infection of Burns and Consequential Toxic Shock Syndromes

Care of burns

Care of burn wounds involves cleaning and dressing at 2- to 3-day intervals. A full sterile procedure is required including a non-touch technique. Wound swabs should be collected on admission and at weekly intervals. Patients with severe burns should be cared for in a clean environment. Wounds should be washed with sterile saline 0.9%; blisters should be deroofed and loose slough removed. Flamazine (silver sulfadiazine) cream or other specialized products can be applied to all burn wounds apart from those on the face. Wounds of the chest and back should be nursed exposed to air but wounds of the limbs should be dressed.

Intravenous fluids are often required and should be administered in accordance with the Muir and Barclay formula. In children, nasogastric or nasojejunal tube feeding is often required at the earliest opportunity using a calorie-fortified milk. Iron and vitamin supplements should be administered, together with fresh frozen plasma or blood transfusions when needed.

A major problem in patients with widespread burns is the risk of septicaemia arising from secondary colonizing organisms, particularly Gram-negative bacteria such as *Pseudomonas aeruginosa*. Experiments with bacterial vaccines to offer protection in this situation have generally been disappointing. The use of topical agents such as silver sulfadiazine is designed to prevent septicaemic complications but regular surveillance swabbing is advisable. Rarely, fungal opportunists such as zygomycetes (*Rhizomucor*, *Absidia* and *Rhizopus* species) may invade burn surfaces to cause severe infection with vascular necrosis.

Dressings for burns have been well reviewed recently by Settle (1996) and wound healing within the burn by Lawrence (1996). Antiseptics, or dressings containing them, including tulle gras are suitable for small burns less than 15% of body surface area and of partial thickness only; suitable products include chlorhexidine, nitrofurazone and povidone-iodine. Multiple antibiotic sprays should *not* be used.

Extensive full-thickness burns require dressing to prevent colonization of the wound particularly with *Ps. aeruginosa*; 0.5% silver nitrate soaks are well documented as being highly effective against *Ps. aeruginosa* colonization. This substance can be applied on absorbent dressings and the wound kept moist with 2-hourly applications of silver nitrate solution poured into the dressings. The disadvantage of this technique is the black stains to skin and surroundings as well as causing further problems with electrolyte imbalance. Flamazine (1% silver sulfadiazine) cream is a more satisfactory product and now considered the best choice for extensive burns. It is applied under absorbent dressings which are changed daily. Mafenide cream is used in the USA but is painful and is associated with acid–base disturbances. Prophylactic systemic antibiotics should not be used but retained for use at the first sign of septicaemia. Routine swabbing of the burns should take place to monitor the microbial flora to assist in choice of an antibiotic combination if needed.

Edwards-Jones and Foster (1994) showed that silver sulfadiazine cream (Flamazine) induced toxin formation earlier than usual in the *S. aureus* growth cycle, with an effect that was long lasting. Further work has suggested that Flamazine may induce transposition of the *tst*-1 element in the genome (Shawcross *et al.*, 1998). Flamazine should therefore be used with caution in hospital wards in which toxic shock syndrome associated with burns has been a problem or in which there has been significant cross-infection.

Toxic shock syndrome (TSS) and toxin-mediated disease (TMD) due to S. aureus and S. pyogenes in children with burns

Toxic shock syndrome due to *S. aureus* has been described in children aged 5–10 years without burns (Wiesenthal and Todd, 1984; Todd *et al.*, 1987) and in children of similar age with burns (Farmer *et al.*, 1985; Frame *et al.*, 1985; Holt *et al.*, 1987), but only once in toddlers.

In the preantibiotic era the sudden development of a severe, generalized erythroderma with mucosal hyperaemia accompanied by hypotension, coma, toxaemia with seizures and diarrhoea was likely to have been caused by *Streptococcus pyogenes* and to have represented toxic scarlet fever (TSF) (Cone *et al.*, 1987; Brook and Bannister, 1988; Shulman, 1993). Its aetiology is the production of pyrogenic exotoxin type A (Hallas, 1985; Johnson *et al.*, 1986; Belani *et al.*, 1991).

A similar syndrome, first recognized in 1927, was thought to be caused by *Staphylococcus aureus* and was called 'staphylococcal scarlet fever' (Stevens, 1927). This syndrome was redescribed in seven children without burns by Todd *et al.* in 1978 and called 'toxic shock syndrome (TSS)'. They described the features of high fever, erythroderma, hypotension, diarrhoea, mental confusion and renal failure (Todd *et al.*, 1987). *S. aureus* was isolated from mucosal swab cultures or foci of infection and shown to produce an exfoliatin-type toxin in newborn mice. This toxin of *S. aureus* has been extensively researched and is now called 'toxic shock syndrome toxin-1 (TSST-1)'. It was previously called 'enterotoxin F' or 'pyrogenic exotoxin'. In addition, the other enterotoxins A to E may be isolated from *S. aureus* strains causing toxic shock, especially when associated with burns or wounds, both alone and in combination with TSST-1. Toxic shock syndrome is a cytokine-mediated disease via T cell activation.

Toxic shock syndrome has been described before in children with burns, as possible and probable clinical cases, but emphasis in the literature has been concerned with tampon-associated disease in women aged 15–25 during the onset of menstruation (Waldvagel, 1990). In non-menses cases, however, isolation of TSST-1 producing isolates of *S. aureus* has been described from other sites, but with little description concerning burn wounds (Harvey Wood *et al.*, 1998).

Diagnosis of the staphylococcal toxic shock syndrome (TSS) has been described for three major criteria (elevated temperature, rash with desquamation and hypotension) and at least three minor criteria (tachypnoea, tachycardia, vomiting or diarrhoea, central nervous system symptoms [confusion or irritability], diminished renal function, raised liver enzymes and polymorphonuclear cytosis [Todd *et al.*, 1987]). Children with toxic shock appear similar to affected adults, with, among other symptoms, pyrexia, rash, hypotension, diarrhoea and convulsions in the absence of bacteraemia. This has been our experience in toddlers with burns but, while the rash may occur as a fleeting generalized erythroderma, it quickly becomes localized to the face, nappy area and knees in a characteristic manner (Figs 7.1 and 7.2). This syndrome can also present in a milder form without the presence of shock and is then known as toxin-mediated disease (TMD) (Harvey Wood *et al.*, 1998). Diagnosis of TSS due to *S. aureus*, and its differentiation from that due to *Streptococcus pyogenes*, is often missed when associated with burns in children.

Over a 1-year period, 107 children were admitted with burns, mostly first-degree scalds, to the Royal Hospital for Sick Children in Glasgow. Three developed TSS (Figs 7.1 and 7.2) and three TMD due to *S. aureus* in children lacking specific immunity. Some 42 out of 100 children without TSS or TMD had burns colonized with *S. aureus* on admission to hospital and 33 of the remaining 58 (57%) became colonized while in hospital. Toxic shock syndrome toxin-1 (TSST-1)-producing isolates of *S. aureus* were cultured from the burns of 28 children, 19 on admission and 9 afterwards (hospital-acquired [32%]) (Harvey Wood *et al.*, 1998). Serum was collected on admission from 63 of these 100 children and tested for antibodies to TSST-1 (Harvey Wood *et al.*, 1998). Of these 63 children, 41 (65%) were non-immune on admission, of whom two-thirds were less than 4 years old. One child with immunity to TSST-1 developed TMD due to *S. pyogenes*, distinguished by a punctate scarlatina rash (Figs 7.3 and 7.4).

Toxic scarlet fever (TSF) mimicking TSS has been reported in adults and in children (Stevens *et al.*, 1989; Begovac *et al.*, 1990; Chomarat *et al.*, 1990; Belani *et al.*, 1991; Torres-Martinez *et al.*, 1992). All developed pyrexia with confusion and a rash typical of scarlatina while most also suffered from hypotension and

141

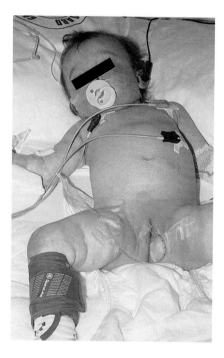

Figure 7.1: Clinical features of TSS in a toddler with scalds.

shock. However, some patients reported in the literature above with TSF had *S. pyogenes* septicaema with streptococci isolated from blood cultures. This situation does *not* satisfy criteria for TSS (Todd *et al.*, 1987) and, in the authors' opinion, cases of TSF should *exclude* patients with bacteraemia. There is confusion, however, in the streptococcal literature, with some authors reporting TSF as a result of TMD alone without bacteraemia (Cone *et al.*, 1987; Brook and Bannister, 1988; Begovac *et al.*, 1990), others reporting TSF and TMD with and without bacteraemia (Belani *et al.*, 1991), while yet others have reported 'streptococcus-associated toxic shock' when *S. pyogenes* bacteraemia has always occurred (Chomarat *et al.*, 1990; Torres-Martinez *et al.*, 1992). When such bacteraemia is present, the shock syndrome observed is due to circulating exotoxin A and other toxins released within the vascular space rather than being absorbed from a burn or focus of infection.

The scarlatina rash, which is classically punctate on the chest, can be macular on the limbs causing confusion with rubella infection. Pastia's sign of accentuation of erythema around puncta and skin creases (Pastia's lines) may be helpful while specific neutralization of toxin in skin to give blanching can also be undertaken. The tongue may have enlarged papillae. Desquamation only occurred in half the reported patients above. Our patient (Figs 7.3 and 7.4) exhibited pyrexia, a typical scarlatina rash, mucosal hyperaemia, diarrhoea, central nervous system irritability and raised C-reactive protein and polymorphonuclear cell

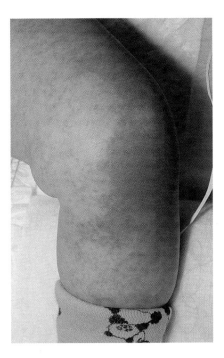

Figure 7.2: Clinical features of TSS in a toddler (close-up of patient in Fig. 7.1).

count, but was not shocked. This is considered toxin-mediated disease, or 'surgical' (or 'burn') scarlet fever, when pyrogenic exotoxin A has been absorbed from the burn wound which was colonized by *S. pyogenes*; blood cultures were negative excluding bacteraemia. The *S. pyogenes* strain was an unusual skin type (M type1658, T11, OF +ve).

The severe and rapid appearance of TSS, within 1 day of a burn occurring, can cause confusion with shock due to electrolyte loss and its severity is often greater than that of the burn itself. TSS and TMD only occurred in children with burns, especially under 4, who lacked immunity to TSST-1, so that identification of specific antibodies to TSST-1 can be useful clinically for excluding the diagnosis (Harvey Wood *et al.*, 1998).

Method for estimating antibody titres to TSST-1

Serum was tested, at dilutions from 1/4 to 1/5120, for antibodies to TSST-1 by a reverse passive latex agglutination test mixing 25-μl aliquots of test serum with 25 μl of filtrate from a known TSST-1-producing isolate of *S. aureus*. The toxin filtrate was diluted to contain a known titre of TSST-1 (approximately 1/32) that would be neutralized if any antibodies were present in the test serum. This mixture was incubated at 4°C for 2 hours and then used as the 'toxin'

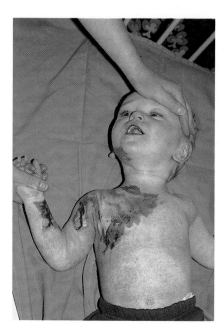

Figure 7.3: Toxic scarlet fever from *S. pyogenes* colonization of a burn in a child.

preparation in the Oxoid kit test (TST-RPLA-TD940) (Harvey Wood *et al.*, 1998). A control preparation of toxin filtrate was included at a titre of 1/32 without the addition of serum. Neutralization of the 'toxin' preparation was shown by finding inhibition of expected agglutination of the coated latex particles, implying the presence of antibody to TSST-1 in the patients' serum. The titre reported is that which gave an end-point of 50% neutralization.

Immunology

It has been estimated that 93% of adults have acquired antibodies to TSST-1 by age 25 (Stolz *et al.*, 1985). This immunity is gained by recurrent infection or colonization with TSST-1-producing strains of *S. aureus* but not by recurrent episodes of TSS. Ritz *et al.* (1984) demonstrated that all individuals with nasal colonization by TSST-1-producing *S. aureus* had high titres of anti-TSST-1 antibodies, while those without such colonization had titres ranging from nil to high. We found that 67% of children (30 out of 45) under 4 years of age lacked immunity to TSST-1, which decreased to 14% by age 11 (Harvey Wood *et al.*, 1998). This is similar to the findings of Bergdoll *et al.* (1990) in children and adults without burns. Children lacking specific immunity are susceptible to develop TSS or TMD if the burn is colonized with TSST-1 producing *S. aureus* before granulation commences. Our experience has been that such TSS can develop as rapidly as 1 day after the burn occurring.

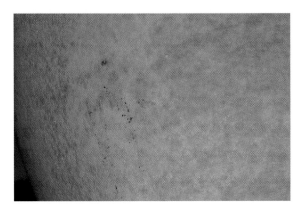

Figure 7.4: Close-up of patient in Fig. 7.3 showing typical punctate erythema. The burn was colonized but not infected by *S. pyogenes*.

Seroconversion to TSST-1 without development of TSS or TMD was recognized in two children with burns, who were both admitted non-immune and had burns colonized with TSST-1 producing *S. aureus* in hospital. This was either the natural response by which silent protective immunity is gained from undetected colonization by TSST-1-producing *S. aureus* or occurred due to toxin modification, during the granulation process, by neutrophil proteinases cleaving off the active site from the toxin. Tissue destruction by neutrophils, within a milieu such as a burn, has been reviewed (Weiss, 1989; Leff and Repine, 1993) when three proteolytic enzymes were considered – the serine proteinase (elastase) and two metalloproteinases (collagenase and gelatinase). These enzymes, which cleave peptide bonds, act in the extracellular matrix under the developing epithelium colonized by bacteria such as *S. aureus*. There is an antiproteinase shield present as well; elastase is neutralized by plasma-derived 52 kDa alpha-proteinase. This will inhibit activity if ready access of serum proteins occurs, but this does not happen in sites of inflammation when exudate fluid has been found to have lost its antiproteinase activity. The two metalloproteinases are synthesized in latent form, being activated by neutrophil-derived oxidants, but their regulation is unknown. While neutrophil proteinases *per se* are not thought important for tissue destruction compared to their oxidants, which can destroy the antiproteinase shield increasing proteolytic activity, their presence in burns needs investigating for an effect on released bacterial toxins. It is from the open, inflamed burn that such modified toxins will be absorbed, or macrophage-ingested, for T cell processing as antigens. This may explain the more likely occurrence of TSS or TMD due to *S. aureus* if the burns are colonized in the first week.

TSST-1 has a molecular weight of 22 kDa comprising 194 amino acids (Edwin, 1989). With papain hydrolysis it has yielded three fragments of 16, 12 and 10 kDa, that of 16 being derived from splitting the peptide bond between tyrosine-52 and serine-53 and the latter between glycine-87 and valine-88. Serologic activity for the whole TSST-1 molecule was shown to relate to the 16- and 12-kDa fragments, but not for the 10-kDa fragment, with monoclonal antibodies suggesting homologous antigenic determinants on both 16- and 12-kDa fragments. The 16-kDa fragment was shown to contain the 12-kDa fragment and to represent 75% of the molecule. Results of biological activity were varied but the 12-kDa fragment gave a better mitogenic effect on proliferation of human peripheral blood lymphocytes than the 16-kDa fragment (although it contained this fragment) whereas the 10-kDa fragment promoted none.

Conclusion

The diagnosis of TSS or TMD, due to S. aureus or S. pyogenes, should be considered in all children with burns, including minor ones, when its severity is often greater than that of the burn itself. Features include rash, mucosal hyperaemia, pyrexia, shock (not present in TMD), central nervous system irritability and diarrhoea; renal and hepatic failure may also be present. Tachypnoea and tachycardia appear more typical of TSS than TSF. General resuscitative measures are required together with antistaphylococcal antibiotics such as flucloxacillin and fusidic acid, or benzylpenicillin for S. pyogenes, although the burn wounds are not clinically infected. Clindamycin inhibits toxin production at sub-inhibitory (bactericidal) concentrations and may be used alone or in combination therapy. Intravenous immunoglobulin (IVIG) can be given as well, which inhibits T-cell activation and contains antibody to TSST-1. TSS and TMD are not new phenomena but their occurrence in children with burns is not always recognized.

8. TROPICAL BACTERIAL, VIRAL AND PARASITIC INFECTIONS

Bacterial infections

Tropical phagedenic ulcer

Streptococcus pyogenes

Severe tropical bacterial pyodermas, which ulcerated similarly to the 'phagedenic' ulcer, were recognized as a particular problem in US troops in Vietnam (Allen *et al.*, 1971). The predominant lesions were ecthymatous ulcers of the legs of which 90% yielded *S. pyogenes* (Fig. 8.1). It was a particular problem of combat-related exposure and the trauma it entailed. In addition up to 50% of the troops were carrying *S. pyogenes* at other sites, which will have contributed to trauma-associated infection. The ulcers were disabling and did not heal quickly. Treatment was given with oral phenoxymethylpenicillin (penicillin V) but intramuscular use of Bicillin (benzyl penicillin and procaine penicillin) is better. Oral therapy with tetracycline does not work because up to 50% of *S. pyogenes* isolates are resistant.

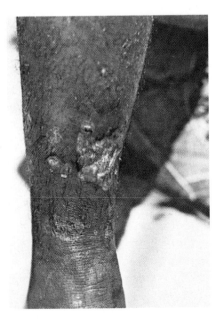

Figure 8.1: Necrotic tropical ulcer due to *S. pyogenes*. (Reproduced from Allen *et al.* 1971, *Arch Dermatol*, **104**, 271–80.)

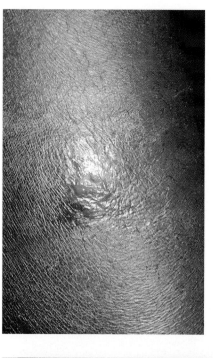

Figure 8.2: Pre-ulcerative phase of a tropical ulcer.

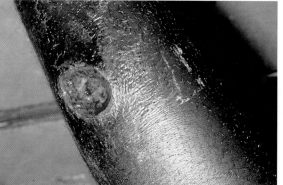

Figure 8.3: Tropical ulcer due to *F. ulcerans*.

Fusobacterium ulcerans

Tropical ulcer or tropical phagedenic ulcer (Figs 8.2 and 8.3) is an acute or chronic ulcer in children or young adults which occurs in endemic areas of the tropics, mainly in the Old World. The onset is rapid and the appearance of the ulcer follows enlargment of a preulcerative papule. Lesions are painful. A consistent finding is the presence of the anaerobe *Fusobacterium ulcerans* and a mixed flora of aerobes and spiral bacteria which are treponemes; such a mixture is

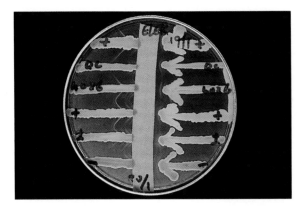

Figure 8.4: Elek plate to test for *Corynebacterium diphtheriae* toxin. (+, toxin producing isolate; −, non-toxin producing isolate; QC, non-toxin producing isolate; 6026, toxin producing isolate)

known to enhance the infectivity of *Fusobacterium* (Smith *et al.*, 1989). The disease may occur in case clusters suggesting exposure to a common source, and contact with stagnant water, mud or flooding is associated with the disease. A small proportion of acute ulcers develop into a chronic phase and various complications such as squamous carcinoma may develop. Treatment is with penicillin or metronidazole and regular dressing to promote healing. However, split skin grafting undertaken at an early stage may be useful.

Diphtheritic ulcer due to *Corynebacterium diphtheriae*

Cutaneous diphtheria (ecthyma diphthericum) commonly presents as an ulcer on the hand or foot. It presents as a chronic non-healing painful ulcer with undermined margins and covered by a thick grey membrane. Spontaneous resolution occurs in 6–12 weeks, but it may last up to 1 year, leaving a depressed concentric scar. Thirty per cent of patients with cutaneous diphtheria carry the organism in their throats and are thus highly infectious for others. A small percentage of patients can develop neurological sequelae, including Guillain–Barré syndrome. Secondary infection of the ulcer with *S. aureus* and other organisms may be present, when the main pathogen of *C. diphtheriae* can be missed.

The possibility of cutaneous diphtheria should be considered in all non-healing ulcers acquired in the Middle East, Russia and the tropical countries, in particular those of the Far East such as the Phillipines. There was a big epidemic of diphtheria in Russia in 1994, while the organism is endemic in southern Russia and Iran (central Asia). Protection can be gained with diphtheria toxoid.

Corynebacterium diphtheriae requires a highly nutritious medium for culture. It grows well on Loeffler's medium (enriched agar with serum). Smears from this

149

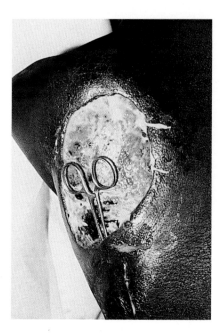

Figure 8.5: Buruli ulcer in West Africa caused by infection with *Mycobacterium ulcerans*. (Courtesy of Abbott Laboratories.)

medium show a Gram-positive rod with Chinese-character palisading. Tests for toxin production can be performed by Elek's method. Antitoxin serum is incorporated into a filter paper strip laid in the middle of a serum-enriched agar plate at right angles to a streak of a control isolate, known to produce toxin, another that does not produce toxin and the test strain. A positive result is given by precipitation lines of toxin/antitoxin joining up between those formed from the positive control isolate and the test strain which should form a 'U' pattern (Fig. 8.4). Duplicate plate cultures should always be performed because this plate test can be unreliable.

Buruli ulcer (*M. ulcerans*)

The environmental saprophyte *Mycobacterium ulcerans* is inoculated into the skin by injury with spiky plants or other vegetable matter. It begins as a small indurated painless lesion that is an itchy nodule. This may resolve but in others increases in size. There is necrosis of the hypodermis and subcutaneous adipose tissue down to the fascial sheath. The overlying skin necroses and ulcerates with release of dead tissue and the formation of a large deeply undermined ulcer (Fig. 8.5). Eyes and other vital organs can be destroyed. Scarring and contractures are frequent. Skin grafting and long stays in hospital may be needed. There is an endemic focus in Ghana (van der Werf *et al.*, 1989).

Numerous acid-fast bacilli are present in the ulcer wall. There is an apparent lack of a CMI response in the tissues. The patients are tuberculin and burulin

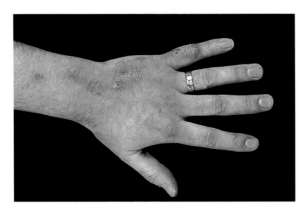

Figure 8.6:
Mycobacterium marinum
infection – 'fish tank'
granuloma.

(extracted from *M. ulcerans*) negative. The infection has a natural history of recovery, led by the formation of CMI with positive reactivity to the antigens above. The numbers of bacilli reduce and the lesion heals with gross scarring. This condition can be treated with rifampicin. A late complication is the development of squamous cell carcinoma so that these patients need to be followed up for further ulceration (Evans *et al.*, 1999).

Mycobacterium marinum and tropical fish tanks

Mycobacterium marinum is another environmental mycobacterium that infects skin. It causes 'fish tank' granuloma or 'fish fancier's' finger which manifests as warty lesions, similar to those of tuberculosis verrucosa cutis, in people handling fish (Fig. 8.6). There may also be sporotrichoid spread with secondary lesions along the lines of dermal lymphatics. People who handle tropical fish in tanks in their homes can become infected (Hay and Seal, 1996a). Treatment is given with systemic anti-tuberculous chemotherapy.

Necrotizing fasciitis due to *Vibrio vulnificus*

Vibrionaceae comprise three genera – *Vibrio*, *Aeromonas* and *Plesiomonas*. These comma-shaped Gram-negative rods are all aquatic organisms associated with shellfish. *Vibrio* spp., except *V. vulnificus*, usually cause intense diarrhoea, but a purulent wound infection has been reported with *V. cholerae* non-01 associated with a tropical fish tank (Booth *et al.*, 1990). *Aeromonas hydrophila* is the predominant clinical pathogen mainly causing wound infection in the summer months in association with minor trauma and exposure to river or sea water. It can also cause septicaemia and necrotizing fasciitis, often in a diabetic or immunocompromised patient (Yoshizuka *et al.*, 1997; Lin and Cheng, 1998; Joynt *et al.*, 1999).

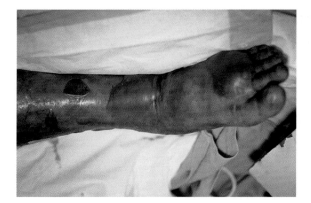

Figure 8.7: Acute necrotizing fasciitis with violaceous ecchymoses typical of *V. vulnificus* infection. (Courtesy of Dr G Joynt, Hong Kong.)

V. vulnificus, first described in 1979, multiplies well in warm water (> 20°C) with a salt concentration of 0.7–1.6%. It is found in warm coastal waters such as the Gulf of Mexico (Penman *et al.*, 1995), South America, Asia (Thailand, Taiwan, Hong Kong) and Australia, but is also reported in small numbers off Belgium and Scandinavia. It is found in oysters, crustaceans and fish which may be the source of infection with or without trauma.

Necrotizing fasciitis due to *V. vulnificus* is severe (Joynt *et al.*, 1999; Halow *et al.*, 1996). It occurs after minor trauma in fishermen and those in contact with fish or sea water. Patients tend to be over 50 and compromised with other conditions, particularly chronic liver dysfunction such as cirrhosis, or diabetes. The infection presents after 1 day with swelling, pain, tenderness, ecchymoses and blistering (Fig. 8.7). Predominant skin lesions have been reported as oedema and subcutaneous bleeding, with ecchymosis and purpura, rather than superficial necrosis as is seen in *S. pyogenes* infection (Fujisawa *et al.*, 1998). Systemically, there are fevers, rigors and hypotension. Septicaemia with *V. vulnificus* is a prominent feature, more so than with *S. pyogenes*. This leads to rapid multi-organ failure within 24 hours, which presents as encephalopathy (Glasgow coma score < 6 off sedation), hepatic failure (bilirubin > 120 µmol/l), renal failure (serum creatinine > 350 µmol/l), respiratory failure (FiO$_2$ < 150) and most importantly DIC (platelet count < 50 000/ml) (Joynt *et al.*, 1999).

Necrotizing fasciitis due to *V. vulnificus* progresses more rapidly than that due to *S. pyogenes* (Fujisawa *et al.*, 1998). Early diagnosis and extensive debridement is essential to save life as otherwise it has an almost 100% mortality. While *Aeromonas* may infect muscle, this is unusual with *V. vulnificus* so that, in principle, debridement and not amputation is needed although this decision must be made uniquely for each case. Computerized tomography and magnetic resonance imaging are useful for locating the site and depth or extension of the infection.

Cultures should be collected from blood, blister fluid, wound and stool specimens. Gram stains show curved bacilli with or without pleomorphic forms.

Antibiotics should be commenced in high dosage but are additional to surgical intervention. A combination of ceftazidime (or cefotaxime) with ciprofloxacin (or another quinolone) or tetracycline should be given in maximum dosage.

Leprosy

Refer to Chapter 4.

Virus infections

Arboviruses

These infections occur primarily in animals as zoonoses with reservoirs in birds or small mammals. They are widely distributed. For every serious illness there are at least 1000 inapparent ones. There are many different arboviruses each taking a name from the region where they were isolated or from the local disease name.

Arboviruses present with fever, arthritis, myositis and itchy maculopapular rashes. A similar clinical syndrome can be caused by: (Togaviridae) O'nyong-nyong and Chikungunya in Africa and India and Ross River in Australia; (Flaviviridae) dengue (four types) throughout tropical Asia, yellow fever, Japanese B encephalitis; (Bunyaviridae) sandfly fever in south Italy and Sicily; (Reoviridae) Colorado tick fever in the USA and eastern Europe and Kemerovo virus in Russia. The vectors for Togaviridae and Flaviviridae are mosquitoes, for Bunyaviridae are sandflies and for Reoviridae are ticks. They cause intense discomfort (break bone fever) but recovery is complete. There are no specific antiviral drugs.

Arboviruses can also cause haemorrhagic fevers with mortality rates of 20%. The initial febrile episode is followed by bleeding into the skin and mucous membranes with haemorrhagic rashes and haemorrhage from body orifices. There is thrombocytopenia and sometimes DIC. Infection by Flaviviridae includes dengue fever (see below), chikungunya (in India) and Omsk (in Siberia, tick-borne) as well as yellow fever causing fever, jaundice, haemorrhage and death in Africa and South America. Infection by Bunyaviridae includes Crimean-Congo fever in central Asia (tick-borne), Rift Valley fever in Egypt (mosquito-borne) and hantavirus fever in eastern Europe, Russia and Korea. Hantan virus causes haemorrhagic fever with renal syndrome in Korea and China. It is carried by small mammals – mice, rats, voles.

Children may suffer from dengue haemorrhagic shock syndrome. It is a dangerous complication with a mortality rate of 12% and is increasing in South-east Asia

153

(Gubler, 1998). It presents with a brief febrile illness followed by collapse, shock and widespread purpura. It is thought to be due to immune enhancement to the virus with a second infection by a heterologous serotype, that is by one of the other four serotypes. In 1998 it was the most important mosquito-borne disease after malaria, with 100 million cases of dengue per year, 500 000 cases of dengue haemorrhagic fever and 25 000 deaths annually (Gubler, 1998). Treatment includes replacing lost fluid, correction of electrolyte balance and transfusion of whole blood if haemorrhage is severe.

Filoviruses

These include Ebola and Marburg viruses, which have a bizarre filamentous morphology. They both present similarly with an abrupt onset after an incubation period of 3–16 days. There is severe headache, high fever and back pains. There is rapid prostration with a transient non-itching maculopapular rash after several days. This is followed by severe bleeding with a high mortality rate of up to 90%.

These viruses are zoonoses, with imported monkeys involved in the Marburg outbreak. Large outbreaks of Ebola virus infection have occurred in the Sudan and Zaïre, where the virus is endemic. Virus is spread by contact with blood and body fluids.

Arenaviruses

Arenaviruses that infect humans include Junin (Argentinian haemorrhagic fever), Machupo (Bolivian haemorrhagic fever) and Lassa (Lassa fever in Africa). These viruses cause persistent symptomless infections in rodents from which humans become infected by contact with the excreta, particularly urine. In endemic areas subclinical infection is common, particularly with Lassa in rural West Africa.

The incubation period is 1–2 weeks. The early signs are non-specific, with fever, headache and sore throat. This is followed by a rash on the face and neck with some prostration. In the second week there is haemorrhage and shock with a mortality of up to 25%.

Parasitic infections

The principal groups of parasites that cause skin disease are:
- protozoa;
- helminths, including nematodes (roundworms), trematodes (flukes), and cestodes (tapeworms);
- insecta.

154

Protozoa

Entamoeba histolytica

Refer to Chapter 5.

Leishmaniasis

Human leishmaniasis is classified as cutaneous or visceral, although skin lesions also occur with visceral disease. Transmission is by sandflies (*Phlebotomus* spp.), which have precise survival requirements for temperature and humidity. It is a zoonotic infection with the human as the accidental host. *Leishmania* spp. is a flagellate protozoa.

The flagellated promastigote stage of *Leishmania* spp. (Fig. 8.8) is found in the proboscis of the sandfly and is inoculated into the skin by a bite, usually at night. These promastigotes are taken up by histiocytes in which they multiply to become the amastigote stage (Fig. 8.9) – this stage only occurs in the human. After time, they are recognized immunologically and a clinical lesion develops. It contains parasitized macrophages, lymphocytes and plasma cells (Fig. 8.9). The epidermis breaks down and there is focal necrosis to produce an ulcer containing live and dead parasites. This activity continues for months, during which time a giant cell granuloma can develop.

Cutaneous leishmaniasis (Fig. 8.10) due to *L. major*, *L. tropica* and others occurs in the Old World. Lesions are usually found on exposed areas in a child. They may be multiple and occur on other members of a family at the same time, probably bitten by the same fly or flies. The various species have different natural histories but they all cause a nodule, crusting and ulceration with healing by scar formation in most cases without treatment. Diffuse cutaneous leishmaniasis and severe mucocutaneous leishmaniasis including the American varieties are discussed in detail by Bryceson and Hay (1998).

Local treatment is unsatisfactory. Systemic treatment is given with sodium stibogluconate or meglumine antimoniate by the intravenous or intramuscular route with a single daily dose of 20 mg antimony/kg until the localized lesion has healed, which may take 15–30 days.

Visceral leishmaniasis or kala-azar is caused by *L. donovani*. It causes a severe systemic infection which may be accompanied by skin lesions. After a long incubation period, fever and lethargy develop with an enlarged spleen, cough and diarrhoea. There is also hepatomegaly, lymphadenopathy and sometimes signs of malnutrition. In a few patients a rash develops after chemotherapy called dermal leishmaniasis or a leishmanoid. In Africa, the rash begins in convalescence on the cheeks, chin and extensor aspects of arms and legs. It comprises discrete papules with a tuberculoid histology and scanty parasites. The leishmanin test is positive. The rash heals spontaneously over a few months. In India, the

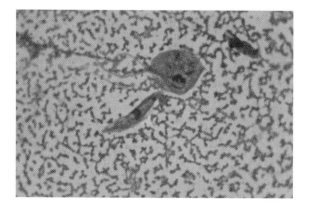

Figure 8.8:
Leishmania
promastigote in
culture (×400).

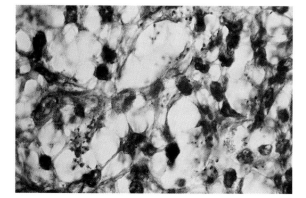

Figure 8.9: Giemsa
stain of scraping
from cutaneous
leishmaniasis showing
histiocytes and
macrophages
containing
amastigotes (×400).

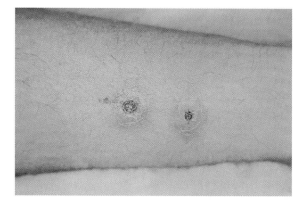

Figure 8.10:
Cutaneous
leishmaniasis (clinical
appearance).

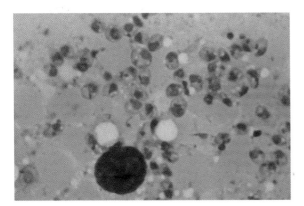

Figure 8.11:
Leishmania amastigotes
in bone marrow
(Giemsa stain)
(×400).

rash begins 1–2 years after recovery as hypopigmented macules with gradual development of diffuse nodulation. This rash is progressive without healing and can involve the tongue, palate and genitalia. These rashes are thought to represent cell-mediated immunity to antigen that remained in the skin. Therapy is similar to that for cutaneous leishmaniasis, employing sodium stibogluconate, an organic pentavalent antimony compound. The dose is 20 mg/kg/day for at least 20 days (10 days for skin lesions) by the IM or IV route.

Amphotericin is used with or after an antimony compound for kala-azar unresponsive to the antimonial alone.

Pentamidine isethionate has been used in antimonial-resistant cases but the relapse rate is high.

Diagnosis of visceral leishmaniasis can be made by aspirates of spleen, bone marrow (Fig. 8.11), liver or lymph node when the amastigote stage can be seen with Giemsa stain. Leishmania promastigotes can be cultured from these aspirates with a special fluid medium but great care should be taken because they are highly infective.

Helminths

Larva migrans

Penetrating larvae of helminth infections such as ancylostomiasis (hookworm) and strongyloidiasis cause a temporary skin eruption, that is variable and transient, with severe pruritus and a papular or papulovesicular rash. This eruption is often at the site of penetration, such as feet.

Cutaneous larva migrans is caused by circulating larvae that fail to develop into the adult worm stages, as in the case of Ancylostoma brasiliensis (the dog hook-

157

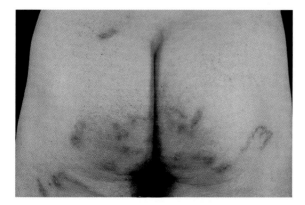

Figure 8.12:
Cutaneous larva
migrans.

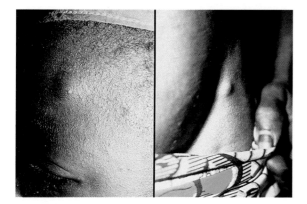

Figure 8.13:
Nodules of
onchocerciasis
showing distribution
in the forehead
(Central America)
and pelvis area
(Africa). (Reproduced
with permission of
Dr Murray McGavin.)

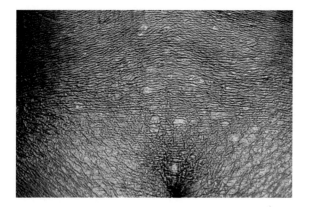

Figure 8.14:
Chronic onchocercal
papulodermatitis.

worm). These larvae end up in the skin (Fig. 8.12), eye and other sites. They may cause a non-specific eruption with features as given above. They may then lie quiet for weeks or months before wandering through the skin at up to 1 cm daily to produce very itchy, raised bizarre serpentine lesions. They produce tracks along which are vesicles causing much scratching, 'dermatitis' and secondary bacterial infection. The disease is self-limiting but can persist for months. Complications occur if these larvae penetrate the eye, particularly the retina (Seal *et al.*, 1998).

Onchocerciasis

This is a filarial disease caused by *Onchocerca volvulus*. It affects 19 million people in tropical Africa, Yemen, and Central and South America. Male worms measure 20–45 mm and female worms 230–700 mm. They produce sheathless microfilariae up to 300 μm long. The vectors are blood-sucking black flies (Simuliidae). Larvae develop in thoracic muscles and 7 days after infection are fully developed in the labium of the proboscis to cause further human infection when bitten.

Mature worms and microfilariae are found in granulomatous dermal nodules (onchocercomata). These are often found on the scalp in Central American patients but near bony prominences on the trunks and limbs in Africans (Fig. 8.13). They measure 3–35 mm in diameter. The adult parasites are contained in an organized fibrous matrix. Microfilariae are found mainly in the dermis, causing a perivascular inflammatory response. With time, fibrosis develops with atrophy of dermis and epidermis. Microfilariae also invade the eye causing keratitis, iritis and posterior choroiditis which often leads to blindness, the most severe effect of onchocerciasis (Seal *et al.*, 1998). Free microfilariae can penetrate superficial lymphatic vessels to be found in urine, tears, sputum and cerebrospinal fluid.

Common features are pruritus, especially with acute onchocercal papulodermatitis (Fig. 1.13). This continues towards chronic papulodermatitis (Fig. 8.14), lichenified papulodermatitis (Fig. 8.15), atrophy and hypopigmentation (Fig. 8.16). There will be onchocercomata and high microfilarial counts. Not all infected persons suffer disease, however, and many patients may have high microfilarial counts in skin snips without disease. The skin changes vary with the age of the patient, location on the skin surface, and region and climate of the area of domicile. In travellers acute onchodermatitis can be difficult to distinguish. However the itching is often strikingly asymmetric, localized to a single limb or body area, and there is a fine diffuse dermal oedema in the same locality.

For several decades diethylcarbamazine (DEC) and suramin have been used systemically in the treatment of onchocerciasis. Both are effective microfilaricidal drugs with a beneficial effect on keratitis and uveitis; they are, however, less effective in posterior choroiditis. The use of DEC may be followed by a severe

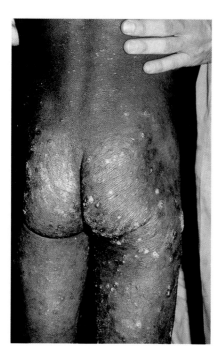

Figure 8.15: Chronic lichenified onchocercal papulodermatitis.

systemic reaction which is largely prevented by the concomitant use of systemic corticosteroids. An appropriate therapeutic regimen has been provided by Taylor and Nutman (1996). DEC was also known to precipitate or exacerbate active optic neuritis in some onchocercal patients as part of a generalized inflammatory reaction (the Mazzotti reaction) (Murdoch *et al.*, 1994).

Therapy has been improved enormously by the introduction of ivermectin which is now the drug of choice. A critical feature of its mode of action involves the adult female worms, in which this drug inhibits reproduction, so that no new microfilariae are produced for several months. It also kills microfilariae in tissue including skin and the eye. Ivermectin (12 mg *single* dose) has been shown to eliminate microfilariae slowly from the anterior chamber of the eye but offers the advantages of minimal ocular inflammation and much less systemic reaction. This agent represents an important advance in the mass therapy of onchocerciasis in endemic areas, by single-dose therapy.

Ivermectin has to be given yearly and the eradication programme is a continuous one. It should not be given to children under 5 years, to pregnant women and to patients with other severe infections such as trypanosomiasis. Ivermectin does not appear to precipitate or exacerbate optic neuritis, at least in the early stages of treatment (Murdoch *et al.*, 1994). The chronic inflammation that occurs in the skin and the eye is a reaction to the dead microfilariae and not to the live ones.

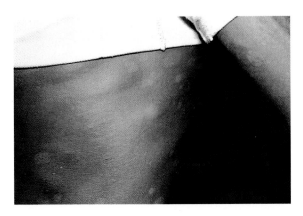

Figure 8.16:
Onchocercal nodule
and hypopigmenta-
tion.

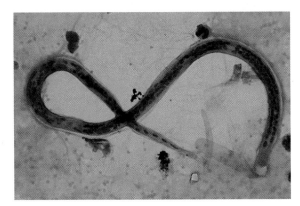

Figure 8.17:
Microfilaria of *Brugia
malayi* (180–290 μm
long × 7.5–10 μm
wide) in human
blood (Harris's
haematoxylin stain,
× 100).

Filariasis

Lymphatic filariasis is a disease due to infection with the filarial worms *Wuchereria bancrofti*, *Brugia malayi* and *B. timori*. It is found in Central Africa, south India and South China in particular. Clinically, the diseases caused by these different genera are indistinguishable. The infection is transmitted by mosquitoes (*Culex*, *Aedes*, *Mansonia* and *Anopheles*) when they ingest human blood containing microfilariae (Fig. 8.17). The microfilaria loses its sheath in the mosquito stomach and in less than 24 hours has entered its thoracic muscles. Metamorphosis proceeds and mature larvae migrate to the labella after 10 days, ready to be inoculated into the next bitten person.

In humans, larvae pass through peripheral lymphatics, migrate and grow into adults which mate in lymphatics proximal to lymph nodes. These adult worms remain coiled up in dilated lymphatics. Fertilized females produce the microfilariae which are found in the peripheral blood (Fig. 8.17) 12 months after initial

161

infection. This discharge is cyclical, occurring mostly at night. Immunity is complex. Exposed individuals from endemic areas can remain healthy and express both antibody and CMI responses. Those with active infections may show reduced CMI.

Clinical illness begins with swelling, tenderness and erythema on the arms, legs or scrotum. Swellings can be firm; nodules and urticaria can also be present. Recurrrent lymphadenitis develops with fever, sweats and painful enlargement of nodes with clinical effects of lymphatic obstruction according to the site affected. Secondary infection by bacteria is rare. This type of lymphangitis must be distinguished from bacterial infection, particularly lymphogranuloma venereum (due to *Haemophilus ducreyi*) if the scrotum is involved.

In the acute stage, microfilaria are demonstrated in the blood in a thick film (Fig. 8.17). Serological tests include indirect immuno-fluorescence and ELISA but they are not species specific. Polymerase chain reaction tests are available as well.

Therapy has relied in the past on DEC. The drug is effective against microfilaria but not adult worms. DEC causes severe side-effects but these are not usually fatal. These include acute allergic reactions on death of the filariae. Ivermectin is also effective but acts much more quickly. It causes similar adverse reactions to DEC. The dose is 400 μg/kg and needs repeating because of recurrent microfilaraemia. Ivermectin paralyses the worms but does not kill them.

Dracunculiasis

Chronic infection due to the nematode *Dracunculus medinensis* occurs in India, Africa, the Middle East and the West Pacific. It infects over 50 million people worldwide and up to 30% of the population in parts of Nigeria. It is a disease of poor rural populations and is spread around by contaminated common water sources.

The worm matures over 1 year in humans and discharges larvae through an ulcerated skin lesion. Millions are produced on contact with water. They survive for several days and develop further in water fleas (*Cyclops*). They pass through two developmental stages before reaching the infective third stage after 2 weeks. Humans are infected by drinking water containing the infected water fleas. The larvae are released from the flea to penetrate the intestine of humans. Maturation occurs in the retroperitoneal space with mating after 3 months. The males die but the females migrate to the lower limbs to penetrate the skin of the leg, when there is ulceration.

Systemic symptoms include fever, urticaria, pruritus, dyspnoea and diarrhoea immediately before the appearance of the female worm through the skin. There is a papule which bursts over 5 days with intense itching. Part of the female worm then emerges through the skin. Secondary bacterial infection of the ulcer and surrounding tissue is common and may be fatal.

Therapy involves removal of the worm. Oral therapy with metronidazole or tiabendazole is effective. The inflammation lessens and the worm can be extracted. Traditional therapy is to wind the free end of the worm around a match stick slowly removing it over several days. If stretched and broken it may cause severe allergic cellulitis.

Loiasis

This is found in damp forests of West and Central Africa and Southern Sudan. It is transmitted by blood-sucking *Chrysops* flies biting by day which inoculate larvae of *Loa loa* into the human. One year after infection, adult worms appear under the skin or in the conjunctiva but microfilariae are not found in the blood for another 5 months. The adult worm moves frequently through the connective tissues of the skin on fingers, trunk, eyelids and conjunctiva and can enter the anterior chamber of the eye (Seal *et al.*, 1998). In Europeans, in particular, transitory oedematous swellings the size of a hen's egg (Calabar swellings) develop on the arm, hand and other sites, which are an allergic reaction to the appearance of a worm. Other allergic manifestations including eosinophilia and angioneurotic oedema are found in non-endemic area residents. The life expectancy of adult worms is 4 years.

One course of DEC is usually curative. Steroid therapy starting 1 day before DEC will prevent severe reactions as for onchocerciasis. Ivermectin has also been used successfully.

Schistosomiasis

Schistosomiasis is caused by the flukes *S. haematobium* (North and East Africa), *S. mansoni* (South Egypt, Central and East Africa and Venezuela) and *S. japonicum* (East Asia). Rashes occur in the invasive stage of this disease, when the skin is penetrated by schistosomal cercariae released from the intermediate host (aquatic snail) into the water. An itchy papular eruption lasts from a few hours to 1 week following invasion. There may also be later involvement at or near mucocutaneous junctions. Urticaria may develop 4–6 weeks after skin penetration by cercariae, which is particularly severe with *Schistosoma japonicum*, together with the systemic disease. In China and Japan this may be prominent and is called 'urticarial fever' or Katayama disease. In areas of high endemicity paragenital granulomata and fistulous tracts develop with adult flukes present in adjacent vasculature. Fistulous tracts with firm masses can be found around the perineum. Ova may be deposited in the skin as well as in other sites to cause ectopic cutaneous schistosomiasis. Treatment is given with praziquantel 40 mg/kg in two divided doses 4–6 h apart on 1 day.

The non-human schistosomes cause cutaneous symptoms only, as above, following penetration of cercariae into the skin – the so-called 'cercarial dermatitis': further development into flukes does not take place because the human is the wrong species for this to happen.

Paragonimiasis

Paragonimus westermani or the 'lung fluke' is found in the Far East and Central Africa. Human infection results from eating inadequately cooked crabs and crayfish. Ingested metacercariae penetrate the intestinal wall and migrate through the diaphragm to the lungs. Adult worms encyst in the lungs and cause a chronic cough with fever, sweats and brown-stained sputum. Flukes can reach ectopic sites such as the skin or conjunctiva to cause large, mobile subcutaneous lesions which develop into cold abscesses. They are painful, up to 10 cm in size and may rupture. This fluke responds well to treatment with two doses of praziquantel at 25 mg/kg given over a single day.

Insecta

Loxoscelism

A rare necrotizing skin lesion, which must be distinguished from necrotizing fasciitis, is caused by the bite of the 'reclusive' spider (*Loxosceles reclusa*) found in North and South America or the black widow spider in Africa. This may be induced during sleep when the spider leaves its hiding place inside furniture, or when dressing in the morning. Unlike the bite of the black widow spider, that of *L. reclusa* remains localized. The necrosis develops into a large slough which may persist for several weeks before healing takes place slowly.

9. TROPICAL FUNGAL INFECTION

Philip A Thomas

Types of tropical fungal infection

Skin and wound infections due to fungi occur in all parts of the world: hence, one may question the need for a separate chapter on tropical fungal infections. This is needed because there are definite differences in the pattern of such infections between tropical and temperate climates. For example, Masri Fridling (1996), in a review of dermatophytosis of the foot, categorically states that tinea pedis is the most common fungal infection worldwide. However, studies in tropical countries such as India and Sri Lanka have consistently shown that tinea corporis and tinea cruris are the commonest types of cutaneous mycoses, while the frequency of tinea pedis is comparatively low (Attapattu, 1997a; Senthamilselvi et al., 1998b). Another important point is that certain fungal skin and wound infections are found almost exclusively in the tropics, for example mycetoma, entomophthoramycoses (subcutaneous and rhinofacial zygomycoses), chromoblastomycosis and lobomycosis.

In the tropics, fungal skin and wound infections may present as:

1. *Superficial mycoses* (refer to Chapter 3)
   These include:
   Pityriasis versicolor (Fig. 3.23)
   Black piedra
   White piedra
   Tinea nigra.
2. *Cutaneous mycoses* (refer to Chapter 3)
   These include:
   Dermatophytosis
   Cutaneous mycoses caused by non-dermatophytes.
3. *Subcutaneous mycoses*
   These include:
   Chromoblastomycosis
   Mycetoma
   Sporotrichosis
   Rhinosporidiosis
   Zygomycoses (mucormycoses and entomophthoramycoses).

4. *Cutaneous manifestations of deep mycoses*
These include:
Phaeohyphomycosis
Dimorphic fungal infections
Hyalohyphomycosis
Infections due to *Fusarium* spp.
Penicilliosis due to *P. marneffei*
Lobomycosis
Cutaneous aspergillosis and cryptococcosis.
5. *Other infections*
These include:
Protothecosis
Adiaspiromycosis
Pythiosis.

Cutaneous mycoses specific to the tropics

Scytalidium dimidiatum (previously *Hendersonula toruloidea*) is a well-recognized plant pathogen in tropical regions causing branch wilt, canker and dieback disease of a wide range of trees, many of them of economic importance. It can infect skin and nails (Figure 9.1).

In a major survey of 399 patients with superficial lesions who had been born outside Western Europe, 32 patients had *S. dimidiatum* infection and 11 patients *Scytalidium hyalinum* (Moore, 1986). Skin lesions from which either *S. dimidiatum* or *S. hyalinum* was isolated were indistinguishable from each other and also from those observed in *Trichophyton rubrum* infections. In an earlier paper, however, Hay

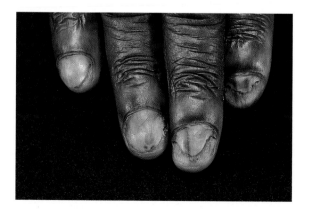

Figure 9.1:
Onychomycosis due to *Scytalidium dimidiatum*.

and Moore (1984) described some differences between the clinical features of these two infecions and those of *T. rubrum*, namely: absence of dorsal infection on the feet; lateral and distal onychomycosis with extensive onycholysis, and the development of paronychia on the fingers. Frankel and Rippon (1989) reported on the first patient with tinea capitis-like infection due to *S. dimidiatum*.

The parallels between the two *Scytalidium* infections are numerous. In their infective phases, both organisms produce similar clinical signs, and their hyphae in the skin are virtually indistinguishable. In culture, they mainly differ in the absence of dark pigment in *S. hyalinum*, but several of the remaining pigments have been shown to be identical biochemically; antigenic composition is also very similar. *S. hyalinum* appears to be geographically more restricted than *S. dimidiatum*, since many of the earliest patients were reported from the West Indies, Guyana and West Africa.

Superficial *S. dimidiatum* and *S. hyalinum* infections often fail to respond to currently available oral and topical therapy. Gugnani *et al.* (1986) reported a favourable response to clotrimazole treatment in patients with *Scytalidium dimidiatum* onychomycosis (these patients had not responded to griseofulvin), but Oyeka and Gugnani (1992) did not have success when isoconazole or clotrimazole was used to treat toenail infections due to these fungi in miners. Rollman and Johansson (1987) reported a successful response of onychomycosis due to *S. dimidiatum* with nail avulsion and topical ciclopiroxolamine. Similarly, Ulbricht and Worz (1994) reported that when ciclopiroxolamine lacquer was used to treat onychomycosis due to non-dermatophyte moulds (including *S. dimidiatum*), the results obtained were as good as when onychomycosis due to dermatophytes was treated.

Subcutaneous mycoses

Chromoblastomycosis

This is a chronic granulomatous infection of skin and subcutaneous tissues caused by species of fungi belonging to the genera *Phialophora*, *Fonsecaea* and *Cladosporium* (Figure 9.2). The disease is mainly encountered in humid parts of tropical and subtropical regions of Central and South America (Restrepo *et al.*, 1988; Quieroz-Telles *et al.*, 1992), especially in barefooted populations. Several authentic cases of chromoblastomycosis have been described from India (cited by Naidu and Singh, 1997). Recently, Attapattu (1997b) described a series of 71 patients with chromoblastomycosis seen in Sri Lanka over a 16-year-period (1978–93); the pathogens identified were *Fonsecaea pedrosoi* (64 patients) and *F. compacta* (2 patients). A high incidence has also been noted in Madagascar, Costa Rica, Maracaibo and the Dominican Republic; Paul *et al.* (1991) reported a patient in French Guyana.

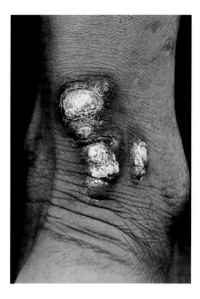

Figure 9.2: Chromoblastomycosis of the ankle.

Several species have been isolated from wood, but the natural environment of others is unknown. Infection is presumed to arise from dermal injury. Male workers in rural areas show the highest incidence of infection. There is no human-to-human transmission.

The lesion develops first as a small papule, or with a smooth or scaly surface, which becomes ulcerated. Growth is very slow and occurs by peripheral extension while the centre of the lesion heals with scar formation. The lesions may remain flat and plaque-like or become raised above the surface on a small stalk. Older lesions may be verrucous, papillomatous or crusted, or simulate the cutaneous forms of other diseases such as tuberculosis, sarcoidosis, leishmaniasis, yaws, syphilis or blastomycosis, from which they must be distinguished. Continued extension produces the characteristic lobulated masses ('cauliflower' lesions). The lesions are generally confined to the skin and subcutaneous tissues of the limbs; however, bone involvement (Lal *et al.*, 1984), disseminated fatal infection and even involvement of the penis have been reported in India.

Although the disease is in itself painless, secondary infection is very common, and pruritus with associated pain may occur. It is often this, rather than the original condition, which causes the patient to seek treatment. Satellite lesions may develop as a result of scratching, and there is also evidence to support a hypothesis of spread via the lymphatic system or the bloodstream. Paul *et al.* (1991) reported neoplastic transformation of lesions of chromoblastomycosis due to *F. pedrosoi*, and stated that although this is extremely rare, three similar observations had been reported in the literature up to that time; another interesting aspect of their patient was the appearance of new cutaneous lesions of chromoblastomycosis in a different site from the original lesion, and presence of an infected synovial cyst.

The most frequently involved aetiological agents are *Fonsecaea pedrosoi* and *Cladosporium carrionii*; *Fonsecaea compacta*, *Phialophora verrucosa* and *Rhinocladiella aquaspersa* (*Ramichloridium cerophilum*) are less common. Both hyphae and spores are pigmented. The organisms can be distinguished by their patterns of sporulation in culture. In tissue (Appendix B), all species are seen as clusters of brown, thick-walled muriform cells (sclerotic bodies) which are often septate, and are found within giant cells or extracellularly among groups of polymorphonuclear leucocytes. The histological picture is of granulomatous nodules containing giant cells and surrounded by a zone of inflammatory cells (plasma cells, lymphocytes, macrophages). In the more advanced lesions, the epidermis becomes greatly enlarged and thickened due to epithelial proliferation and the influx of inflammatory cells. If secondary infection occurs, an acute pyogenic reaction is superimposed upon this granulomatous reaction.

In endemic areas, the presence of unilateral vegetative, trophic and scarred lesions on a lower limb should suggest chromoblastomycosis. However, it is necessary to exclude other fungal infections (blastomycosis, paracoccidioidomycosis, phaeohyphomycosis, sporotrichosis and, in certain areas, rhinosporidiosis and sporotrichosis) and protothecosis, leishmaniasis, podoconiosis (endemic non-filarial lymphoedema), mossy foot, verrucous tuberculosis and syphilis. This necessitates performing mycological and histopathological tests (Appendix B, Tables B2–4).

Direct examination of pus or scales (from the surface of the lesion) digested in KOH frequently reveals the causal organisms as sclerotic cells. Isolation of the causal organisms from infected scales, pus or biopsy specimens should be attempted by inoculation on to glucose-neopeptone agar containing an antibacterial (not cycloheximide, to which these fungi are sensitive). Histopathological studies of biopsy material should aim to demonstrate the presence of the sclerotic bodies.

Chromoblastomycosis is a difficult condition to treat (Appendix A). Several therapeutic approaches have been used, including heat, surgery, tiabendazole, amphotericin B (intravenously) combined with flucytosine, and azole derivatives, but their success has been modest (Restrepo, 1994). When ketoconazole (200–400 mg/day orally) was given for up to 90 days, marked improvement was noted in 2 and a moderate improvement in 4 of 7 patients with chromoblastomycosis (Cuce *et al.*, 1980). Restrepo *et al.* (1988) reported that itraconazole (100-200 mg/day for 12–24 months) was effective in reducing the number, size and severity of lesions in 9 of 10 Colombian patients with active chromoblastomycosis (although the fungus was totally eradicated in only 3 patients); all the patients were infected with *F. pedrosoi*. Quieroz-Telles *et al.* (1992), in Brazil, reported that itraconazole (200–400 mg/day) achieved clinical and biological cure in 8 of 19 patients with *F. pedrosoi* infection after a mean duration of therapy of 7.2 months; clinical cure was achieved in another 7 patients and clinical improvement in the remaining 4 patients. Kumar *et al.* (1991) reported that 2 Indian patients with chromoblastomycosis due to *F. pedrosoi* (that were poorly responsive to amphotericin B and/or ketoconazole) responded very well to itraconazole (200 mg/day) while Yu (1995) reported that oral itraconazole (100 mg/day for 15 months) effected a cure of chromoblastomycosis due to *C. carrionii* in a Chinese patient. Paul *et al.* (1991) were of the opinion that although itraconazole could be used as an alternative to classic therapy for chromoblasto-mycosis, large lesions did not respond satisfactorily. Terbinafine in a dose of 250 mg daily is also very effective. Recently, Ijima *et al.* (1995) reported that high-dose oral amphotericin B resulted in clinical and mycological cure in a Japanese patient. Perhaps the way forward is a combination of therapeutic options. One such combination is flucytosine (200 mg/kg in four divided doses IV for not more than 7 days) with oral tiabendazole (25 mg/kg orally every 12 h for 3 days). Extended therapy under clinical supervision for up to 1 month may be needed for clinical cure (Richardson and Warnock, 1993). Another combination is oral itraconazole and cryotherapy or cryosurgery. In a series of 10 Thai patients with chromoblastomycosis due to *F. pedrosoi*, itraconazole alone (200 mg/day for 3 months) effected a cure in 2 patients while itraconazole (400 mg/day) with monthly liquid nitrogen cryotherapy for 5–10 months was highly effective in 7 patients (Kullavanijaya and Rojanavanich, 1995). Similarly, Bonifaz *et al.* (1997) reported that in Mexican patients with chromoblastomycosis due to *F. pedrosoi*, the combination of itraconazole (to reduce the size of lesions) with subsequent cryosurgery was useful for large lesions, with few side-effects.

Mycetoma

'Mycetoma' is a term used to describe a chronic, granulomatous, subcutaneous 'tumour' resulting from invasion by certain species of true fungi (eumycetoma) and aerobic actinomycetes (actinomycetoma). It may be characterized by enlargement, deformity and destruction of the affected organ. The parasite vegetates as a compact mycelial colony, often having a radial structure with the peripheral zone occupied by more resistant, thick-walled cells. The whole structure is embedded in an amorphous cement derived from the breakdown of tissue elements, and is called the 'grain'.

About 23 species of fungi and 10 species of actinomycetes are believed to cause mycetoma (Rippon, 1988). The principal aetiological agents include:

1. Fungi: *Acremonium* (*A. falciforme, A. kiliense, A. recifei*), *Aspergillus nidulans, Curvularia* (*C. geniculata, C. lunata*), *Exophiala* (*E. jeanselmei*), *Fusarium* (*F. monil-iforme, F. solani*), *Leptosphaeria* (*L. senegalensis, L. tompkinsii*), *Madurella* (*M. grisea, M. mycetomatis*), *Neotestudina rosatii, Pyrenochaeta romeroi* and *Scedosporium apiospermum* (*Pseudallescheria boydii*).

2. Actinomycetes: *Actinomadura (A. madurae, A. pelletieri), Streptomyces (S. somaliensis, S. paraguayensis), Nocardia (N. asteroides, N. brasiliensis, N. otitidis-caviarum).*

The predominant organisms vary from country to country. Eumycotic infections appear to take a longer time to evolve than do actinomycotic infections, which may develop within 5 years.

This disease is mainly distributed in the tropical and semitropical areas of the world, but isolated cases occur virtually everywhere. Mycetomas are frequent in the northern tropical zones of America (Mexico, Venezuela and the Caribbean), Africa (Senegal, Mauritania, Sudan) and Asia (India, Sri Lanka) but can also be observed beyond these areas (Mahgoub, 1989; Serrano *et al.*, 1994; Develoux *et al.*, 1995; Attapattu, 1997a; Serrano *et al.*, 1998a). In Africa, a high endemicity has been noted in regions where there are long dry seasons and short rainy seasons (Develoux *et al.*, 1995), and presumably similar conditions prevail in other endemic areas. Rainfall is believed to influence the distribution of these agents in Africa, with *Streptomyces somaliensis* being found more often in desert areas and *Actinomadura pelletieri* in areas with more rainfall (Develoux *et al.*, 1995). In Venezuela, *Actinomadura madurae* is the most frequent aetiological agent of actinomycetoma, followed by species of *Nocardia* and *Streptomyces* (Serrano *et al.*, 1994, 1998a); the most comnmon causes of eumycetomas are *Pyrenochaeta mackinnonii*, *P. romeroi* and *Madurella grisea* (Fig. 9.3) (Serrano *et al.*, 1998b). In India, 65% of mycetomas are believed to be actinomycotic in origin, while others are due to fungi, mainly *Madurella mycetomatis* (Fig. 9.4) (Rippon, 1988). This has been confirmed in a recently published retrospective analysis of 212 patients with mycetoma, where 161 (75%) were due to aerobic actinomycetes; the principal aetiological agents were *N. brasiliensis*, *N. asteroides*, *N. caviae* (otitidis-caviarum), *Actinomadura* and *Streptomyces* (in actinomycetomas) and *Madurella grisea*, *M. macadamia*, *P. romeroi* and *Scedosporium apiospermum* (in eumycetomas) (Maiti and Haldar, 1998). Interestingly, 67% of mycetomas on 'exposed areas' of the body were actinomycetomas while 94% of those on 'covered areas' were due to actinomycetes. Campbell (1987) reported the isolation of a new hyphomycete, which he designated *Polycytella hominis (gen. et sp. nov.)*, from an Indian patient with pale-grain mycetoma; the fungus formed elongate multiseptate conidia in culture, while the grains it formed in tissue closely resembled those of *Scedosporium apiospermum* in having a prominent 'eosinophilic fringe' and in having many swollen hyphal cells.

Nocardia asteroides has been isolated from soil in the Sudan: *Scedosporium apiospermum*, *Acremonium* and *Fusarium* are also found in the soil. Similarly, other causal organisms are believed to have a saprobic existence in soil or vegetation.

The highest incidence of mycetoma occurs in men engaged in agricultural occupations. Maiti and Haldar (1998) observed that in patients suffering from mycetomata on exposed parts of the body, the male:female ratio (3:1) was significantly higher than that (1:1) in patients with mycetomas on 'covered' parts of

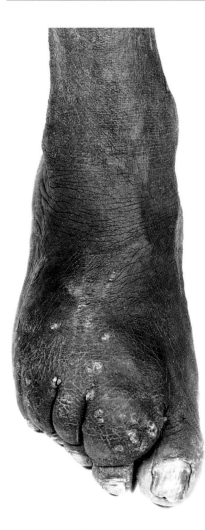

Figure 9.3: Eumycetoma of foot due to *M. grisea* in a Caribbean patient.

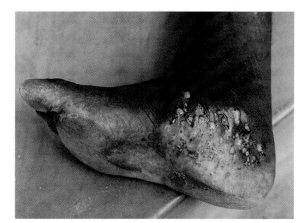

Figure 9.4: Nodules and sinuses of eumycetoma on the medial aspect of the right foot of a male patient in India. (By courtesy of Prof. G Senthamilselvi, Chennai.)

the body; the 'exposed areas' were also significantly more prone to trauma than the 'covered' areas. The nature of the trauma, the virulence of the organisms, the temperature of the anatomical region affected and the presence of associated bacterial flora are all believed to determine the occurrence of this condition. A local traumatic incident, such as an insect bite or thorn prick, is the usual mode of infection. About 25% of patients will give a history of injury at the site of the lesion. Occasionally, thorns have been found in the centre of grains. Feet and lower parts of the leg are usually affected but any part of the body may be invaded, such as the scalp (Peerapur and Inamadar, 1997), thumb (Anandi et al., 1997), exposed parts of upper limbs, abdomen, chest, back, neck and shoulder, buttock, upper thigh and upper arm (Maiti and Haldar, 1998).

Maiti and Haldar (1998) noted that in persons with mycetomas on 'exposed areas' of the body, the lesions were principally on the feet of barefooted individuals and cultivators or on the backs of workers who used to carry sacks contaminated by soil or sugar cane; conversely, in persons with mycetomas on 'covered areas', the lesions usually occurred after a chance accident due to different types of injuries.

The period of incubation varies from a few weeks to several years. The first sign of infection is a painless swelling, which may be ill-defined or hard, colourless or dark-coloured, depending upon the causal agent. Growth and spread are usually extremely slow, but continuous. Extension occurs along tissue planes, and eventually the deeper tissues are invaded, including bone, but muscle is less often affected. In the majority of cases, nodules develop on the surface of the lesion and open to reveal sinuses discharging a purulent fluid; this is formed by tissue breakdown and contains the characteristic grains. As the disease progresses, some of the sinuses heal with scar formation and fresh ones open up. Actinomycetoma lesions tend to be ill-defined and very extensive, and do not produce the enlargement characteristic of eumycetomas; the disease usually spreads rapidly and bone is readily destroyed. The disease is characteristically painless and without constitutional symptoms, unless secondary bacterial infection develops. Breakdown of the granuloma and transport of fragments within phagocytes to neighbouring sites is thought to be the main method of dissemination. Occasionally, lymphatic spread may occur.

In tissues, the fungal/actinomycete colony or grain is surrounded by an inner zone of polymorphonuclear leucocytes, and outer zones of granulation tissue and macrophages. The whole granuloma is enclosed in a fibrous capsule (Appendix B).

In establishing the diagnosis, clinical findings, and colour and size of the discharged grain, are useful. Conventional radiographs and magnetic resonance imaging (MRI) may be helpful in indicating the extent to which bone and deeper tissues are involved. Knowledge of the geographical location may help to indicate the most probable causal agent.

Crushing of the grain and direct examination under the microscope (Appendix B) will reveal the filaments: broad (fungi), or narrow (actinomycetes). If the grain is very hard, it may be soaked first in 10–20% potassium hydroxide. However, a definitive diagnosis of the aetiological agent involved can only be made by culture of the organism from the grain (Appendix B). The best results are obtained from biopsy specimens collected under sterile conditions, since discharged grains are often non-viable or heavily contaminated with bacteria. Fungal grains may be cultivated on glucose-neopeptone and glucose nutrient agars, with antibiotics. Actinomycete grains may be cultured on glucose-neopeptone agars without antibiotics, but blood agar or Löwenstein–Jensen medium is often better for primary isolation. A high proportion of pale grain fungi produce sterile (no spores) growth in culture and cannot be identified.

Histopathology is a very important aid to diagnosis, particularly when culture is impossible (Appendix B). The shape and size of the grain, staining properties, type and arrangement of hyphal elements, and pigmentation are used to identify the causal agent, at least to generic level (see Appendix B). Patients with well-established mycetoma may produce circulating antibody, which may be detected by simple immunodiffusion techniques, by counterimmunoelectrophoresis (CIE) and, more recently, by ELISA. Molecular methods may also play a role in future in diagnosis (Serrano et al., 1994).

Surgery has been used extensively in the past and is still widely used, particularly if the lesions are small and localized. If any part of the organism remains in the tissue, recurrence is certain and thus amputation, at a point higher than the visible lesion, is necessary.

Actinomycetoma frequently responds to dapsone (adult dose about 100 mg, three times a day) given over a period of 6–24 months. Sulfonamides and co-trimoxazole have also been used successfully. The drug of choice is now strepto-mycin sulphate (1000 mg/day) given intramuscularly; this should be combined with co-trimoxazole (960 mg twice daily) in cases caused by S. somaliensis, A. pelletieri and N. brasiliensis (Richardson and Warnock, 1993). Early actinomycetomas (and some late and advanced cases) usually respond well to this treatment. If no response is seen after 3 weeks, other regimens (for example, streptomycin and rifampicin) can be given. In favourable situations, oedema and tenderness regress, and there is a diminution of secretion and grain formation. Treatment should be continued even after there is no longer clinical or laboratory evidence of infection.

The response of eumycetoma to antifungal treatment is disappointing (Appendix A). S. apiospermum mycetoma may respond to intravenous miconazole or oral ketoconazole (400 mg/day); 70% of patients with M. mycetomatis respond to prolonged treatment with ketoconazole; griseofulvin has been tried in non-responders with partial success (Restrepo, 1994). Long-term treatment with itraconazole has resulted in some improvement in M. grisea mycetoma, while limited data in patients with eumycetoma due to Fusarium species indicate good responses to itraconazole (Restrepo, 1994). According to certain workers (Bourrel et al., 1989; Shafei et al., 1992; McGinnis, 1996), combined surgical and medical therapy with ketoconazole may present the best outcome.

174

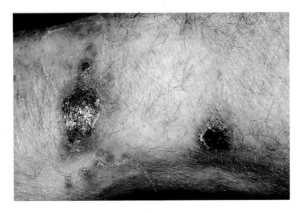

Figure 9.5:
Sporotrichosis of the forearm.

Sporotrichosis

Sporotrichosis is caused by the dimorphic fungus *Sporothrix schenckii*. This disease generally causes lesions in the cutaneous and subcutaneous tissues (Fig. 9.5), and is characterized by the formation of nodular lesions that suppurate, ulcerate and drain. Sporotrichosis commonly presents as the lymphocutaneous form (in about 75% of patients) while the other varieties, fixed cutaneous, mucocutaneous, extracutaneous and disseminated, are less common. However, Kusuhara *et al.* (1988) reported a preponderance of fixed cutaneous lesions in their series of 150 Japanese patients, and so did Cuadros *et al.*(1990) in their small series of patients in Peru.

Sporotrichosis is worldwide in distribution, including tropical and temperate regions. In Central and South America, it has been reported from Mexico, Brazil, Peru, Venezuela, Colombia and Bolivia (see Cuadros *et al.*, 1990). Many patients have been studied in Japan (Kusuhara *et al.*, 1988; Eisfelder *et al.*, 1993), China (Li *et al.*, 1997b) and various parts of India (Khaitan *et al.*, 1998). This mycotic infection has also been noted in Sri Lanka (Attapattu, 1997a), Nepal (Rajendran *et al.*, 1990), Thailand (Kwangsukstith *et al.*, 1990) and South Africa. However, the largest number of reported cases is from the Americas (Richardson and Warnock, 1993).

Sporothrix schenckii is saprophytic on decomposing vegetation, and is frequently isolated from soil, fertilizer, grass, insects and from a variety of animals, including rats, horses, camels and iguanas. In humans, traumatic injuries, such as cuts, animal and insect bites, thorn pricks or splinters, create breaks in the integrity of the skin, which are then contaminated by materials bearing the fungus, which subsequently enters the tissues. The occupational group principally at risk is that of manual labourers, particularly those in the plant industry. Forestry workers and laboratory workers are at risk, as are those who handle contaminated sphagnum moss (DiSalvo et al., 1987). In a recent report, Hajjeh et al. (1997) described an outbreak of lymphocutaneous sporotrichosis in 65 workers involved in the production of sphagnum moss topiaries. Choong and Roberts (1996) reported on a Samoan male who developed cutaneous sporotrichosis after tattooing.

In a statistical survey of 150 patients with sporotrichosis in Kurume (Japan), Kusuhara et al. (1988) observed the following: a male:female ratio of 1:1.45; an age range of 4 months to 92 years (with two peaks in the first and fifth decade); presentation mostly during the winter and autumn seasons; a definite history of trauma in 42% of patients. The fixed cutaneous variety of sporotrichosis (especially on the upper limbs and face) was the most frequent presentation, followed by the lymphocutaneous variety (possibly because patients presented early for treatment, before progression to the lymphocutaneous type). Sporotrichin skin test was strongly positive in most of the patients. Some parasitic forms of S. schenckii were seen in 69% of patients. In India also, a female preponderance has been noted in some studies, whereas in Peru, males predominated (Cuadros et al., 1990).

Sporotrichosis tends to affect the exposed parts, particularly the limbs, and especially the hand and fingers of the right side. The primary and most common manifestation is a subcutaneous nodule, which becomes ulcerated and produces pus. It may remain localized (fixed cutaneous type), but usually extension occurs along the lymphatic system (lymphocutaneous type). Secondary ulcers develop on the lymph nodes, and the lymphatics become hardened and cord-like. The overlying skin becomes pigmented and inflamed. Multiple small subcutaneous lesions and superficial dermal lesions also occur. Dissemination, either by haematogenous or lymphatic spread, to mouth and upper respiratory system, bones and viscera, is very rare but usually fatal. Widespread skin lesions are the most characteristic feature of disseminated sporotrichosis but lesions of the mucous membrane of the mouth and nose are also common. Primary cutaneous lesions may heal spontaneously, leaving behind unsightly scars, which may impair function. Secondary lesions may persist for years.

In tissues (Appendix B), the fungus appears as small, spherical, oval or elongated budding yeast cells with irregular-stained cytoplasm, or the yeast cells may appear cigar-shaped. They may be found in histiocytes or giant cells, or may occur free in the granulomatous material. 'Asteroid bodies' may occur, consisting of a central spherical or oval basophilic cell (3–5 μm in diameter), surrounded by a thick, radiate eosinophilic substance (which is believed to be a mass of antigen–antibody complexes). The asteroid body is characteristic of sporotrichosis only if the fungal cell within is typical of S. schenckii (Fig. 9.6), since similar bodies may be observed in other mycoses. In cutaneous and subcutaneous lesions, ulceration and thickening of the epidermis is associated with

176

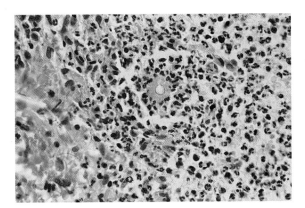

Figure 9.6: Asteroid body containing a single yeast phase - *Sporothrix schenckii* (PAS stain) (× 400).

infiltration by lymphocytes, plasma cells and neutrophils, and giant cells. The tissue reaction is of the epithelioid cell granulomatous and suppurative types. Small foci of histiocytes or pyogenic microabscesses surrounded by inflamed tissue are found; in older lesions, the central area becomes necrotic.

For diagnosis (Appendix B, Tables B2–4) pus, skin scrapings and swabs from ulcers are obtained. Although direct microscopy of pus or tissue is generally not considered to yield good results (since the organisms may be present only in small numbers), others have reported good results with direct microscopy. However, definitive diagnosis depends on the isolation of the aetiological agent in culture. *Sporothrix schenckii* is dimorphic and grows as a mould at room temperature and in yeast phase at 37°C.

In tissue sections stained by periodic acid–Schiff (PAS), Gomori's methenamine silver stain (GMS) or Calcofluor white (CFW), elongated budding yeast cells can be detected (Appendix B).

The drug treatment of choice (Appendix A) for cutaneous sporotrichosis in developing countries remains potassium iodide (KI), since it is easy to administer and relatively inexpensive. Oral therapy is given with 250 mg up to 1 g or more three times daily up to the limit of tolerance for therapy and at least 1 month after cure. Therapy needs to be given for 2–4 months for cure, and for a month thereafter. Li *et al.* (1997b) in China reported that most of their 400 patients with sporotrichosis, who had an average duration of the disease of 6 months, responded satisfactorily to KI administered for 4–6 weeks; similar good results have been reported by Cuadros *et al.*, (1990) in Peru, and by others in the past. However, Kauffman (1995) has expressed the view that the 'old' therapies for sporotrichosis – saturated solution of KI and amphotericin B – have now been supplanted by the currently available oral imidazoles, particularly itraconazole; this is because KI administration is frequently associated with side-effects.

Response rates of > 90% are obtained with itraconazole therapy for lymphocutaneous sporotrichosis (Kauffman, 1995, 1996; Li *et al.*, 1997), and there are many case reports of patients with sporotrichosis showing favourable responses to itraconazole (Grant and Clissold, 1989; Choong and Roberts, 1996). Terbinafine is also effective when used in a dose of 250 mg daily. Kauffman *et al.* (1996) reported that fluconazole therapy (400 mg/day) cured 71% of 14 patients with lymphocutaneous sporotrichosis, but a smaller percentage of extracutaneous disease; these workers concluded that fluconazole is only modestly effective for treatment of sporotrichosis, and should be considered as second-line therapy for the occasional patient who is unable to take itraconazole. Finally, Bargman (1995) reported successful treatment of 3 patients with cutaneous sporotrichosis by using liquid nitrogen, and suggested that cryotherapy might be useful in treating some patients with this disease.

Rhinosporidiosis

Rhinosporidiosis is a chronic granulomatous infection caused by *Rhinosporidium seeberi*, which is generally considered to be a fungus. This disease has been reported from virtually every continent (Kameswaran, 1991); however, the disease is endemic in India and Sri Lanka, and also in some parts of South America and Africa. The disease is most prevalent in rural areas, and seems to be a sequel to working in rice fields or bathing in stagnant water (in large ponds used by the general public in villages for bathing). The causative organism possibly spends part of or its entire life-cycle in water; the organism is also possibly airborne since, in South Africa, where dust storms are common, the disease has been found mainly to affect the eye.

Rhinosporidium seeberi causes the production of large polyps or wart-like lesions that occur predominantly on the nasal mucosa. Cutaneous rhinosporidiosis appears to be very rare. The cutaneous disease arises as a result of spread from a neighbouring mucosal focus; the lesions are similar to those seen on mucous membranes, that is, initially minute papillomas which gradually become large and pedunculated; the surface is irregular and polypous. Although cutaneous lesions are generally asymptomatic, they may cause pain if located in a part of the body subjected to friction or frequent movement. If very friable, these may bleed on touch. Ulcerated rhinosporidiosis lesions are found to be dotted with white spots which can be easily seen by the naked eye; these spots are, in fact, the sporangia.

When the lesions are present on the nasal mucosa or the conjunctiva, the diagnosis is fairly straightforward. However, since cutaneous rhinosporidiosis is an unusual presentation, it needs to be distinguished from cutaneous tuberculosis, lepromatous leprosy, cutaneous leishmaniasis, treponematoses, and cutaneous manifestations of cryptococcosis.

The diagnosis is established by histopathological examination of clinical material (haematoxylin and eosin staining suffices) (Appendix B, Tables B2–4). In infected tissue, spherical bodies (spherules or sporangia) are present, varying in size from 6 to 300 μm. The presence of well-defined spherical bodies of varying size in a rather dense stroma covered by hyperplastic epithelium is a distinctive feature. The young spherule has a vesicular nucleus, granular cytoplasm and a well-defined chitinous wall. Later, it becomes multinucleate, with the development of numerous endospores at the centre and periphery of the spherule. The endospores are released by rupture of the mature sporangia in the region of the pore; mature spores are 8–9 μm in diameter. *R. seeberi* has yet to be cultivated in vitro. Serological tests have not been found useful for the diagnosis of the condition (Naidu and Singh, 1997).

This condition is treated by surgical excision of the lesions. No drug treatment has proved effective for the condition.

Zygomycoses (mucormycoses and entomophthoramycoses)

Zygomycoses (formerly called phycomycoses) refers to infections caused by fungi belonging to the class Zygomycetes.

Some of these fungi cause rhinocerebral, lung, gastrointestinal, cutaneous or disseminated infection in predisposed individuals; this group of infections is commonly referred to as 'mucormycosis' (to differentiate it from entomophthoramycosis) and occurs worldwide. At present, 'cutaneous zygomycosis' is the term used when the skin is affected by fungi of this class (Wirth *et al.*, 1997; Chakrabarti *et al.*, 1997; Dickinson *et al.*, 1998; Linder *et al.*, 1998). Other fungi, namely *Conidiobolus coronatus* and *Basidiobolus ranarum*, can cause chronic subcutaneous infection of the trunk or limbs or the face; this group of infections is commonly referred to as 'entomophthoramycosis', or subcutaneous or rhinofacial zygomycosis, and occurs mainly in tropical regions in Africa, South and Central America and Southeast Asia.

Cutaneous zygomycosis. This may present in either indolent or acute fulminating forms (Adam *et al.*, 1994). Cutaneous zygomycosis is a fulminant form of the disease and affects mainly immunocompromised patients. Since premature infants with perinatal complications are immunocompromised, they are at risk for cutaneous zygomycosis. Primary cutaneous zygomycosis has been associated with multiple nosocomial outbreaks caused by contaminated elastic bandages.

Secondary cutaneous zygomycosis usually occurs in immunosuppressed patients where haematogenous dissemination of the fungus leads to an erythematous nodular, painful cellulitis which then evolves into ulcers covered with a black eschar.

179

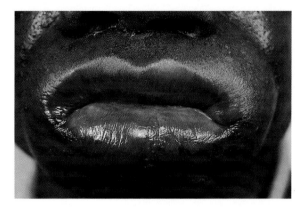

Figure 9.7:
Subcutaneous
zygomycosis due to
Conidiobolus –
infection around the
lips.

Subcutaneous zygomycoses. These are the second most common group of deep mycoses encountered in southern India (after mycetoma). They present in two clinical forms: rhinofacial and subcutaneous.

Infection due to *Conidiobolus* (conidiobolomycosis, rhinoentomophthoramycosis) originates in the nasal sinuses, and spreads to the adjacent subcutaneous tissue of the face, causing disfigurement (Fig. 9.7).

The disease has been found to occur in the tropical rainforests of Africa and South and Central America. In Tamilnadu State of Southern India, conid-iobolomycosis accounted for 2 of 10 patients with entomophthoramycoses encountered over a 4-year period (Krishnan *et al.*, 1998). Mukhopadhyay *et al.* (1995) also reported this infection in a middle-aged woman in Calcutta. In Sri Lanka, rhinofacial zygomycosis due to *C. coronatus* was reported by Attapattu (1997a).

The causal organism is *Conidiobolus coronatus*, which lives as a saprophyte in soil and on decomposing plant matter in moist warm climates; it can also parasitize certain insects. The disease is most common among adult males, particularly those living or working in tropical rainforests. In the study by Krishnan *et al.* (1998) in Tamilnadu, India, both patients with conidiobolomyco-sis were more than 45 years old, and had had the disease for 3 months.

Infection is acquired through inhalation of conidia or their introduction into the nasal cavities by soiled hands. It generally begins with unilateral involvement of the nasal mucosa, so that nasal obstruction is the commonest initial symptom; epistaxis and the development of a nasal polyp may also occur. There may be limited spread, in which instance subcutaneous nodules develop in the nasal and perinasal regions and may be associated with epidermal lesions. Usually, there is slow but relentless spread with invasion of the subcutaneous tissue occurring from the inferior turbinate, which becomes swollen. Gross facial swelling involving the forehead, periorbital region and upper lip is very distinctive. The lesions are usually smooth, with distinct margins, firmly adherent to the underlying tissue but sparing the bone. The skin remains intact. Spread to lymph nodes may occur.

Although the diagnosis may be fairly obvious from the clinical findings, mycological and histological tests are essential. Organisms grow readily on Sabouraud's glucose-neopeptone agar.

In tissue sections, broad thin-walled branching and occasionally septate hyphae are found. They have a varied morphological appearance, stain poorly and are surrounded by eosinophilic cellular debris.

Treatment of this condition is difficult. Potassium iodide by mouth (see page 177) or amphotericin B IV can be given but long-term results are poor. Amphotericin is toxic (Appendix B). Surgical resection of infected tissue is risky, since it may actually hasten the spread of infection. Mukhopadhyay *et al.* (1995) reported that a combination of oral ketoconazole and potassium iodide proved effective in their patient with conidiobolomycosis. Kumar *et al.* (1991) reported that their patient with rhinofacial zygomycosis, who had responded only partially to amphotericin B therapy, responded well to itraconazole, with eradication of the fungus from the lesion.

Gugnani *et al.* (1995) in Nigeria reported that 2 out of 4 patients with zygomycosis due to *C. coronatus* were completely cured, while the other 2 patients were considerably improved following treatment with oral fluconazole. Attapattu (1997a) in Sri Lanka reported that one of her patients responded to potassium iodide while the other responded to oral ketoconazole. Krishnan *et al.* (1998) reported that one patient who did not respond to KI responded to ketoconazole.

Infection due to *Basidiobolus* is a chronic subcutaneous infection of the trunk and limbs. This disease is encountered chiefly in tropical regions in East or West Africa and Southeast Asia. Attapattu (1997a) has reported the isolation of *Basidiobolus ranarum* from 2 Sri Lankan children presenting with subcutaneous lesions. There have been several reports from southern India (Krishnan *et al.*, 1998).

The causal organism is *Basidiobolus ranarum*. This zygomycete has been isolated from soil and decaying plants, and from the faecal material of frogs, reptiles, fish and bats. It is still not clear how humans acquire the disease and what is the length of the incubation period. Trauma and subsequent contamination of the wound by the fungal conidia are the probable mechanisms.

The majority of cases have been reported from children or adolescents and the disease sometimes shows spontaneous regression. It is characterized by

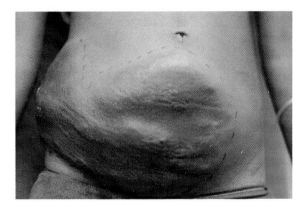

Figure 9.8:
Entomophthoramycosis
(basidiobolomycosis)
on the abdomen of a
female child. (By
courtesy of Prof. G
Senthamilselvi,
Chennai.)

induration and swelling of the subcutaneous tissues over extensive areas, particularly of the limbs, trunk or buttocks (Fig. 9.8).

The lesion is sharply demarcated, very hard but painless and can be raised
above the underlying tissues. In basidiobolomycosis, there is no adherence to
underlying tissue, unlike the situation in conidiobolomycosis. Although the infection causes much disfiguration, there is no ulceration of the skin. Sometimes,
there may be invasion of the lymph nodes by the fungus or hyperplastic
lymphadenopathy. Visceral involvement is very rare.

In tissues, *B. ranarum* is found in microabscesses or in giant cells as short broad
hyphal fragments, usually branched and non-septate. Very often, the hyphae
appear in cross-section as holes in the tissue surrounded by an eosinophilic cuff.
They stain deeply with haematoxylin. The tissue reaction is a granulomatous one
and the massive infiltration of eosinophils is the most significant feature.
Although the disease can be diagnosed by clinical features alone, microbiological and histological examination is also recommended. Once again the organism
is cultivable on conventional media.

In the tropics, oral potassium iodide (KI) appears to be the drug of choice
for treatment of subcutaneous zygomycosis (basidiobolomycosis). Krishnan *et al.*
(1998) reported that 9 of their 10 patients with entomophthoramycosis (all 8
with basidiobolomycosis) responded to oral potassium iodide in a dose of
40 mg/kg body weight per day till the lesions resolved and for 4–6 weeks thereafter. Attapattu (1997a) reported that both her patients responded to oral KI.
Others, in Indonesia, have reported a good response of subcutaneous zygomycosis (basidiobolomycosis) to oral itraconazole. Hence, this new triazole could
be tried in patients with subcutaneous zygomycosis that does not respond to KI.

Cutaneous manifestations of deep mycoses

Phaeohyphomycosis

This refers to superficial, cutaneous, subcutaneous and deep-seated infections due to dematiaceous filamentous fungi that appear as pigmented, septate fungal hyphae in tissue; there are no grains (as in eumycetomata) or sclerotic bodies (as in chromoblastomycosis). Phaeohyphomycosis has a worldwide distribution, but cutaneous and subcutaneous infections appear to occur more frequently in tropical parts of Central and South America, in India and other tropical countries.

The more important aetiological agents include species of *Alternaria*, *Bipolaris*, *Curvularia*, *Exophiala*, *Exserohilum* and *Phialophora* and *Xylohypha bantiana* and *Wangiella dermatitidis*. The primary factor unifying the dematiaceous fungi is the dark pigmentation, which has been identified as dihydroxynaphthalene melanin; there is increasing evidence that melanin itself may serve as a virulence factor in pathogenic fungi (Polak, 1990). While many of these fungi are saprobes on wood pulp and decaying vegetable matter, others are plant pathogens. Cutaneous and subcutaneous infections generally arise due to traumatic implantation of the fungus.

Phaeohyphomycosis can be divided into a number of distinct forms (based on tissue involvement and clinical presentation) as superficial, cutaneous and corneal, subcutaneous and systemic (Dixon and Polak-Wyss, 1991). Localized superficial infections of the stratum corneum by dematiaceous fungi occur in tinea nigra.

Cutaneous phaeohyphomycosis usually follows traumatic implantation; the arms and legs are the commonest sites of infection. Small plaques or ulcers are the main clinical features. Subcutaneous phaeohyphomycosis usually follows traumatic implantation of the fungus from the soil into the subcutaneous tissue (Jha *et al.*, 1996); even minor trauma (cuts or wounds due to thorns or wood splinters) is often sufficient. Lesions occur mainly on the arms and legs. The initial lesion is a firm, sometimes tender, subcutaneous nodule which may enlarge slowly to form a painless cystic abscess; although lesions are attached to the skin, they are not attached to the underlying tissue or bone (Richardson and Warnock, 1993). Subcutaneous phaeohyphomycoses have rarely been reported in organ transplant recipients.

The lesions of subcutaneous phaeohyphomycosis have to be distinguished from the cutaneous lesions of other fungal infections (chromoblastomycosis, sporotrichosis, blastomycosis, coccidioidomycosis, paracoccidioidomycosis) and cutaneous leishmaniasis. In sporotrichosis, lymphatic spread is usually seen, while in the other mycotic infections referred to above, the cutaneous lesions are usually verrucous.

For diagnosis (Appendix B, Tables B2–4), direct microscopy of wet preparations of clinical material (pus, skin scrapings, etc.) in KOH mounts permits the demonstration of the characteristic brown-pigmented septate fungal hyphae.

Histology is helpful in the diagnosis. These fungi are often difficult to identify in haematoxylin and eosin-stained sections because of variability in the amount of pigment in the walls. This difficulty can be overcome by lowering the microscope condenser, to make the hyphae more refractile, or by staining with melanin-specific stains such as Fontana–Masson (Jha *et al.*, 1996). Culture is essential to confirm the diagnosis and to initiate the appropriate treatment.

Medical management alone is usually ineffective and surgery, either on its own or combined with IV amphotericin B or oral itraconazole in immunocompromised patients, is the usual approach.

Dimorphic fungal infections

Blastomycosis

This is caused by the dimorphic fungus *Blastomyces dermatitidis*; the chief endemic zone is North America, but cases have also been reported from South America, South Africa, Tunisia, Saudi Arabia and India (Nouira *et al.*, 1994; Desai *et al.*, 1997). This fungus is believed to be saprobic, it has been isolated from soil and wood debris.

The primary infection is always pulmonary. The characteristic cutaneous lesions (found particularly on the face and extremities) are often the presenting symptom; they may follow local infection, or be secondary to the pulmonary form, probably arising as a result of haematogenous spread (Nouira *et al.*, 1994; Desai *et al.*, 1997). Haematogenous spread is reported to lead to cutaneous lesions in up to 70% of patients with the disseminated disease (Richardson and Warnock, 1993). An ulcerating pustule first develops, which then spreads to become an ulcerated granule with an indurated edge. Both base and edge of the ulcer contain numerous small abscesses. The underlying bone may become involved, in which instance the patient presents with a discharging sinus. Dissemination to subcutaneous tissue occurs rarely; multiple skin lesions are usually associated with the disseminated form.

The tissue reaction is a combination of suppurative and epithelioid cell granulomata with giant cells. In cutaneous lesions, the epidermis is severely inflamed and enlarged; yeasts are found in microabscesses or in giant cells. In lesions in deeper tissues, yeasts may occur freely in the necrotic tissue or in giant cells.

For diagnosis, pus and granulomatous material from cutaneous lesions is obtained (Appendix B, Tables B2–4). Direct smears (KOH) reveal the characteristic yeasts with broad-based buds. Sen *et al.* (1997) described non-invasive, rapid diagnosis of dermal lesions by the Papanicolaou technique, where a smear from a leg ulcer stained by this method revealed fungi within giant cells. Histopathology and culture (Appendix B) are important in establishing the diagnosis.

Amphotericin B is the drug of choice for serious systemic illness. For more indolent disease (such as cutaneous lesions), the oral imidazoles can be used. Of these, itraconazole 200–400 mg daily was found effective (Dismukes et al., 1992), and the results were better than those obtained with ketoconazole 400–800 mg/day (Kauffman and Carver, 1997). Nouira et al. (1994) in Tunisia reported a favourable outcome with ketoconazole, while Chodorowska and Lecewicz-Torun (1996) (in Poland) reported the best improvement in a patient with cutaneous blastomycosis when fluconazole was used.

The differential diagnosis includes scrofuloderma, keratoacanthoma, nodular syphilis, leprosy, pyoderma, atypical mycobacterial disease and epithelioma. Frean et al. (1993) described two patients with disseminated blastomycosis (including skin lesions) masquerading as tuberculosis.

Paracoccidioidomycosis

This is caused by the dimorphic fungus *Paracoccidioides brasiliensis*, which is endemic to Latin America from Mexico to Argentina (Lima et al., 1997; Negroni et al., 1997). The individual is usually infected by inhalation.

Mucocutaneous paracoccidioidomycosis is the second most common clinical form of this disease. Cutaneous lesions often appear on the face around the mouth or nose, due to contiguous spread from these sites; however, in patients with severe infection, there can be widespread scattered lesions. Small papular or nodular lesions enlarge over weeks or months into plaques with an elevated, well-defined margin; verrucous lesions or ulcers with a rolled border may develop.

The tissue reaction is of the epithelioid granulomatous type with associated pyogenic inflammation. Microabscesses and collections of phagocytes are found in inflamed and enlarged epidermal tissue; necrosis may or may not occur, and there may be fibrosis in older lesions. The characteristic yeasts with multiple buds are found in giant cells or in abscesses, or are free in the granulomatous tissue (Appendix B).

For diagnosis (Appendix B, Tables B2–4), pus is taken from the lesions. Direct microscopy (KOH) is used to demonstrate the yeasts. The fungus is dimorphic and grows on mycological media. Histology is usually necessary to demonstrate the parasite in the tissue. Serological tests are useful to establish the diagnosis as well as to monitor response to treatment.

The differential diagnosis includes leishmaniasis, scrofuloderma, chromoblastomycosis, sporotrichosis and syphilis.

This infection must be treated, because spontaneous resolution does not occur; late relapses may occur in up to 25% of patients. In the past, amphotericin B and sulfonamides were the mainstays of therapy. Sulfonamide required prolonged therapy which was suppressive rather than curative, whereas use of amphotericin B was associated with a significant degree of toxicity. At present, itraconazole is the drug of choice (Restrepo, 1994); the dose is 50–100 mg/day for 6–12 months. Van Tyle (1984) reviewed 158 patients with the disease treated with ketoconazole and stated that this imidazole, in doses of 100–400 mg/day for up to 1 year, effected cure or noticeable improvement in 97% of those treated; at present, ketoconazole and fluconazole are considered to be less effective than itraconazole in treating this condition.

Coccidioidomycosis

This is caused by the dimorphic fungal pathogen *Coccidioides immitis*. This disease is found to be endemic in the dry subtropical climate of the southwestern USA and the tropical climates of Mexico, northern Argentina and Venezuela. It may also occur in persons who had earlier resided in or visited these places (Chen *et al.*, 1991).

The natural habitat of the fungus is in its mycelial phase as a saprobe in the dry and arid desert soil. This mycelium fragments into arthroconidia.

Infection occurs when soil dust contaminated with the arthroconidia is inhaled. The lungs are the usual site of infection. There may be sharp upsurges in the number of patients, due to dust storms (Stevens, 1995). This disease is not contagious, the only person-to-person transmission occurring indirectly – for example, infected pus draining into a dressing (Stevens, 1995). People with diabetes mellitus or a compromised immune system are very susceptible to chronic or disseminated forms of the infection, which includes a variety of skin lesions.

The primary illness is a respiratory infection, either asymptomatic or mild. Fewer than 1% of infected individuals (generally immunosuppressed or other groups) develop disseminated disease (Richardson and Warnock, 1993). Cutaneous and subcutaneous lesions are among the most common manifestations of the disseminated disease. Cutaneous lesions may be single or multiple, persist for long periods and present as verrucous papules, ulcers, erythematous plaques and nodules (Galgiani, 1991; Richardson and Warnock, 1993). Cutaneous lesions may also follow direct inoculation, often presenting as an indurated nodule with central ulceration; lymphangitis may supervene. Arsura *et al.* (1998) reported that patients with facial lesions were more likely to develop meningitis than those without. Quimby *et al.* (1992), in a study of 6 patients with specific cutaneous manifestations of disseminated coccidioidomycosis, reported solitary granulomatous plaques, multiple papular, nodular or pustular and subcutaneous abscesses as the lesions; the histopathologic features showed various degrees of three primary patterns: (1) abscess formation with necrosis;

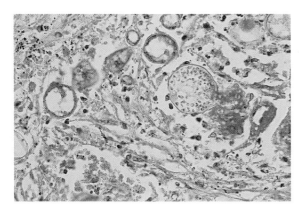

Figure 9.9:
Spherules of
Coccidioides immitis
(PAS stain) in lung
(disseminated
infection) (× 400).

(2) epithelial hyperplasia and granuloma formation with microabscesses; and (3) vascular and perivascular proliferative inflammatory cell reactions. Tissue eosinophilia was present in all patients. The authors concluded that cutaneous manifestations of disseminated coccidioidomycosis may be more common and varied than usually recognized.

The parasitic (tissue) phase of the organism (Appendix B) is characterized by the presence of large multinucleate, thick-walled cells (spherules) filled at maturity with spores which escape by rupture of the cell wall; these are usually found in giant cells. There is a granulomatous type of tissue reaction with histiocytes and giant cells.

For diagnosis of cutaneous/subcutaneous lesions (Appendix B, Tables B2–4), pus or other material is taken for direct microscopy (to demonstrate the characteristic spherules – Fig. 9.9), and for culture on cycloheximide-containing media *in tubes or bottles* (to prevent dissemination of the mycelial arthroconidia) at 26°C (for the mycelial phase). Histology should be done to demonstrate the spherules in tissue. The coccidioidin skin test, which demonstrates delayed-type hypersensitivity, becomes positive 1–3 weeks after onset but is negative in the early and the final fatal stage.

Serological tests are helpful in diagnosis of this condition (although there may be cross-reactions in patients with other dimorphic fungal infections). Tests to detect IgM antibodies against *C. immitis* are most useful for diagnosis of acute infection (appears within 4 weeks of infection but disappears after 2–6 months), while IgG antibodies are best for the later stages of the disease, appearing 4–12 weeks after infection. In disseminated infections, IgG titres persist till death or recovery, rising with progression of the infection and declining as the patient improves. The IgG titre in cerebrospinal fluid may be used to monitor meningeal disease.

In patients with disseminated disease, prolonged chemotherapy is always indicated (Stevens, 1995) (Appendix B). Amphotericin B (1–1.5 mg/kg body weight per day intravenously) could be given till the disease becomes inactive, or for 2–3 months. Amphotericin B, in a lipid-complex formulation, may be advantageous. The oral imidazoles are a good alternative to amphotericin B, since they are less toxic and the response rates appear to be similar; itraconazole (200 mg twice daily with meals), ketoconazole (400 mg/day) or fluconazole (400–600 mg/day) are the suggested doses (Stevens, 1995). Ketoconazole has been shown to be moderately efficacious for the treatment of a variety of different forms of coccidioidomycosis (Kauffman and Carver, 1997). The Mycoses Study Group trial revealed that 57% of patients responded to itraconazole (Graybill et al., 1990). Diaz et al. (1991) in Mexico obtained good results with itraconazole (excellent or very good response in 94% of patients). Similar results have been obtained with fluconazole, but use of this drug leads to remission rather than cure of the infection (Dewsnup et al., 1996).

Histoplasmosis

The classic form (small form) of this disease is caused by the dimorphic fungus *Histoplasma capsulatum*, while a variant form known as African histoplasmosis or large-celled histoplasmosis is caused by *H. duboisii*. This disease has a global distribution apart from Europe, but is most prevalent in the central region of North America and in Central and South America (Borges et al., 1997; Nasta et al., 1997; van Gelderen de Komaid and Duran, 1995); other endemic regions include tropical areas such as Africa (Maresca et al., 1987) and parts of east Asia, especially India (Padhye et al., 1994; Naidu and Singh, 1997), Malaysia (Ng and Siar, 1996), China (Wen et al., 1996) and Taiwan (Kao et al., 1997). Histoplasmosis was first detected in Sri Lanka in 1975, and a subsequent skin test survey found positive skin test reactivity in 4% of healthy adults and 6.3% of patients with chronic lung disease (Attapattu, 1997a); in India, positivity rates vary from 0.6 to 12.3% of population samples (Mukherjee et al., 1986; Naidu and Singh, 1997).

Mucosal lesions (ulcers) are seen in classic or small form histoplasmosis. Cutaneous and subcutaneous disease appears to be more a feature of African histoplasmosis than the classic variety. The mode of infection is presumably by inhalation or by entry through broken skin surfaces.

Two clinical types of histoplasmosis are recognized:

1. a localized form, affecting only one tissue, such as skin or bone. This type may persist for a long period and there is a tendency to spontaneous regression;
2. a disseminated form involving skin, bone, lymph nodes and viscera. Typically, multiple foci occur in bone and cold abscesses in subcutaneous tissue, and

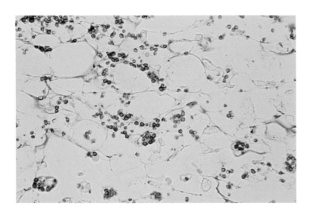

Figure 9.10:
Histoplasma capsulatum (Gomori's methenamine silver stain) in lung (disseminated infection) ($\times$ 400).

there is an enlarged liver and spleen and pleomorphic skin lesions. The resemblance to blastomycosis is noteworthy; *H. duboisii*, however, seldom affects the lungs.

The pathogen particularly attacks the reticuloendothelial system. In the parasitic (tissue) phase (Appendix B), large round-oval thick-walled yeasts (similar to those of *Blastomyces dermatitidis* in size) are found in giant cells or histiocytes or lying free in abscesses (Fig. 9.10). There may be very little tissue reaction but, when present, it resembles an epithelioid cell granuloma. The yeasts bud on a narrow base, and paired cells are often found. The differential diagnosis includes other deep mycoses and tuberculosis.

The diagnosis of cutaneous and subcutaneous disease (Appendix B, Tables B2–4) is established by obtaining material from cutaneous or mucosal lesions (and other sites if necessary). Direct microscopy of wet preparations is not suitable; all material should be examined as stained smears. Organisms tend to be much more abundant in peripheral blood smears and bronchial washings from AIDS patients. The definitive diagnosis depends on isolation of the fungus in culture.

Demonstration of the pathogen in histological sections may be necessary (Appendix B). Haematoxylin and eosin is not always satisfactory, but fungus stains (periodic acid–Schiff, Gomori's methenamine silver etc.) are useful to demonstrate the fungus.

The histoplasmin skin test is not recommended for diagnosis of histoplasmosis but serological tests are useful. The immunodiffusion (ID) and complement-fixation tests (CFT), with histoplasmin as antigen, are positive in about 80% of patients (lower positivity in disseminated disease). The CFT is more sensitive than ID but ID is more specific. Antigen detection is a sensitive method for diagnosis of disseminated disease in AIDS patients.

189

Amphotericin continues to be the mainstay therapy of life-threatening or central nervous system (CNS) infections, particularly in AIDS patients. In less severe disease (such as cutaneous disease), one of the oral azoles can be used since all have demonstrated activity in histoplasmosis (Kauffman and Carver, 1997). The standard therapy of histoplasmosis in AIDS patients has become itraconazole (200 mg twice daily) for mild-to-moderate infection not involving the CNS. Therapy must be continued for life as the relapse rate is extraordinarily high in this population.

Hyalohyphomycosis

The term 'hyalohyphomycosis' was proposed by Ajello and McGinnis (1984) to refer to 'opportunistic' mycotic infections caused by non-dematiaceous fungi whose tissue form consists of hyaline hyphal elements. The term was not intended to replace well-established names, such as aspergillosis, but to be used in place of such terms as fusariosis, penicilliosis or paecilomycosis (Castro *et al.*, 1990).

Infections due to *Fusarium* spp.

Species of *Fusarium* are commonly found in the soil and are also important plant pathogens. *Fusarium* species have been known as important causes of fungal keratitis for many years (Thomas, 1994). In the past 15 years, there has been an increasing number of reports regarding *Fusarium* infections in other parts of the body, such as the nails (Hemashettar and Patil, 1989), skin and subcutaneous tissues (Barrios *et al.*, 1990; Helm *et al.*, 1990; Schneller *et al.*, 1990). Cutaneous or subcutaneous infections due to *Fusarium* may be primary (due to infection of skin ulcers, surgical wounds or burns) or secondary (due to disseminated infection). Cutaneous lesions have been noted in 70% of patients with disseminated *Fusarium* infections (Richardson and Warnock, 1993), and this is thought to be due to their predilection for vascular invasion, resulting in thrombosis and tissue necrosis.

Penicillium marneffei

Penicillium marneffei is a dimorphic fungus that can cause systemic mycosis in humans. Eight human cases of naturally acquired, progressive, disseminated *Penicillium marneffei* infection were reported in Guangxi, China, in 1984 and 1985 (Deng *et al.*, 1986). Five other patients were described from Thailand in 1984 (Jayanetra *et al.*, 1984). In 1986, Deng *et al.* reported an additional 6 human patients with this disease in Nanning, Guangxi. It is now well-established that *P. marneffei*, the aetiologic agent of this systemic mycosis, is endemic to Southeast Asia and the southern region of the People's Republic of China, Hong Kong and Taiwan: patients have also been seen in Malaysia, Myanmar (Sirisanthana, 1997) Thailand (Supparatpinyo *et al.*, 1994) and India (Singh *et al.*, 1999).

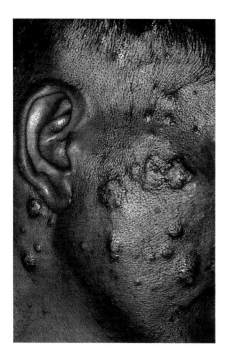

Figure 9.11: Papules with central umbilication due to disseminated infection with *P. marneffei*. (By courtesy of Dr Rataporn Ungpakorn, Bangkok.)

Prior to the epidemic of HIV, penicilliosis was a rare event; the marked increase in the incidence of this fungal infection in the past few years has paralleled the incidence of HIV infection. In fact, in Thailand, *P. marneffei* is the third most frequent AIDS-defining infection in HIV-infected persons (after tuberculosis and cryptococcosis) (Chariyalertsak *et al.*, 1996). The magnitude of the problem in endemic areas such as Thailand can be gauged from the fact that at a large hospital in northern Thailand, between 1991 and 1994, a diagnosis of *P. marneffei* infection was made in 550 patients (male:female ratio being 9:1), while cryptococcosis was diagnosed in 793 patients (male:female ratio being 6.8:1).

In the progressive disseminated form of *P. marneffei*, spread to many organs, principally the lungs, liver, intestines, spleen and lymph nodes, is noted. Fever, leucocytosis and multiple abscesses of the internal organs are among the clinical signs of the disease. The skin is affected during the final stages of the disease, with the development of papules, nodules and abscesses.

The source of the infection is uncertain. Although Deng *et al.* (1986) reported that 18 of 19 bamboo rats (*Rhizomys pruinosus*) yielded cultures of *P. marneffei* from one or more of their internal organs, they eliminated the possibility that individuals who eat infected bamboo rats could be insidiously affected; these authors were of the opinion that both humans and bamboo rats are probably infected from a common environmental source. During each year, *P. marneffei*, but not cryptococcosis, was found to present more frequently in the rainy season than in the dry season at a large hospital in northern Thailand (Chariyalertsak *et al.*, 1996). It was hoped that this observed seasonal variation could provide valuable information in determining the important reservoirs and types of exposure to the organism causing the disseminated disease. Although *P. marneffei* is predominantly an Asian pathogen, it must be recognized in international travellers.

The patients usually present with fever, anaemia, weight loss, skin lesions, generalized lymphadenopathy and hepatomegaly. About 80% of the patients who present are immunocompromised in some manner (Duong, 1996); the average number of CD4+ T-lymphocytes at presentation is 64/cu.mm. The skin lesions are most commonly papules with central necrotic umbilication (Fig. 9.11); nodules and abscesses may also be noted. These skin lesions are observed in about 71% of the patients (Sirisanthana, 1997). The diagnosis of *P. marneffei* infection is easily made when the typical skin lesions are present, but is frequently missed in their absence (Kantipong *et al.*, 1998). This fungus is thermally dimorphic (tissue phase in yeast forms) and grows well on mycological media (in hyphal form).

The disease may clinically resemble histoplasmosis. Other entities to be excluded include tuberculosis, molluscum contagiosum and cryptococcosis.

The diagnosis of *P. marneffei* infection is easily made when typical skin lesions appear, but when these are not present, other investigations are needed. A blood culture can be performed; a positive blood culture from patients in endemic areas is now considered to be an HIV marker. The organism is easy to culture from various clinical specimens on Sabouraud's agar when it gives a red pigment (Fig. 9.12); bone marrow is most sensitive (100%), followed by skin biopsy (90%) and blood culture (Sirisanthana, 1997). After isolating the organism in culture, definitive identification is made by demonstrating dimorphism and/or by the exoantigen procedure (Sutton *et al.*, 1998).

Serological tests are useful for demonstrating circulating antibodies and/or antigens in the patient's serum (Imwidthaya *et al.*, 1994b). Cao *et al.* (1998) described a specific ELISA-based test to detect antibody against M_p1_p, a purified recombinant antigenic mannoprotein of *P. marneffei*. Desakorn *et al.* (1999) found that urinary antigen was detected by enzyme immunoassay in all patients with *P. marneffei* infection; at a titre of 1:40, the assay had a sensitivity of 97% and a specificity of 98%. These workers were of the opinion that this test could be used as a rapid method of diagnosing *P. marneffei* infection in patients with AIDS, and could be a useful adjunct to conventional methods of diagnosis (Appendix B).

Histology can be used to demonstrate this fungus in the lesions (Appendix B). In tissue, this fungus forms characteristic yeast-type cells which divide by a central septum (Fig. 9.13); there is no budding. Most cells in biopsy material are intracellular small oval structures resembling the tissue phase of *Histoplasma capsulatum*; occasionally, large banana-shaped 'bullet' cells are seen.

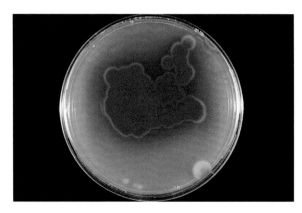

Figure 9.12: Hyphal phase of *P. marneffei* showing red pigment when grown on Sabouraud's agar at 22°C. (By courtesy of Dr Donald Lyon, Hong Kong.)

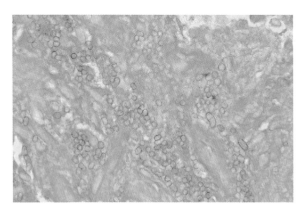

Figure 9.13: Bullet-shaped yeast cells of tissue phase in the gastrointestinal tract of *P. marneffei* (methenamine silver stain). (By courtesy of Dr John Chow, Hong Kong.)

Limited in vitro susceptibility data suggest that *P. marneffei* is susceptible to amphotericin B, 5-fluorocytosine, itraconazole, ketoconazole and miconazole, and relatively less susceptible to fluconazole (Sutton *et al.*, 1998). Radford *et al.* (1997) reported that both voriconazole and itraconazole showed comparable good activity against *P. marneffei*. The response to antifungal therapy is usually good if treatment is started early. Sirisanthana *et al.* (1998) reported that 97% of their patients responded well to a regimen of intravenous amphotericin B (0.6 mg/kg/day) for 2 weeks, followed by oral itraconazole 400 mg/day for 10 weeks. After initial treatment, it is recommended that itraconazole 200 mg/day be continued as secondary prophylaxis for life, since even after successful primary treatment, the relapse rate is as high as 50%; such a regimen was reported to be useful and well tolerated in all 36 patients treated (who were also infected with HIV), in comparison to 57% of patients on placebo who relapsed after successful primary treatment (Supparatpinyo *et al.*, 1998).

Lobomycosis (keloidal blastomycosis)

This slowly progressive infection of the skin and subcutaneous tissue is caused by a fungus that has never been cultured *in vitro*. The causative agent was initially designated *Loboa loboi*, and later *Paracoccidioides loboi*, but has recently been renamed *Lacazia loboi* gen. nov., comb. nov. (Toborda *et al.*, 1999). There is no involvement of internal organs or mucous membranes. Most infections have occurred in men aged 30–40 years who reside in or have travelled frequently through the tropical forests of South America (Amazon region of central Brazil, Colombia, Surinam) and Central America. This fungus has also been found recently in the Atlantic blue-nosed dolphin (Rodriguez and Barrera, 1997). The natural habitat of the fungus remains unknown. The organism is believed to gain entry through skin lesions caused by trauma (insect or snake bites, cuts, abrasions). There is no human-to-human transmission (Fuchs *et al.*, 1990). All cases of human infection acquired from the environment have occurred in geographic zones where the temperature exceeds 24°C and the annual rainfall 2000 mm.

Lobomycosis is an indolent infection which starts as a small papule or nodule and then proliferates to form extensive lesions. These lesions are keloid-like, and leathery in appearance and in consistency; they can be hyperchromic or depigmented. The normally smooth and shiny epidermis of the face or trunk, when involved, can become vegetative, with verrucous and keratotic elements (Pradinaud, 1991). The lesions are found in areas of the skin which are easily traumatized, namely, lower limbs, ear (unilateral) and upper limbs. There is neither localization on the scalp or nose nor involvement of the viscera (Pradinaud, 1991). It is important to distinguish between the stable, localized form of the disease (where patients have one or several confluent lesions) and the disseminated form (where there are hundreds of lesions all over the body).

The lesions of lobomycosis need to be distinguished (particularly in tropical areas) from other cutaneous infections (lepromatous leprosy, cutaneous leishmaniasis, chromoblastomycosis) and cutaneous neoplasia and true keloids. Squamous cell carcinoma was found to appear in old lobomycosis scar lesions.

Direct microscopy (Appendix B, Tables B2–4) reveals the presence of numerous hyaline, round or oval cells (9–10 μm diameter) enclosed in a double-contoured membrane; the cells are capable of budding, and are often present in giant cells or macrophages. The cytoplasm is often shrunken, and the cell wall is poorly stained. The cells are connected by isthmuses in short three-dimensional chains. The cells have to be distinguished from those of *P. brasiliensis* and *H. duboisii*. *Lacazia loboi* has never been successfully cultured.

Histological sections (Appendix B) show the epidermis to be atrophic or hyperkeratotic and vegetative; often, a clear band of collagen may be seen under a normal basal membrane (Pradinaud, 1991). The dermis reveals hypertrophic and partly hyalinized bundles of connective tissue, between which can be seen granulomatous infiltrates containing numerous yeast cells (Rodriguez and Barrera, 1997). There is typically no necrosis or suppuration, and evolution leads to fibrosis.

Antifungal drugs are not effective. The improvement sometimes seen with clofazimine is only a reflection of anti-inflammatory action. No reduction of lesion size or change in character has been seen even after 6 months' treatment with ketoconazole (Lawrence and Ajello, 1986). Repeated cryotherapy may help.

Cutaneous aspergillosis

This may be primary or secondary. Primary cutaneous aspergillosis usually involves sites of skin injury, for example, at or near intravenous access catheter sites or sites of traumatic inoculation, and at sites associated with occlusive dressings, burns or surgery. Secondary cutaneous lesions result either from contiguous spread to the skin from infected underlying structures or from widespread blood-borne seeding of the skin (van Burik *et al.*, 1998). These authors have provided an extensive review of cutaneous aspergillosis occurring in HIV-infected populations. Primary or secondary cutaneous aspergillosis may also arise in immunocompromised non-HIV-infected patients such as burn victims, neonates, individuals with cancer and transplant recipients.

Cutaneous cryptococcosis

Cryptococcus neoformans is a true yeast with a global distribution, often found in bird faeces. It can cause systemic infection with skin lesions in immunocompromised individuals. It can be recognized in a skin biopsy (Fig. 9.14) and cultured on cornmeal agar (Appendix B).

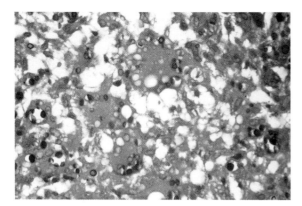

Figure 9.14:
Cryptococcus neoformans in a skin biopsy. (PAS stain) ($\times$ 400).

195

Other infections

Protothecosis

Protothecosis refers to an uncommon infection caused by species of *Prototheca*, which are considered to be achlorophylous algae. Although not fungi, these organisms have been traditionally considered in textbooks of mycology. The first case was reported in an otherwise healthy rice farmer in Sierra Leone (Davies *et al.*, 1964, cited by Emmons *et al.*, 1977); since then, nearly 80 human cases have been reported in the literature (Huerre *et al.*, 1993). Protothecosis manifests as a verrucous cutaneous or disseminated disease. Protothecosis has been reported from Europe, Asia (China, Hong Kong, Japan, Taiwan, Thailand), Oceania and the USA (particularly the southeast USA).

Prototheca is a ubiquitous inhabitant of sewage, and is found in slime flux and animal wastes contaminating different aquatic systems. The infection is believed to be transmitted to humans or animals by traumatic inoculation. *Prototheca* is also found in the digestive system of humans and animals; however, it has not been found to invade the epithelium or mucosae from this site (Huerre *et al.*, 1993). The pathogenicity and virulence of this organism is moderate, and it is considered to be a rare opportunistic pathogen. Protothecosis is caused by *Prototheca zopfi* and *P. wickerhamii* and, perhaps, other species.

Clinically, the disease manifests in three different ways: cutaneous lesions, such as papules, plaques or eczematoid, papulonodular areas of the extremities; olecranon bursitis; and disseminated protothecosis.

Immunosuppression (renal allograft recipients, patients on long-term prednisolone treatment or anticancer chemotherapy) has been observed in some affected individuals (Tsuji *et al.*, 1993; Huerre *et al.*, 1993). However, protothecosis has also been detected in an immunocompetent French individual who had visited southeast Asian countries (Pierard *et al.*, 1990) and from the cheeks of 2 otherwise healthy Japanese women (Matsumoto *et al.*, 1996).

Protothecosis must be differentiated from chromomycosis, from chronic crusted papular skin lesions of various aetiologies, and from verrucoid cutaneous lesions of the foot caused by lymphostasis. McAnally and Parry (1985) reported on a patient whose protothecosis mimicked a relapse of chromoblastomycosis following response to local excision and ketoconazole therapy for this condition.

Disease diagnosis is made by demonstration of the alga in tissue or its isolation in culture. *Prototheca* is large enough to be found easily in histologic preparations; its tendency to grow profusely in groups in the lesion makes it conspicuous, and the organism is stained by periodic acid–Schiff, Gomori's methenamine silver and the mucicarmine stain (Huerre *et al.*, 1993). Histology reveals a dermal granuloma, often with little cellular reaction, with endospores. The characteristic feature of protothecosis in tissues is the presence of specific mature sporangia of *Prototheca* species, with a morula-like pattern, with symmetrically arranged endospores (Kuo *et al.*, 1987).

Prototheca grows easily in culture on ordinary media at temperatures between 25 and 35°C.

Various modes of treatment have been tried for cutaneous protothecosis. Otoyama *et al.* (1989) reported non-responsiveness of a patient to flucytosine, which necessitated surgical resection. Combined amphotericin B and tetracycline therapy has been found useful (McAnally and Parry, 1985) and also amphotericin B alone (Tsuji *et al.*, 1993). Although oral ketoconazole was found ineffective by McAnally and Parry (1985), use of this drug has been found efficacious by other workers (Kuo *et al.*, 1987; Matsumoto *et al.*, 1996). Itraconazole has also been found useful (Pierard *et al.*,1990; Tang *et al.*, 1995). If the lesions fail to respond to therapy, death can result.

Adiaspiromycosis

This is a disease found commonly in the lungs of animals and can cause pulmonary infection in humans. Cutaneous adiaspiromycosis has been recorded caused by *Emmonsia crescens* in 2 female adults (Kamalam and Thambiah, 1979). The disease presented with cutaneous plaques over the gluteal region and neck, as whitish yellow papules over the neck, shoulder, upper arm and cubital fossa in one and as a plaque on the left knee in the other. In both, the lesions had exuded cheesy and chalky material which had shown adiaspores microscopically. *Emmonsia crescens* with classical barrel-shaped arthrospores, conidia or conidiospores were observed and on raising the incubator temperature above 37°C adiaspores were obtained in culture. On these findings and histological demonstration of spherical thick-walled adiaspores with multiple nuclei a diagnosis of adiaspiromycosis was made. Associated calcinosis cutis at the site was characteristic.

Histologically, multinucleated dermal cells with hyperchromasia and mitotic figures, which are usual in adiaspiromycosis, may be misinterpreted as sarcoma and the patient subjected to unwanted amputation. Hence, increasing awareness of this condition by clinicians and pathologists is desirable.

Pythiosis

Pythium insidiosum is a cosmopolitan aquatic organism and causes diseases in plants and animals. In certain countries, particularly Thailand, it has been found to cause a unique human infection of three types (Imwidthaya, 1994a):

- A subcutaneous lesion in thalassaemic patients, with the pathological findings of a granulomatous reaction, diffuse infiltration and oedema of the vessel walls; patients suffering from this type usually respond to saturated solution of potassium iodide.

* Chronic inflammation and occlusion of blood vessels, mainly in the lower extremities, which results in gangrene or aneurysm formation; this type is found only in thalassaemic patients. Amputation of the affected extremity or resection of the involved arteries may need to be done.
* Keratitis.

One explanation for the large number of patients reported from Thailand could be that Thailand is an agricultural country in which there are many swampy areas and plants to support the life-cycle of *Pythium*; furthermore, many Thais suffer from thalassaemia (Imwidthaya, 1994a).

Diagnosis may be established by culture. In culture mounts, the most significant diagnostic feature is the induction of biflagellate/motile asexual zoospores. This can be done by placing small pieces of *P. insidiosum* grown on agar into water and incubating at 37°C in the dark; such water cultures are examined by light microscopy after 1, 2 and 24 hours of incubation to look for encysted zoospores (after 1 hour) and numerous zoosporangia (after 24 hours). Zoospores are filamentous and, at maturity, sporangial protoplasm flows into a discharge tube and forms a hyaline, globose to subglobose vesicle (Sutton *et al.*, 1998).

Serodiagnosis of human and animal pythiosis can also be performed. Conventionally, the immunodiffusion test is used, and although this is specific for human and animal pythiosis, it has limited sensitivity and may be negative in some culture-positive patients. Recently, Mendoza *et al.* (1997) reported that the ELISA is a reliable serodiagnostic test for pythiosis since it is as specific as immunodiffusion but more sensitive.

Treatment of this condition is difficult. Oral potassium iodide (page 177) is beneficial only in the subcutaneous form of the disease, and is not of use in the vascular or ophthalmic forms, for which surgical removal of the source of infection needs to be carried out (Thianprasit *et al.*, 1996). A combination of itraconazole and terbinafine appeared curative in one patient from the USA who suffered from particularly aggressive orbital cellulitis.

Acknowledgements

I wish to thank the following for their assistance: Dr P Geraldine (my wife); Dr J Kaliamurthy (my student); Dr G Senthamilselvi, Chennai; Dr Arunaloke Chakrabarti (Chandigarh); Dr SM Singh (Jabalpur); and Dr BM Hemashettar (Belgaum).

10. Epidemiology of Skin and Wound Infection

Terminology

In order to investigate risk factors for infectious diseases, a basic understanding of epidemiological method is required. This is important in order to avoid misinterpretation when comparing the results of one study with another. Crude rates should not be used to compare populations of different structure without definition. Similarly, it is not appropriate to draw population-based conclusions from studies of limited size and power; this includes single-site case-control studies which do not provide suitable data for studies of a population. Definitions can be summarized as follows.

- *Epidemiology*: is the study of disease in relation to populations. All findings must relate to a defined population. Epidemiology relates the pattern of disease to the population in which it occurs and requires study of both diseased and healthy persons. For epidemiology, incidence and prevalence rates form the basis for comparison between defined population groups.
- *A population*: is a defined group of people including both diseased *and* healthy subjects, about whose health some statement is to be made.
- *Group orientation*: clinical appearances determine decisions about individual patients. Epidemiological observations determine decisions about groups and are the basis for preventive medicine.
- *Incidence*: is the proportion (1 in $n1000$) or percentage (%) with *new* disease of a defined group occurring within a given time period. It is annualized unless otherwise expressed, but may be stated over any time period.
- *Prevalence*: is the proportion or percentage with disease, including both *old* and *new* cases, of a defined group occurring at or over a specific time. This may take place over a day, week or month, etc.
- *Error*: statistical inference is valid only if the sample, for which each individual has defined criteria, is *random* and the control groups have no inherent bias. Important factors for variability in epidemiology include random error and biased error.
  - In *random error*, individuals are apt to be misassessed or misclassified – this is serious in clinical practice but is not so serious in epidemiology, which is concerned with group decisions.

- In *biased error*, the wrong groups are selected, usually the controls, which then distorts comparisons – an epidemiological disaster which cannot be corrected by statistics! Using hospital-based instead of community-based controls, for patients admitted from the community to the hospital, often causes bias and should be avoided.
- *Morbidity (sickness rate)*: is the number of persons suffering from a given disease in relation to the total population (expressed per 100 000 persons) and/or age group and/or sex during a specified time interval.
- *Mortality (death rate)*: is the number of persons dying from a given disease in relation to the investigated population.
- *Case–fatality rate*: is the ratio of deaths from a given disease to existing cases of that disease (usually given in %).
- *Manifestation ('showing the disease') index*: is the number of persons presenting with the clinical disease in relation to the number of persons infected with the causative agent.
- *Endemic*: signifies the continued presence of an infectious disease in an area (such as leprosy in Southeast Asia and South America).
- *Epidemic*: is the increased occurrence of an infectious disease limited in locality and time.
- *Pandemic*: is the worldwide occurrence of an infectious disease limited in time but not in locality.

In epidemiology, computed information is usually used. This can have errors from:

- *Imprecision* – information correctly entered into the computer but data are wrong.
- *Unreliability* – correct data entered into the computer incorrectly.

Disease outcome has to be assessed accurately. Clinical experience alone cannot predict prognosis and outcome. There will be biased case selection and incomplete follow-up.

Epidemiological methods can be represented as follows:

1. Descriptive studies
   (a) Populations (comparison studies)
   (b) Individuals
       (i) Case reports
       (ii) Case series
       (iii) Cross-sectional (or prevalence) surveys.

2. Analytical studies
   (a) Observational studies

    (i)   Non-interventionist – audit studies of existing practice
    (ii) Case-control studies – retrospective or prospective
    (iii) Cohort (or longitudinal) studies - retrospective or prospective.
  (b) Interventional studies
    (i)   Clinical trials.

Examples

Descriptive studies

Populations

Comparison can be made of infectious disease outcome between different groups within a population. Kalter (1986) demonstrated in Houston, Texas, that *Trichosporon beigelii* infection of genital hairs (the cause of white piedra) was more common amongst black patients (54% culture positive) than white patients ($P < 0.001$), with a 6.4 times greater risk by odds ratio analysis. The study also showed that the infection was common, endemic and, for the first time, occurred in females. Confounding factors and bias must be considered, however. Comparisons drawn provide preliminary data only, which require confirmation in analytical studies.

Individuals

Case reports are of value for identifying new, unusual or rare cases such as *Vibrio vulnificus* gangrenous infection of the foot (Yip *et al.*, 1996) or clostridial necrotizing fasciitis as opposed to myositis (Schreider and Chatoo, 1997), but are of little relevance in epidemiology, which relates to the study of populations.

Case series. A number of cases of infection are recorded, for example, of *new* cases of cutaneous infection in meat workers (Shanahan, 1997) in a particular place over a time period, which may suggest a variety of different causes. In the above example, conducted in an abbatoir in Adelaide, Australia, cutaneous infection was considered common at 0.65 per 1000 working days; the workers handling animal hides had the highest infection rates compared to other workers. It can be a useful start to the study of a particular problem. This type of descriptive study may record incidence (if new cases are involved) or prevalence (if new and old cases are included) in the population but the assessment of risk factors is open to bias within the population studied. This type of study can provide a useful basis on which to plan an analytical study.

    Another example is a retrospective review (descriptive study) of a defined condition presenting to a referral hospital. Sellers *et al.* (1996) reviewed their experience in the management of patients with necrotizing fasciitis from 1991 to 1995. They had 8 patients of whom 6 developed streptococcal toxic shock with 2 deaths. This led to their conclusion that aggressive diagnosis and surgical treatment was still very important to manage their cases.

Cross-sectional (or prevalence) surveys measure the prevalence of health outcomes in a population at a point in time or over a short period. This has been pursued in particular for leprosy on the basis of trying to find *M. leprae* in nasal swabs and by serological testing (van Beers *et al.*, 1994) as opposed to relying on clinical diagnosis of disease. The cross-sectional or prevalence study considers *existing* disease in a descriptive format, as contrasted with the *development* of new disease in an analytical study. Care is required in detecting known existing cases of disease, since they may not be representative of all cases of the disease. In the above example (van Beers *et al.*, 1994), the rate of finding clinical cases of leprosy was 1% (the prevalence) but *M. leprae* was found in 7.8% of the population by polymerase chain reaction testing of nasal swabs and 31% by serological-based diagnosis. This gave a manifestation index of 3–12.5%, depending on the test used. Furthermore, cases of chronic disease of long duration, such as leprosy, are overrepresented in a cross-sectional study. A cross-sectional (or prevalence) study may be used as a pilot study to a cohort study by defining the population at risk, but it does not replace the cohort study, which is usually structured to measure the incidence and risk factors of *new* cases of the disease under study.

Prevalence studies have been used to assess skin diseases in various climates and countries, including Mali (Mahe *et al.*, 1995). In order to estimate the importance of skin diseases as a public health problem, Mahe *et al.* investigated the prevalence and severity of skin diseases in a representative sample of children in Mali: 1817 children were randomly selected in 30 clusters by probability-proportional-to-size sampling in Koulikoro region. The mean prevalence ($\pm$ 2 standard deviation) of skin diseases was $34 \pm 4\%$. The most frequent dermatoses were pyoderma ($12.3 \pm 1.6\%$), tinea capitis ($9.5 \pm 2.5\%$), pediculosis capitis ($4.7 \pm 1.4\%$), scabies ($4.3 \pm 1.5\%$), and molluscum contagiosum ($3.6 \pm 1\%$). The most troublesome dermatoses were scabies and severe pyoderma. Pyoderma was the only dermatosis associated with poor individual or household hygiene. Public health services were little used by the population for skin diseases, partly because of the high cost of treatment. The high prevalence and severity of many lesions make pyoderma and scabies a significant public health problem in Mali (Mahe *et al.*, 1995).

Analytical studies

Observational studies

The non-interventionist type of study is often carried out for audit purposes and involves observing current practice to assess whether, and by how much, it is beneficial for the patient. The observations are then assessed to decide if the particular practice could be improved as better medicine and whether the same treatment could be performed in a way that would represent better value for money. Such studies are carried out as part of hospital practice and are not usually published as scientific papers. Large non-interventionist studies can, however, be conducted to record specific types of infection and their associated characteristics. This can be performed on a prospective basis, as in the case of Paraskaki *et al*. (1996), who investigated the number of times (218) *Ps. aeruginosa* was isolated from 6859 clinical samples and where the isolates came from (chronic otitis media 75%, appendicitis 10%, osteomyelitis 9%, skin or hypodermis 6%). This type of study can also be conducted on a retrospective basis, as in the case of Aebi *et al*. (1996), who investigated retrospectively bacterial complications of varicella infection in 84 patients younger than 16 years of age who required hospitalization between 1985 and 1995. The purpose of the study was to describe demographics, clinical manifestations, bacteriology and outcome. Secondary bacterial skin infections occurred in 61 patients (73%), and deep-seated infection and/or shock in 23 (27%). The latter complications were significantly associated with thrombocytopenia ($P = 0.01$) and bacteraemia ($P = 0.02$) at the time of admission, prolonged fever ($P = 0.001$), prolonged hospitalization ($P < 0.0001$), intensive care management ($P < 0.0001$), and fatal outcome ($P = 0.02$). *S. pyogenes* represented 59% of bacterial isolates and *S. aureus* 28%, illustrating their role in secondary infection of chickenpox (VZV) lesions. These data are biased, however, because only patients sufficiently ill to be admitted to hospital were selected – no conclusions can be drawn from this study on the frequency of such secondary bacterial infection with VZV in the community.

The case-control study compares those with and without the disease who are suitably matched. The study should include only incident cases of disease, that is *new* cases of infection that develop during the study and not chronic cases of long duration from before the study started. Diagnostic criteria must be well defined and, for cases of infection, *should* be culture-positive or involve microbial antigen recognition. Patients who develop a disease are compared with controls who have not developed the disease. This permits estimation of odds ratio statistics but not of the population attributable risk (Friedman, 1994). In addition, allowance must be made for potential confounding factors. The most important point to note is that the controls *must* match the patients. If patients enter the hospital from a countrywide community, for example the UK, then the controls must be selected likewise or there will be bias from the local population selected, as in the case of hospital-based controls. Controls are best matched to each patient for age, sex, location of residence and educational status.

An example of a population-based case-control study is that of van den Eeden *et al*. (1998), who compared men aged 18 or over, who were seen for genital condyloma, with controls matched for clinic site, age and race. Interviews were conducted with patients and controls to ascertain their exposure histories. Recurrent condylomata were reported by about one-third of their patients. Men with multiple partners were strongly associated with development of the disease. Other behavioural activities, such as recreational drug use, were also related to the occurrence of recurrent condyloma.

A case-control study can be used to compare different types of infection. It is effective for investigating risk factors within a defined group, but does *not* identify the frequency of the infection in the population, that is, neither the number of new cases (incidence) nor the proportion present at any time (prevalence) is measured. This is because of confounding factors that not only characterize or influence the method of referral of the patients to hospital but also include possible bias in the way that the controls are selected. This is especially important when a tertiary referral hospital is involved. It is dangerous to extrapolate the findings of a case-control study into the population at large – the results only apply to the precise population studied and other inferences can be unreliable.

The cohort or longitudinal study examines associations between exposure to suspected causes of disease and morbidity (the actual disease). The simplest type of longitudinal study is the cohort study, when those subjects exposed to one or a number of risk factors related to the development of the disease and those not exposed are followed up prospectively in a defined, community-based population over a period of time. Incidence of disease is measured in each group in the community together with the relative risk of the different exposures and the population-attributable risk. Cohort studies are time-consuming and costly and are therefore reserved for testing precisely formulated hypotheses, which have been previously explored by cross-sectional, case-control or other studies.

The duration of the study depends on the number of new cases of disease and on the induction period between risk and the occurrence of the disease; sufficiently large numbers are needed to gain statistical significance, with usually a minimum of 50 new cases. Retrospective cohort studies may be possible if the necessary data have already been collected from the population.

Kaul *et al*. (1997) performed a prospective cohort study in Ontario, Canada with surveillance for *S. pyogenes* necrotizing fasciitis. They wished to measure the incidence of the disease and to assess its risk factors. They collected data from all cases of necrotizing fasciitis from November 1991 to May 1995 in Ontario, for which purpose they used a combination of clinical, bacteriological and histopathologic criteria. With this properly conducted cohort study, they found an incidence of necrotizing fasciitis in 1994/95 of 0.4 per 100 000 population. This is interesting and much higher than other, less well conducted studies depending on reports of bacteriologically proven cases (Chapter 5, Incidence of necrotizing fasciitis, p.106). Their results demonstrate the need for population-based cohort studies instead of descriptive figures from reference laboratories or tertiary referral facilities. Risk factors identified included old age, while for mortality, the presence of toxic shock syndrome (Chapter 4), hypotension and septicaemia were more important; mortality did not relate to S. *pyogenes* M type or, surprisingly, the presence of exotoxins.

Intervention studies

Clinical trials. Randomized, placebo-controlled, double-blind (neither investigator nor patient knows whether drug or placebo is being used), cross-over (or partial cross-over) trials are required to establish the effectiveness of new antibiotics or their formulations on infectious disease. These types of trials are especially important for investigating chronic disease such as the blepharitis of rosacea (Seal *et al.*, 1995). The importance of study design is reflected in this example (Seal *et al.*, 1995), when the beneficial effect of topical fusidic acid (Fucithalmic) was demonstrated for patients suffering with rosacea and blepharitis but not for those with blepharitis alone. This result had not been anticipated at the start of the intervention study, which thus identified a subpopulation of those with blepharitis (those with adjunctive rosacea) that benefited from the treatment. This benefit was probably due to the cyclosporin-type effect of fusidic acid reducing inflammation in rosacea blepharitis secondary to cell-mediated immunity to colonization of lid margins with S. *aureus*.

Other uses of epidemiological methods

Epidemiology can also be used to investigate other aspects of therapy for different purposes. For instance, epidemiological methods have been applied to the investigation of the costs attributable to failed treatments as a measure of inefficient health care. In a study in rural Mexico, Hay *et al.* (1994a) showed that the cost of failing to treat scabies within families was approximately US$34 per family per 3 months, a large proportion of the family's disposable income.

Assessment of statistical associations

When a significant result is gained, there should always be consideration of:

- *has the result been due to bias?* Is there bias in patient selection or in patient referral to the hospital? Is there bias in the selection of the controls? Have the wrong controls been selected? Have hospital controls been used for community patients?
- *could the result be due to chance?* Always calculate the confidence intervals and consider the degree of statistical significance. Statistics define the degree of chance but do not abolish it altogether.
- *are there unsuspected confounding factors at play?* This may involve unsuspected secondary microbial contamination. Always consider where and why patients become infected. Is the organism or the host at fault?
- *does the significant association calculated represent a real effect for a risk factor or a confounding one?* A confounding risk factor may be associated with the infection but is not the primary cause of it. Have the correct statistical methods been used? Should the results have been stratified before analysis? Is there a better statistical model by which to analyse the results of the study? Are the results suitable for analysis by multivariate or logistical regression analysis?

11. PREVENTION OF HOSPITAL-ACQUIRED SKIN AND WOUND INFECTION

Cross-infection may occur in the out-patient clinic, the ward and the operating theatre.

The out-patient clinic or surgery

Patients receiving treatment within a medical environment are at risk of contracting an infection from another patient or from a health care worker. Such an unexpected outcome can arise from contact with the practitioner's hands or from equipment used to examine the patient. The courteous act of shaking hands with a patient is sufficient to transfer organisms, so that hand-washing, preferably with an antiseptic soap, between examining patients is considered important.

The following disinfection regime is suggested to reduce the chances of hospital-acquired infection (HAI).

- Hand-washing – perform after handling the skin or wound of any infected patient, using an antiseptic-impregnated liquid soap preparation from an elbow- or floor-operated container. Such hand-wash preparations include 10% povidone-iodine (Betadine scrub), which is bactericidal and virucidal, or 4% chlorhexidine (Hibiscrub), which is only bactericidal. For patients suspected of presenting with acute HIV or hepatitis infection, disposable gloves should be worn with hand-washing using povidone-iodine (refer to hand-washing section at end of chapter). Disposable gloves can also be worn at other times and there should be a plentiful supply available at all times.
- Sterilizers – it is better for clinics to use a Central Sterile Supply Service Department (CSSD) than to have each clinic carrying out its own sterilization procedures, but this is not always possible. The clinic should avoid all use of disinfectant 'soaking' solutions if possible. Autoclaving is required for sterilizing equipment, for which purpose small units are produced for clinics. Equipment that cannot be autoclaved can be sterilized by ethylene oxide or,

if suitable, by gas plasma sterilization with ionized oxygen. There is still a place for gluteraldehyde, peracetic acid and others such as chlorine dioxide.

The hospital ward

Dermatology patients can be colonized with *S. aureus* due to their underlying medical condition such as severe eczema or rosacea. They may be profuse 'shedders' and are therefore a risk to other patients, such as those with open wounds or those who are immunocompromised in some way. If these patients have made frequent trips to the hospital or a neighbouring one, they may also have acquired colonization with MRSA (methicillin-resistant *S. aureus*) or staphylococci with other transferable resistance mechanisms (Zafar *et al.*, 1995; Brun-Buisson 1998). These patients should be subjected to surveillance cultures and, if colonized with multiply resistant staphylococci, care taken with their management in hospital to avoid serious cross-infection to others. Unfortunately, this ideal type of situation can only be achieved with use of an isolation facility equipped with air-locked single rooms and a nursing staff separate from that of the general hospital. Sharing of wards should not take place between dermatology and surgical patients but may occur with medical patients.

Most hospital wards allow airborne spread of *S. aureus* between patients, staff and their immediate environment. This has been shown recently for the acquisition of TSST-1- producing *S. aureus*, when 32% of such isolates were cultured from children with burns *after* their admission to hospital (Chapter 7). There are numerous other incidents described in the medical literature. Much work has been performed in the past to reduce this airborne spread to a minimum, involving types of blankets (woollen blankets harbour staphylococci) and types of floor cleaning that disperse skin scales containing staphylococci into the immediate environment (wet mop cleaning is required). Ward design with cubicles may help achieve privacy for the patient but does not unfortunately prevent staphylococci riding in and out of cubicles on air currents every time doors are opened and closed. An additional problem is the survival of *S. aureus*, including MRSA, for prolonged periods of weeks or months in dust (shed skin scales) on all horizontal surfaces in wards such as tops of fluorescent lights, cubicle walls and cupboards. The old adage that 'cleanliness is next to godliness' is indeed true for the hospital ward setting, as frequent damp dusting will remove dirt and with it most of the environmental sources of staphylococci.

Staff or patient carriers of MRSA should be offered antistaphylococcal soap such as Hibiscrub (chlorhexidine 4%) for showering and shampooing hair, and suppression of nasal carriage of staphylococci with mupirocin nasal ointment (Appendix A).

Streptococcus pyogenes can also be spread within the ward setting, causing considerable morbidity to patients. An example is given in Fig. 11.1, which shows how *S. pyogenes* spread throughout the patients in a geriatric ward causing

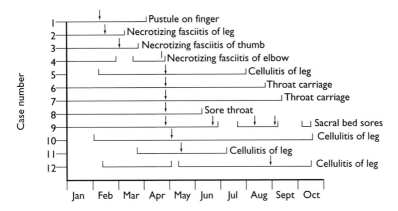

Figure 11.1: Hospital ward outbreak of skin sepsis due to *S. pyogenes.*

a variety of symptoms from sore throats in the staff to necrotizing fasciitis in two patients (geriatric patients are very susceptible), to cellulitis and coloniza-tion of bedsores. This is a particular problem for the dermatology and geriatric wards and involves spread of beta-haemolytic streptococci via air currents, handling of infected patients and fomites. Indeed, such infected patients may require isolation in single room cubicles on an infectious diseases ward until colonization with a virulent organism such as *S. pyogenes* has been eliminated. Use of air-beds with 'fluidized' beads, such as the 'Clinitron' bed, for immobile patients with open colonized wounds is controversial and may result in further airborne spread of streptococci within the ward.

Occlusive bandages lead to increased growth of bacteria and yeasts on the skin surface underneath them. Their use has been followed by serious hospital-acquired infection (HAI) with *Candida albicans* in a neonatal unit (Marples *et al.*, 1985). Occlusive dressings should not be used in situations predisposing to cross-infection but should be replaced with porous materials instead.

Topical medications must *never* be shared between patients. Each patient must be provided with their own preparation of drugs or be given topical drug therapy by single-use sachets. This stringency is necessary to avoid the risk of cross-infec-tion from one patient to another. This situation is best exemplified on the derma-tology ward when a patient is admitted with unrecognized Norwegian scabies and is managed with a common jar of skin emollient for dry scaling skin; such action will transfer the scabies mite to all the patients and staff! There is also the need to avoid transfer of highly infectious viruses such as hepatitis B and HIV in body secretions, since the patient with denuded or damaged epithelium is at risk of rapid virus absorption.

The operating theatre

Dust on theatre shelves and other horizontal surfaces consists predominantly of shed skin scales, which harbour staphylococci, from staff and patients. Hence, a standard of excellence for the theatre demands good cleanliness and that a minimum of dirt be brought into the theatre on shoes, trolley wheels or equipment (such dirt also harbours clostridial spores). If ward trolleys enter the theatre, their wheels must be disinfected but ideally a bed/trolley transfer system should be used.

In addition, all modern operating theatres should be serviced by dirty corridors, for removal of used equipment for sterilization. They should be supplied with the services of a central TSSU – theatre sterile supply unit – that is maintained by staff experienced in sterilization techniques who clean, disinfect and sterilize equipment for the next operation. This should no longer be performed on site at the back of the theatre by the nurses and orderlies but often occurs in practice due to shortage of equipment.

All staff undertaking surgery should change into operating theatre clothing in designated areas and must *not* leave the clean theatre area wearing operating clothing and shoes. If they leave the theatre area, they must discard theatre clothing for outside clothing and *change into new theatre clothing on return* – hence the need to provide food for meal breaks within the theatre common room. All staff should wear hats, and masks fully covering nose, mouth and chin, to reduce staphylococcal shedding and aerosolized mouth droplets as much as possible. Showers should not be taken before surgery because this increases staphylococcal shedding. Beards should *not* be worn by surgeons when performing surgery, as they are considered a major risk factor for staphylococcal shedding into the surgical wound.

All operating staff should perform intensive hand-washing with a surgical disinfectant hand scrub such as Betadine (10% povidone-iodine) or Hibiscrub (4% chlorhexidine); both these solutions contain detergent, to which some staff can become allergic. An alternative regime is use of a hypoallergenic soap, from a dispenser, followed by an alcoholic hand rub.

Before surgery commences, the operating theatre doors should be shut, and kept shut, and there should be a minimum movement of staff. This will assist the function of the artificial ventilation system to produce adequate air changes within the operating theatre and to produce air flow over the operating site to remove shed skin scales – this will not happen if the theatre doors are left open!

Theatre air flow engineering to prevent HAI

While the majority of postoperative infection occurs from the patient's own microbial flora, the minority (approximately 5%) is probably acquired from the theatre staff. This can be reduced, but not abolished, by operating on the patient in the presence of adequate air flow to carry airborne skin squames containing staphylococci, or aerosolized droplets containing beta-haemolytic streptococci (if the surgeons or scrub nurse have a sore throat), away from the surgical wound towards the periphery of the theatre and through vents or gaps in the theatre doors towards the theatre corridors. To achieve this aim, the operating theatre needs to be kept at a positive pressure greater than 10 pascals compared to its neighbouring rooms and corridors, which can be easily monitored.

The air flow distribution within the theatre should be arranged so that the filtered air on entry progresses across the operating field before leaving the theatre. Unfortunately, this primary aim of theatre air flow is often not achieved in practice! Problems abound but mainly consist of placing air flow entry ports in the wrong site so that most of the air flow crosses the ceiling, missing the surgical wound altogether, and hits the walls opposite instead, drops down to floor level to collect staphylococci shed by staff and then circulates up towards the surgical wound area as 'dirty' air. A modern theatre should maintain a minimum of 20 air changes per hour, but this is often breached by staff leaving doors open and continually walking in and out – this must not be allowed! Air flow can be easily monitored, and should be on a routine basis, using smoke tests. For more sophisticated analysis, the electronic particle counter has been found particularly useful (Seal and Clark, 1990). Ultra-clean air systems have been perfected in the UK for orthopaedic surgery in particular.

Theatre-acquired HAI

When infection involves *S. aureus*, advice of professional microbiologists should be sought, as it may indicate that a staff member is carrying the organism. The unit may need to be temporarily closed to surgery and staff investigated to identify the carrier. With staphylococcal or streptococcal infection, staff with sore throats or exacerbations of eczema or other dermatoses are usually involved. Theatre staff with skin disease such as atopic dermatitis or psoriasis may be heavily colonized with *S. aureus*.

When the organisms causing wound infection are different, there should be a review of the surgical techniques used and a consideration of ways to reduce the chances of infection. Past pseudo-outbreaks have occurred in summer when operating theatre fans have broken, or conditions have been excessively hot, which considerably increases staphylococcal shedding by staff and its deposition into the wound. When these problems have been corrected, the outbreaks usually stop.

Management of the atopic individual

The atopic individual has a symbiotic relationship with *S. aureus*, which colonizes the skin extensively (Tuft *et al.*, 1992; Noble, 1997) (Chapter 3). *S. aureus* also

211

colonizes, and may infect, eczematous skin. Care is therefore needed when planning surgery if the patient is atopic. Whole body bathing, including shampooing hair, with 4% chlorhexidine impregnated liquid hand scrub (Hibiscrub) is recommended for 72 hours prior to surgery. If the patient is allergic to this preparation then an alternative can be used such as povidone iodine. Postoperative prophylaxis should be considered with oral fusidic acid 750 mg three times a day (enteric-coated tablets) or trimethoprim 200 mg twice daily for 5 days.

Classification of surgical wounds for audit of HAI

Hospitals should keep records of their wound infection rates. Surgical wounds have been classified into four risk categories (1–4):

1. Class 1 'clean' wounds are performed on non-contaminated skin and expected to have < 1% postoperative sepsis. Procedures include clean surgery such as cosmetic surgery, removal of non-inflamed cysts or biopsies.
2. Class 2 'clean-contaminated' wounds occur with operations on contaminated areas such as the mouth, respiratory tract or perineum. The wound infection rate should be < 5% for uncomplicated cases.
3. Class 3 'contaminated' wounds include major accident trauma. The infection rate may reach 20–30% but can be reduced to 10% with judicious use of prophylactic intravenous antibiotics at the time of surgery.
4. Class 4 'dirty' wounds are those which are grossly contaminated such as emergency operations on the unprepared gastrointestinal tract. The serious wound infection rate reached 50% before the use of short-course high-dose intravenous antibiotic regimens for aerobic and anaerobic bacteria such as ceftazidime (or cefuroxime) and metronidazole. This type of regime has reduced the postoperative wound infection rate to 10%, so that it is not ethical to operate without them.

Hand-washing

The skin flora of hands contains a permanent and transient microbial flora, the latter being amenable to reduction by hand-washing, depending on the technique used. There are, however, notable instances, particularly with multiply resistant *Klebsiella* spp., when an expected reduction in the microbial flora fails to occur. Frequent use of thin disposable gloves should be made, since they represent an impermeable barrier between the skin flora and the surface to be handled.

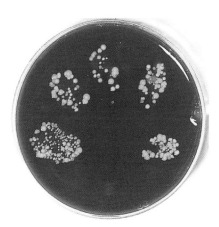

Figure 11.2: Finger imprints on blood agar of unwashed hands, showing multiple colonies of bacteria isolated from each finger.

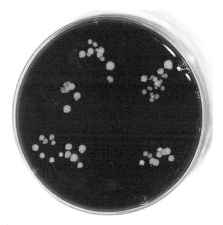

Figure 11.3: Finger imprints on blood agar of hands washed with liquid soap, showing some reduction in the numbers of bacteria isolated.

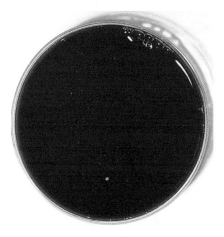

Figure 11.4: Finger imprints on blood agar of hands washed with liquid soap followed by an alcoholic hand rub – only one bacterial colony-forming unit was isolated.

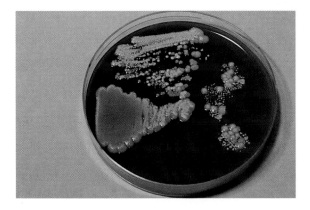

Figure 11.5: Finger imprints on blood agar (right half of plate) after handling a contaminated solution (left half of plate).

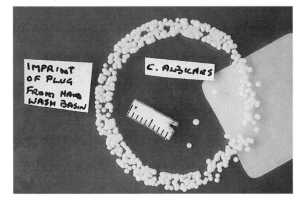

Figure 11.6: Laboratory agar culture of a washbasin plug contaminated with *Candida albicans* in a neonatal unit with nosocomial candidiasis.

Figure 11.2 illustrates the numbers of bacteria that can be cultured on blood agar as an impression plate from unwashed fingers. If hands are washed with liquid soap, then there is some reduction in numbers of bacteria removed from the skin (Fig. 11.3). The best technique involves washing with liquid soap followed by an alcoholic hand rub – only one bacterial colony-forming unit was isolated on the impression agar plate (Fig. 11.4). This latter technique is thus the favoured method but can cause the skin to become dry. This is compensated for by the industry adding an emollient to the product, although this can result in the hands becoming sticky.

The acquisition of transient flora by fingers is well illustrated by Fig. 11.5. This impression plate photograph shows the bacterial growth on fingers acquired from handling a contaminated solution. This situation is occurring on the hospital wards all the time when staff handle patients, particularly their contaminated excreta such as infected urinary drainage bags. Hands can also become colonized by organisms contaminating hospital wash basins or their associated equipment such as bar soap, soap dishes or washbasin plugs (Fig. 11.6).

214

Appendix A
MODES OF DELIVERY, AND FORMULATIONS, OF ANTIBIOTICS AND ANTIFUNGAL DRUGS

Some modes of delivery discussed here are outside the specifications of the product licence for the agent and are therefore used at the clinician's responsibility.

Topical preparations

Creams and ointments are the standard means of administering antibiotics to the surface of the skin either for prophylaxis or treatment (Tables A.1 and A.2). Ointments prolong contact time and therefore permit less frequent application and are less likely to be washed away. They also provide a barrier to water loss and may be more acceptable for those with dry skin lesions, although less cosmetically acceptable.

Systemic preparations

For full details of systemic antibacterial therapy with oral, intravenous or intramuscular antibiotics, the reader is referred to O'Grady *et al.* (1997). Metronidazole has been found effective for treatment of rosacea, for which purpose there is a topical preparation. In rosacea-associated blepharitis, topical fusidic acid will be effective in 90% of patients and oral tetracycline 250 mg twice daily or doxycycline 100 mg once daily in 50% (Seal *et al.*, 1995).

Table A.1 Topical antibacterial antibiotics.

Antibacterial antibiotic	Trade name	Commercial preparation
Creams		
Neomycin sulphate	Neomycin cream BPC	0.5%
Silver sulfadiazine	Flamazine	1%
Fusidic acid	Fucidin	2%
Gentamicin sulphate	Cidomycin Topical	0.3%
Metronidazole	Novitate	1%
Ointments		
Mupirocin	Bactroban	2%
Chlortetracycline	Aureomycin	3%
Fusidic acid	Fucidin	2%
Gentamicin	Cidomycin Topical	0.3%
Tetracycline hydrochloride	Achromycin Topical	3%
Gels		
Fusidic acid	Fucidin	2%
Metronidazole	Metrogel	0.75%
	Rozex	0.75%

Table A.2 Antibacterial combinations.

Antibacterial antibiotics	Trade name	Commercial preparation
Creams		
Neomycin sulphate + bacitracin zinc	Cicatrin	3300 U + 250 U/g
Ointments		
Framycetin sulphate + gramicidin	Soframycin	1.5% + 0.005%
Polymyxin B sulphate + bacitracin zinc	Polyfax	10 000 U + 500 U/g

Table A.3 Topical antiseptic preparations.

Antiseptic compounds	Trade name	Commercial preparation	Hospital preparation
Cetrimide	Cetrimide Cream BP	–	0.5%
Chlorhexidine + cetrimide	Savlodil/Tisept Savlon	Solution/Cream (0.1% + 0.5%)	–
Proflavine	Proflavine Cream BPC	–	0.1%
Povidone-iodine	Betadine	10%	–
Hydrogen peroxide	Crystacide	1%	–
Hexachlorophane	Dermalex	0.5%	–
Silver sulphadiazine	Flamazine	1%	–
Magnesium sulphate	Magnesium sulphate paste BP	45%	45%
Sugar paste with hydrogen peroxide	Sugar paste NPH	–	Thick and thin

Table A.4 Topical antiviral compounds.

Antiviral substance	Trade name	Commercial preparation	Indication
Skin creams			
Aciclovir	Zovirax	5%	Herpes infections
	Avert	5%	Herpes infections
Penciclovir	Vectavir	1%	Herpes infections

Table A.5 Topical parasiticidal compounds.

Parasiticidal compounds	Trade name	Commercial preparation
Creams and lotions		
Carbaryl	Carylderm	0.5% (alcoholic base)
	Clinicide	0.5% (alcoholic base)
	Derbac C	1% (aqueous base)
Malathion	Prioderm	0.5% (alcoholic base)
	Suleo-M	0.5% (alcoholic base)
	Derbac-M	0.5% (aqueous base)
	Quellada M	0.5% (aqueous base)
Permethrin	Lyclear	1% (alcoholic base)
		5% (cream base)
Phenothrin	Full Marks	0.2% (alcoholic base)
		0.5% (aqueous base)

Table A.6 Topical antifungal antibiotics.

Antifungal compounds	Drug type	Commercial preparation	Indications
Creams			
Amorolfine (Loceryl)	Morpholine	0.25%	Dermatophytoses
Clotrimazole (Canesten, Masnoderm)	Imidazole	1%	Dermatophytoses; candidosis
Econazole nitrate (Ecostatin, Pevaryl)	Imidazole	1%	Dermatophytoses; candidosis
Ketoconazole (Nizoral)	Imidazole	2%	Dermatophytoses; candidosis
Miconazole nitrate (Daktarin)	Imidazole	2%	Dermatophytoses; candidosis
Sulconazole (Exelderm)	Imidazole	1%	Dermatophytoses; candidosis
Nystatin (Nystan)	Polyene	100 000 U/g	Candidosis
Terbinafine (Lamisil)	Allylamine	1%	Dermatophytoses; candidosis
Naftitine	Allylamine	1%	Dermatophytoses
Solutions for nail infections			
Tioconazole (Trosyl)	Imidazole	28%	Onychomycosis
Amorolfine lacquer	Morpholine	5%	Onychomycosis
Combinations			
Nystatin + tolnaftate (Tinaderm-M)	Polyene + tolnaftate	100 000 U/g + 1%	Dermatophytoses with secondary candidosis
Nystatin + chlor-hexidine (Nystaform)	Polyene + bisbiguanide	100 000 U/g + 1%	Candidosis with secondary bacterial infection

218

Table A.7 Principal antifungal drugs used for therapy

Drug and route of administration	Advantages	Disadvantages
A. Nystatin i. Macrocyclic polyene. ii. Variably fungistatic and fungicidal (depending on concentration). iii. Available as oral tablets (200 000 U, 500 000 U), suspension (100 000 U/ml) and ointment (100 000 U/g). iv. Primarily used to treat cutaneous, mucosal and oral candidosis.	a. Good in vitro activity against *Candida*, *Cryptococcus*, some dermatophytes (*Trichophyton*, *Microsporum*), *Histoplasma*, *Blastomyces* and *Penicillium*. b. Generally non-toxic. c. Not absorbed orally.	1. Poor in vitro activity against certain key fungal pathogens causing skin and wound infection. 2. Not effective in *Candida* onychomycosis. 3. No antibacterial activity. 4. Too toxic for systemic use. 5. Stains yellow.
B. Amphotericin B i. Macrocyclic polyene. ii. Variably fungistatic or fungicidal. iii. Available in oral, topical and parenteral forms. iv. Intravenous amphotericin is the drug of choice when cutaneous lesions are due to deep mycotic infections by *Aspergillus*, *Blastomyces* and other dimorphic fungi. Dose *Adults*: start with 0.1 mg/kg body weight per day and increase gradually to 1.0 mg/kg body weight per day. *Children*: 0.1 mg/kg body weight per day increasing to 0.3 mg/kg body weight per day. Liposomal amphotericin B can be administered at 3 mg/kg body weight per day or higher by titration with toxicity.	a. Broad spectrum of action against *Aspergillus* spp., *Blastomyces dermatitidis*, *Candida* spp., *Coccidioides immitis*, *Cryptococcus neoformans*, *Histoplasma capsulatum*, *Paracoccidioides brasiliensis*. Most of the usual pathogenic fungi (especially yeasts) are susceptible to MICs of 0.1–1.0 μg/ml, while certain filamentous fungi are susceptible to 1–5 μg/ml. b. Emergence of resistant mutants is rare. c. Liposomal amphotericin B can be given to patients who are unable to tolerate or who have failed to respond to conventional amphotericin. d. Effective in certain forms of hyalohyphomycosis and phaeohyphomycosis.	1. Fungi such as *Scedosporium* sp. and *Trichosporon* spp. are frequently resistant in vitro. 2. Often find only marginal clinical improvement in fungal mycetomas, chromoblastomycoses, entomophthoramycoses, the dermatophytoses. 3. Conventional intravenous therapy is very toxic when deoxycholate is used as the vehicle. Liposomal amphotericin B is much better tolerated. 4. The most serious toxic effect of intravenous amphotericin is renal tubular damage. Renal function must be monitored, especially for low serum potassium levels.

Table A.7 *continued*

Drug and route of administration	Advantages	Disadvantages
C. Flucytosine (5-fluorocytosine) i. A synthetic fluorinated pyrimidine. ii. Available as oral tablets and as an intravenous infusion. iii. Oral dose is 50–150 mg/kg per day in four divided doses. iv. Principally used to treat *Candida* infections and may be used to treat chromoblastomycosis.	a. Active against *Candida*, *Cryptococcus neoformans*, *Cladosporium carrionii*, *Fonsecaea*. b. Most useful as adjunctive therapy (topical) for *Candida* infection. c. Effective against some strains of *Aspergillus* and *Torula*.	1. Cannot be administered alone in treating serious *Candida* or *Cryptococcus* sepsis due to rapid emergence of resistance. 2. Limited spectrum of activity against filamentous fungi. 3. Best avoided in AIDS patients since many of these develop significant bone marrow suppression.
D. Itraconazole i. Synthetic dioxolane triazole ii. Oral capsule – dose 200–400 mg/day (200 mg once daily for superficial skin infections and pityriasis versicolor, 400 mg daily for dermatophytoses, 400 mg daily for 2–3 weeks for onychomycosis). Oral solution for oral candidosis at 200 mg daily. IV formulation for systemic mycosis at 200–400 mg daily. iii. Used for treatment of chronic dermatophytoses. iv. An effective alternative treatment to ketoconazole for (lympho)cutaneous sporotrichosis (100 mg only daily for 3–6 months).	a. Broad spectrum of activity against *Candida* (including mucocutaneous infection), *M. furfur*, all *Aspergillus* species, dermatophytes, most dimorphic fungi, and fungi that cause chromoblastomycosis. b. Well absorbed after oral administration. High tissue levels are found in skin and liver with a half-life of 15–24 hours. c. Excellent safety profile when given orally. d. IV formulation useful for treating AIDS patients and others with mucositis. e. There are no known differences in the efficacy of fluconazole and itraconazole in candidosis. f. There are strains of *C. albicans* that are resistant to fluconazole but sensitive to itraconazole. g. No interactions with oral diabetic drugs.	1. Ineffective against some Zygomycetes, *Fusarium* spp. 2. Care needed in patients with previous liver disease. 3. Absorption affected by antacids and H_2 receptor antagonists. 4. Fluconazole may give better treatment results for *Cryptococcus* infections. 5. May interact with cyclosporin, rifampicin, terfinadine, cisapride, astemizole, simvastatin, lovastatin, atorvastatin, oral triazolam and midazolam which are contra-indicated.

Table A.7 *continued*

Drug and route of administration	Advantages	Disadvantages
E. Fluconazole i. Synthetic bistriazole. ii. Oral (50–200 mg/day). Often used in weekly pulses of 150–300 mg. iii. Intravenous preparation at 2 mg/ml (give 100 mg/day). iv. Active in dermatophytosis. Very effective in mucocutaneous candidosis and in cryptococcosis.	a. Excellent safety profile and good tissue penetration. Good bioavailability after oral administration, stable, evenly distributed between tissues and body fluids; long half-life. b. Broad spectrum of activity against *Candida* spp., *Cryptococcus neoformans*, *Histoplasma capsulatum*, *Paracoccidioides brasiliensis*, *Blastomyces dermatitidis*. c. Increasingly available worldwide. d. Well tolerated.	1. Ineffective for *Aspergillus*, the *Mucorales*, most subcutaneous infections and *Candida krusei* and *C. glabrata*. 2. Emergence of resistant strains of *C. albicans* in AIDS patients has been reported. 3. Only moderately effective in lymphocutaneous sporotrichosis. 4. May interact with cisapride, oral diabetic drugs and phenytoin.
F. Miconazole i. Synthetic phenylethyl imidazole. ii. Topical 1–2% ointment, oral tablets and intravenous preparation (10 mg/ml). iii. Used for treatment of dermatophytoses, candidosis. iv. Intravenous treatment used for serious sepsis due to *Scedosporium apiospermum* at 200–2400 mg/day (localized *S. apiospermum* can be treated with oral itraconazole or fluconazole).	a. Broad spectrum of activity in vitro against many types of fungi including *Aspergillus*, *Candida*, *Scedosporium sp.*, *Histoplasma capsulatum*, *Blastomyces dermatitidis*, *Sporothrix* and *Coccidioides immitis*.	1. Use of intravenous preparation is occasionally associated with toxicity due to the vehicle used. 2. Variable results obtained when treating *Fusarium* infections. 3. May not be effective clinically for treatment of *Aspergillus*, chromoblastomycosis or mycetoma.
G. Ketoconazole i. Synthetic dioxolane imidazole. ii. Oral tablets (200–400 mg/day).	a. Broad spectrum of activity against dermatophytes and *Candida* spp.	1. Poor in vitro activity against *Aspergillus fumigatus* and *Fusarium* species.

Table A.7 *continued*

Drug and route of administration	Advantages	Disadvantages
iii. Topical 2% cream, effective for pityriasis versicolor (2–3 weeks) and dermatophytosis (3–6 weeks). iv. Shampoo is available for treatment of seborrhoea	b. Moderate activity against *Cryptococcus*. c. Onychomycosis responds to oral ketoconazole but requires 6 months' treatment.	2. Oral administration may be associated with a transient rise in levels of some serum enzymes. 3. Requires acid pH for absorption. 4. High doses may cause impotence, gynaecomastia and loss of hair.
H. Terbinafine i. Synthetic allylamine. ii. Oral tablets 250 mg and topical preparations – dose 250 mg once daily. iii. Oral therapy effective for dermatophytosis (2–6 weeks), onychomycosis (3 months fingernails, 6 months toenails), sporotrichosis and chromoblastomycosis. iv. Topical therapy with 1% cream for common superficial mycoses including candidosis.	a. Good in vitro activity against dermatophytes. b. Lipophilic drug that concentrates in the epidermis, dermis and adipose tissue. Secreted in sebum and hence appears in stratum corneum within a few hours of oral administration. There is also diffusion from the nail bed. c. Well tolerated. d. May be useful in chromoblastomycosis and sporotrichosis.	1. Ineffective orally for pityriasis versicolor. 2. Fungistatic for *C. albicans*. 3. Transient mild allergic skin reactions and nausea may occur. Taste loss is rare.

Appendix B
SAMPLING, MICROSCOPY, IDENTIFICATION AND CULTURE OF BACTERIAL, FUNGAL AND ACANTHAMOEBAL PATHOGENS

This book is not intended to be a textbook of microbiology – numerous such books exist – but a manual for the investigation of skin and wound infection; the reader interested in a particular microbe should refer to a specialist text for details. Useful stains and culture media for isolating bacteria and fungi from skin specimens are summarized below, while more specific and detailed techniques are given for those many different types of fungi known to cause disease in temporal and tropical climates.

When skin scrapings or nail clippings are taken, it is important to ensure that: (a) adequate amounts of material are selected; and (b) they are sent to the laboratory in a suitable packet – dark-coloured card is best. Swabs should be moist, and not dry, otherwise bacteria will not survive the passage to the laboratory; transport medium should be used whenever possible. For viruses, the techniques for taking specimens will depend on local facilities; it is important to contact the virology department to ensure that the best methods are used.

Bacteria

Common stains used to identify bacteria on heat-fixed smears or skin scrapings include:

Gram: methyl violet 1% (*must* be filtered) 1 minute, rinse with water, iodine 2% 1 minute, rinse with water, acetone 5 seconds, rinse with tap water and counterstain with carbol fuchsin 1% or neutral red 1%. View under light microscopy but do not include a blue filter (used by haematologists to examine blood films). Observe under low power at × 4, to identify a small sample, and under × 10, 20 and 40. Then add oil and observe under high power (× 100 objective lens); this is *essential* to identify bacteria especially if small numbers are present as often occurs. Record bacteria as Gram-positive (black), or negative (red), cocci or rods, and whether in pairs, tetrads, chains, clusters, pallisades or diffusely spread. Yeasts stain brown/black and fungal mycelium stains with carbol fuchsin.

Acridine orange: stain with 0.1% dissolved in phosphate buffer at pH3 for 10 minutes. Wash with tap water. View under ultraviolet light in a dark room when bacteria, fungi and protozoa that have taken up the stain fluoresce yellow. This is a useful non-specific stain for these microbes including *Nocardia* but does not stain mycobacteria.

Modified Ziehl–Neelsen: (for *Nocardia*, *M. leprae*. and *Mycobacteria* spp.) Add concentrated carbol fuchsin and heat slide with a taper, until the stain begins to boil, for 20 minutes. Wash with tap water. Add 5% acetic acid for 2 minutes. Wash with tap water and counterstain with malachite green 2% for 5 minutes. Wash with tap water. View with light microscopy, and observe for long, possibly branching bacilli (*Nocardia*) or slightly curved shorter bacilli (*Mycobacteria*), both of which stain red against a green background. If present, *Nocardia* and *M. leprae* may be found in large numbers. Differentiate by decolourizing the slide with acetone for 10 seconds, and treat the slide with concentrated sulphuric acid (20% solution)-95% alcohol for 15 seconds. Counterstain with malachite green 2%. *Nocardia* and *M. leprae* will promptly decolourize, while *Mycobacteria* will retain the carbol fuchsin stain, being acid-alcohol fast bacilli.

Collect a skin smear for *M. leprae* by squeezing the selected site between thumb and forefinger and make an incision 7 mm long through the epidermis just into the dermis. Turn the scalpel blade through 45° and scrape along the gaping edge of the incision. Spread on a clean slide and dry fix in a flame.

Culture of skin and wound swabs

Inoculate blood and chocolate agars and incubate at 37°C in 4% CO_2 for 48 hours. Identify colonies and perform sensitivity tests – ignore coagulase-negative staphylococci in the immunocompetent host. Wound swabs should be cultured as well for anaerobic bacteria using both solid medium such as pre-reduced blood agar incubated in an anaerobic tent or jar for 2 days and a fluid medium such as thioglycolate broth incubated at 37°C for 2 weeks. Beware that *Propionibacteria* require a minimum of 14 days' culture.

Culture specifically for *S. aureus* using selective agar viz. mannitol salt, or use selective broth, such as salt cooked meat, and incubate at 37°C for 48 hours. If sensitivity tests are performed for CNS against teicoplanin, or vancomycin, these should follow the methods given by Kennedy and Seal (1996). Include brain–heart infusion (BHI) or thioglycolate broths for all 'culture-negative' specimens, especially tissue that has been exposed to antibiotics (Fig. B.1). These broths will support the growth of fastidious bacteria, actinomycetes, anaerobic bacteria, saprophytic mycobacteria and most fungi.

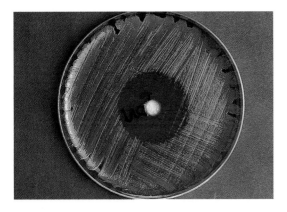

Figure B.1: Agar plate with inhibition of *S. aureus* from penicillin diffusing out of a central well containing tissue removed from necrotizing fasciitis treated with penicillin; such tissue is culture-negative for BHS unless inactivated with betalactamase.

Serology testing for *S. pyogenes* and *S. aureus* infection

Serological tests that should be performed to diagnose infection by the beta-haemolytic streptococci include: the antistreptolysin O (ASO) test, which cross-reacts between Lancefield groups A, C and G; the antihyaluronidase (AHL) test, which is specific for group A or, as a separate test, is shared betweeen groups C and G; and the anti-DNAse B (ADB) test, which is specific for group A. Research-based tests can measure antibody to the individual M proteins, to suggest infection by a particular type, as well as to the Opacity Factor, produced predominantly by skin strains of *S. pyogenes*. Molecular-based tests for toxin production, such as streptococcal pyrogenic exotoxin, are given in Appendix C.

Throat infection causes a high titre in only the ASO test with slightly elevated AHL and ADB titres. Skin infection causes higher AHL and ADB titres, while necrotizing fasciitis due to *S. pyogenes* elevates the ADB test up to a titre of 1/6000 to 10 000. Such high titres in the ADB test are almost pathognomonic of this condition.

There are no suitable tests for acute infection by *S. aureus*. Chronic infection by *S. aureus* can be assessed by measuring the anti-staphylolysin titre, which is usually elevated. Research-based tests involve measuring antibody by ELISA to the teichoic acid of the cell wall (Ficker *et al.*, 1992), which is usually raised with chronic infection.

Fungi

Collection of material

Disposable scalpel blades held vertically to the skin are used to obtain scrapings. Cleaning of skin with alcohol may be useful in the presence of ointment or powder. If the lesion has a definite edge, the material should be taken from the active margin. When blisters are present, fine scissors may be used to cut off the roof for microscopy and culture; such samples are often packed with hyphae. Ears should be sampled with swabs, collecting as much material as possible.

Skin scrapings should be transported in folded paper, which keeps the specimen dry and prevents contamination. Plastic containers are unsuitable as the skin adheres to the sides and is difficult to remove. Dermatophytes in skin scrapings may remain viable for months and yeasts for several weeks. Scrapings from the external auditory canal should be supplemented with swab samples, for both bacteria and fungi.

Hairs to be examined for the presence of dermatophytes or black or white piedra can be cut off at skin level. If dermatophytosis is suspected, the hairs should be plucked out with the roots intact using fine forceps; cut hairs are not suitable. The affected hairs may be recognized because they are dull and broken or they remove easily. This is useful for examining scalp or beard kerions caused by *Trichophyton verrucosum*, where little fungus may provoke a severe reaction. It may be necessary to test many hairs before an infected hair is found. Examination of lesions with Wood's light (365 nm) may aid selection of the best material for culture in appropriate cases of small-spored ectothrix infection or favus; samples should be collected with disposable toothed forceps and plated out directly onto agar.

In onychomycosis it is more difficult to isolate the fungus than in infection affecting the skin or hair. In most nail infections the material for examination is collected from the distal end of the nail, where the fungus is less likely to be viable, despite the fact that the infection is advancing proximally. It is not usually practicable to take deep samples from the proximal advancing edge with minimum discomfort to the patient. The full thickness of the nail should be sampled as most infections start in the hyponychium. Superficial scrapings are inadequate except in cases of superficial white onychomycosis. Debris may be scraped out from under the nail, using the flat end of a dental probe, and this can be culture positive. In paronychia, the nail fold should be moistened and the flat end of a probe inserted into the fold to withdraw material.

Mucous membranes may be sampled with a blunt scalpel or swabs. Swabs should be stored in transport media as yeasts rapidly die in dry conditions.

Examination of material

For routine examination, specimens are mounted in 10–30% potassium hydroxide; the higher the percentage, the faster the specimen will clear. Infected hairs are delicate and should be examined as soon as possible after mounting or the characteristic arrangement of the arthroconidia will be obscured. Beware of overilluminating the slide, especially at low power, as it will render the fungal elements invisible.

Use of alternative techniques can make observation of fungal elements easier. Phase-contrast and dark-field microscopy can produce good results but require the specimen to be thin and will need a longer period of softening. Stains such as Congo red, methylene blue and cotton blue have been recommended to enhance the contrast between fungus and skin, but these require a fully softened specimen. Parker's stain is particularly useful for pityriasis versicolor as *Malassezia furfur* takes up the stain immediately to become bright blue, whereas *Candida* spp. and dermatophytes only do so after a period of hours. It is made by mixing equal volumes of Parker's blue-black Quink ink with 10% potassium hydroxide.

Fluorescence microscopy using either acridine orange or Calcofluor white, which specifically stain polysaccharides in the fungal cell wall, is becoming popular. Histological processing of nail material and staining with a fungus-specific stain such as PAS (periodic acid–Schiff reagent) can be more sensitive and confirms that the nail plate is invaded by the fungus.

Culture of material

For some superficial mycoses (pityriasis versicolor, black and white piedra and tinea nigra), the appearance of the fungal elements is so characteristic that culture is not required, while for otomycosis it is essential. Fungi grow readily on simple media containing glucose and preferably on an organic nitrogen source. They are not fastidious but not all fungi, particularly plant fungi, will grow on a rich medium such as Sabouraud's dextrose agar (4% glucose, 1% peptone, pH 5.4) or Emmon's modification (2% glucose, 1% peptone, neutral pH). Such fungi prefer media such as cornmeal agar. Antibacterial antibiotics such as gentamicin (0.0025%) and/or chloramphenicol (0.005%) can be added to reduce contamination. If a dermatophyte-type infection has been diagnosed, the addition of 0.04% cycloheximide will inhibit the growth of non-dermatophyte moulds. This antibiotic must be excluded, however, if infection by a non-dermatophyte mould such as *Scytalidium* or candidosis is suspected. Although *C. albicans* is not affected, other species of *Candida* which are found particularly in nail and mucous membranes will be inhibited. Fungi should be investigated and cultured as given in Tables B.1–4. Typical examples are illustrated in Figs B.2–10. A flow chart for identification is given in Fig. B.12.

Tissue specimens and host/graft material

Tease out the tissue with a sterile needle and blade, and divide into two halves. Use one for histology and electron microscopy (place in glutaraldehyde fixative), and use the other for smears (make at least three) and culture for microbes as given above.

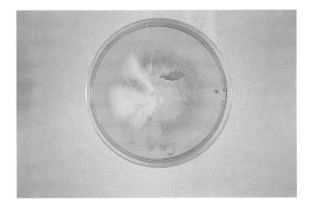

Figure B.2: Plate culture of *Microsporum canis*.

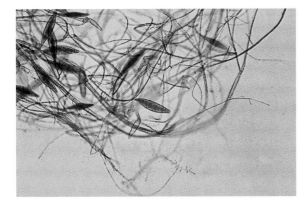

Figure B.3: Lactophenol cotton blue stain of macroconidia of *Microsporum* spp (×200).

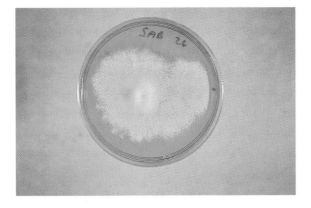

Figure B.4: Plate culture of *Trichophyton mentagrophytes*.

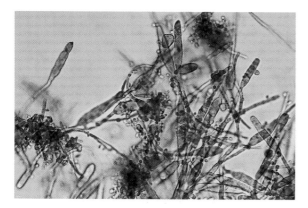

Figure B.5:
Lactophenol cotton blue stain of macroconidia of *Trichophyton mentagrophytes* (×200).

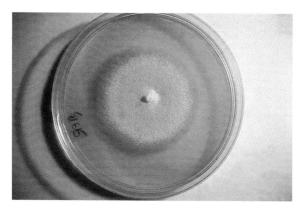

Figure B.6: Plate culture of *Epidermophyton floccosum*.

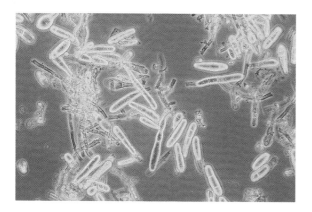

Figure B.7: Phase-contrast microscopy of macroconidia of *Epidermophyton floccosum* (×200).

229

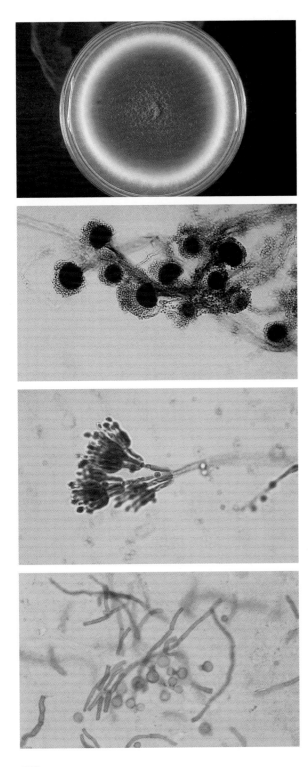

Figure B.8: Agar plate culture of *Aspergillus fumigatus*.

Figure B.9: Microscopy of *Aspergillus* conidiophore (×200).

Figure B.10: Microscopy of *Penicillium* conidiophore (×200).

Figure B.11: Microscopy of *Malassezia globosa* cultured in olive oil (×400).

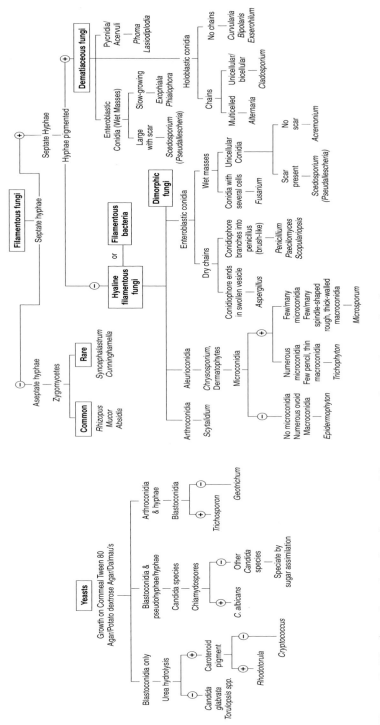

Figure B.12: Flow chart for identification of fungi causing skin and wound infection.

231

Table B.1 Cultural conditions for isolation of superficial and cutaneous fungal pathogens (from Hay and Moore, 1998).

Disease	Fungi	Media		Antibiotics		Temperature		Length of incubation (days)
		GP	MEA	Cyc	Chlor	26/28	37C	
Black piedra	Piedraia hortae	+	+	+	+	+	–	28
White piedra	Trichosporon spp.	+	+	–	+	+	–	14
Tinea nigra	Phaeoannellomyces	+	+	–	+	–	–	21
Dermatophytosis	Trichophyton spp.	+	+	+	+	+	–	21–28
	Microsporum spp.							
	Epidermophyton spp.							
Dermatomycoses	Scytalidium spp.	+	+	–	+	+	–	21
Onychomycosis (non-dermatophytes)	Scopulariopsis spp.	+	+	–	+	+	–	21
	Acremonium spp.							
	Fusarium spp.							
Candidosis	Candida spp.	+	+	–	+	–	+	7
Otomycosis	Aspergillus spp.	+	+	–	+	–	+	21

GP: glucose-peptone agar; MEA: malt extract agar; Cyc: cycloheximide 0.4 g/l; Chlor: chloramphenicol 0.05 g/l; + recommended; – not recommended.

Table B.2 Diagnosis of fungal infections of skin and wounds.

Clinical entity and samples to be collected	Direct microscopy KOH	Gram	Other	Culture	Histopathology H & E	Other	Skin tests	Serological tests Antibodies	Antigen
Tinea nigra	+	–	–	Dark yeast-like colonies	–	–	–	–	–
Pityriasis versicolor	+	–	–	Unnecessary	–	–	–	–	–
Ringworm	Skin scraping, Hair: +	–	–	Necessary for specific identification	–	–	–	–	–
Onychomycosis	+	+ (for Candida)	–	Necessary for specific identification	–	–	–	–	–
Candidosis (superficial)	±	+	Special fungus stains	Necessary for specific identification	–	–	–	+ (DD, Aggl)	+ (LPA)
Sporotrichosis	±	±	Special fungus stains	At 37°C (to isolate yeast phase) and 25°C (to isolate mycelial phase)	±	Fungus stains	+[b] in association with leishmaniasin and PPD	+ (Aggl., LPA)[b] (CIE, DD, ELISA)	–
Chromoblastomycosis	+	+	Special fungus stains	Dark colonies	+	Fungus stains	–	+ (DD)	–
Phaeohyphomycosis	+	–	Special fungus stains	Dark colonies	+	1. Fungus stains 2. Melanin stain	–	–	–

Samples to be collected:
- Tinea nigra: Skin scraping
- Pityriasis versicolor: Skin scraping
- Ringworm: Skin scraping, Hair
- Onychomycosis: Nail scraping/clipping
- Candidosis (superficial): Skin scraping, pus, exudates
- Sporotrichosis: Crusted scales, exudates, pus, biopsy
- Chromoblastomycosis: Scales, crusts, pus, biopsy
- Phaeohyphomycosis: Skin scraping, pus, biopsy

Table B.2 Continued

Clinical entity and samples to be collected	Direct microscopy KOH	Gram	Other	Culture	Histopathology H & E	Other	Skin tests	Serological tests Antibodies	Antigen
Hyalohyphomycosis	Skin scraping, pus, biopsy	+	−	Special fungus stains	Necessary for specific identification (*Fusarium*, *Paecilomyces*, *Penicillium*)	+	Special fungus stains	−	−	−
Penicillium marneffei	Pus, biopsy	+	+	Fungus stains	Culture at 37°C and 25°C	+	Fungus stains	−	+	+
Mycetoma										
Actinomycotic	Pus, grains, skin scrapings, biopsy	+	+	AFB	Filamentous bacteria	+	Gram, AFB, FA	±	+ (DD, CIE)	−
Eumycotic	Pus, grains, skin scrapings, biopsy	+	−	Fungus stains	Fungal colonies +	+	Fungus stains, FA	±	+ (DD, CIE, ELISA)	−
Entomophthoramycosis	Skin scrapings, pus, biopsy	+	−	Fungus stains	Necessary for specific identification	+	Fungus stains	−	−	−
Lobomycosis	Material from cutaneous lesion and biopsy	+	−	+	Cannot be cultured	+	Fungus stains	−	−	−
Rhinosporidiosis	Biopsy only	−	−	−	Cannot be cultured	+	Fungus stains	−	−	−
Mucormycosis (cutaneous)	Biopsy, pus	−	−	Fungus stains	Very difficult to culture	+	Fungus stains	−	−	−

Disease	Specimen		Direct exam		Culture		FA		Serology	
Cryptococcosis (cutaneous)	Pus, biopsy	−	Fungus stains	+	Mucoid colonies	+	Fungus stains, FA	−	+ (Aggl, LPA)[b]	+ (LPA)
Aspergillosis (cutaneous)	Skin scraping, pus, biopsy	+	Fungus stains	−	Grows well in culture	+	Fungus stains, FA	+[b]	+ (DD,[b] LPA, ELISA)[b]	+ (LPA)[b]
Blastomycosis[a]	Skin, mucous membrane, pus, biopsy	+	Fungus stains	+	Culture at 37°C and 25°C	+	Fungus stains, FA	−	+ (DD, LPA, CFT, ELISA)[b]	−
Paracoccidioidomycosis[a]	Skin, mucous membrane, pus, exudate, biopsy	+	Fungus stains	+	Culture at 37°C and 25°C	+	Fungus stains, FA	±[b]	+ (DD, CFT, CIE, IFA, MELISA)[b]	−
Classic histoplasmosis[a]	Exudate, biopsy	+	Fungus stains	+	Culture at 37°C and 25°C	+	Fungus stains, FA	+[b]	+ (DD, CFT, LPA)[b]	+
African histoplasmosis[a]	Pus, exudate, skin scrapings or scales	+	Fungus stains	+	Culture at 37°C and 25°C	+	Fungus stains, FA	−	+ (DD, CFT, LPA)[b]	−
Coccidioidomycosis[a]	Mucous membrane, skin, pus, biopsy	+	Fungus stains	+	Culture at 37°C and 25°C	+	Fungus stains, FA	+[b]	+ (DD, CFT)[b]	−

Fungus stains = periodic acid–Schiff, Gomori's methenamine silver stain, Calcofluor white. H & E = haematoxylin-eosin. FA = fluorescent antibody. +: very useful. ±: may or may not be useful. DD: immunodiffusion. CIE: countercurrent immunoelectrophoresis. Aggl: tube agglutination. LPA: latex particle agglutination. CFT: complement-fixation test. IFA: indirect fluorescent antibody. ELISA: enzyme-linked immunosorbent assay. MELISA: magnetic ELISA. PPD: purified protein derivative (M. tuberculosis). AFB: acid fast bacilli.

[a] If the skin/wound infection is a cutaneous manifestation of systemic mycosis, other samples (blood, sputum, etc.) need to be collected.

[b] Although skin tests/serological tests are available for these diseases, they may or may not be indicated or may not be of value in skin and wound infections caused by these fungi.

Table B.3 Techniques for detection of fungi in skin and wound infections by direct microscopy.

Method	Advantages	Disadvantages
A. Potassium hydroxide (KOH 5–30%) mount i. Very sensitive in superficial and cutaneous fungal infections. ii. Modifications include ink-KOH mount (ink has fine particles that attach to fungal cell walls) and KOH-dimethyl sulfoxide (for better digestion of tissue).	a. Single-step, inexpensive, rapid (usually 5 minutes) method. b. Specimens cleared to make fungi more readily visible by digesting tissue. c. After initial digestion of tissue, counterstain (PAS, acridine orange, Calcofluor white) can be used. d. Oil immersion magnification not required.	1. Experience required since background artifacts may cause confusion. 2. Clearing of some specimens may take an extended time. 3. When KOH alone is used, sufficient contrast may not be obtained by routine brightfield microscopy. 4. *Candida* and other yeasts may escape detection.
B. Gram staining i. Takes 3–5 minutes to perform. ii. Commonly used to detect bacteria in samples; most fungi are also detected. Filamentous bacteria (*Nocardia*, *Actinomyces*) are detected. iii. Several modifications, for staining fluids, pus and exudates and tissue sections (Brown and Brenn, Brown–Hopps).	a. Stains *Candida* blastoconidia and pseudohyphae, yeast forms of dimorphic fungi, hyphae of filamentous fungi. b. Bacteria stained and differentiated c. Preparations can be restained with Gomori's methenamine silver (GMS).	1. Stains fibrous protein, causing opacity of the preparation. 2. Crystal violet precipitation may obscure detail and cause confusion. 3. Some fungi (e.g. *Cryptococcus*) may show only stippling or no staining. 4. Some *Nocardia* isolates stain weakly or not at all.
C. Giemsa staining i. Rapid method, takes 1 hour. ii. Can be used to detect fungi in blood smears, bone marrow and body fluids, pus and exudates.	a. Permits differential staining of tissue and cellular elements. b. Stains yeast cells and fungal hyphae. c. Stains viral inclusions, protozoa (e.g. *Leishmania*), chlamydiae.	1. Disadvantages similar to those of Gram's stain. 2. Tissue cells also stain, resulting in opaque areas in thick preparations. 3. Buffer and working solutions require careful preparation.

Table B.3 *Continued*

Method	Advantages	Disadvantages
D. Acid-fast stain (modified Kinyoun's, modified Fite–Faraco) i. Takes 15–20 minutes to perform. ii. Used to detect mycobacteria and some species of *Nocardia* in body fluids, pus and exudates.	a. Permits detection of *Nocardia* and *B. dermatitidis*. b. Can be used to stain smears and tissue sections.	1. Tissue homogenates are difficult to observe because of background staining. 2. Working solutions require careful preparation. 3. *Nocardia* in tissues is sometimes not acid-fast. Fungi are not acid-fast.
E. Papanicolaou stain i. Takes 30 minutes to perform. ii. Used to detect fungi in body fluids, pus and exudates and tissue sections.	a. Fungal structures can be detected in fluids, pus and exudates. b. Some protozoa can be detected.	1. Cannot be used for tissue homogenates. 2. Working solutions require careful preparation.
F. Periodic acid–Schiff (PAS) i. Takes 20–30 minutes to perform. ii. Used to detect fungi in body fluids, pus and exudates and tissue sections.	a. Fungal structures stain well (reddish). b. Hyphae of filamentous fungi and yeast cells can be readily distinguished.	1. *Nocardia* species do not stain well and *B. dermatitidis* appears pleomorphic. 2. Does not allow determination of innate colour of a fungus. 3. Working solutions require careful preparation. Procedure requires careful standardization.
G. Methenamine silver staining (GMS) i. Takes 1 hour to perform.	a. Stains fungal cell wall clearly; no interference from background (fungi stained black-brown and background stained light green).	1. Excessive silver deposition may obscure cell walls and septa.

Table B.3 Continued

Method	Advantages	Disadvantages
ii. Conventional technique used to detect fungi in histologic sections while a modified technique can be used to detect fungi in fluids, pus and exudates. iii. GMS can be combined with haematoxylin-eosin (H & E) staining to permit study of tissue responses in addition to delineating fungi.	b. Positives more frequent and reliable than in methods A–F. c. Negatives more reliable. d. Can detect *Pneumocystis*, protozoa and filamentous bacteria.	2. Stains cellular debris and melanin. 3. Controls needed; reagents and procedure need standardization.
H. Calcofluor white (CFW) i. Takes I minute to perform. ii. Can be mixed with KOH 5–30% for better digestion of tissue prior to viewing. iii. Fluorescent dye has a high affinity for poly-saccharides, e.g. chitin of fungal cell walls.	a. Detects fungi rapidly because of bright fluorescence. b. Yeast cells and hyphae are clearly stained and distinguished. c. Can also detect protozoa, *Pneumocystis*. d. Material from KOH mounts can be used for subsequent CFW staining.	I. Fluorescence microscope needed. 2. Background fluorescence prominent, but fungi exhibit more intense fluorescence. 3. Reagents and procedure require standardization and expertise.
I. Immunofluorescence i. Allows rapid detection and identification of both viable and non-viable fungi in cultures and in most types of clinical materials, including tissue sections. ii. Can be used to detect and measure antibodies in sera and other body fluids. iii. Reagents available to detect tissue forms of dimorphic fungi and of *Aspergillus*, *Candida*, and *Cryptococcus*	a. Detects fungi rapidly because of bright fluorescence. b. Very sensitive and specific technique. c. Able to detect the aetiological agent (fungi) in clinical material or tissue even if the presentation is atypical. d. Can be used to detect and identify fungi in sections previously stained by H & E, Giemsa or Gram stains.` e. Can be used to diagnose fungal infection in retrospect.	I. Fluorescence microscope needed. 2. Reagents and procedures require standardization and expertise. 3. Cannot be used to identify fungi in sections previously stained by GMS or PAS. 4. Specific reagents to detect mycelial forms of dimorphic fungi not readily available.

238

Table B.4 Guide to recognition of fungi and actinomycetes in clinical specimens from skin and wound infections.

Morphological form found	Fungi	Direct microscopic appearance
A. Hyaline septate hyphae	a. Dermatophytes 1. Skin and nails	Hyaline septate hyphae (3–15 μm width) commonly seen; chains of arthroconidia may be seen.
	2. Hair	Arthroconidia on periphery of hair shaft producing sheath (ectothrix) or those produced by fragmentation within the hair shaft (endothrix) can be seen; 3–15 μm width. Long hyphal filaments (unfragmented) within hair shaft indicate 'favus'.
	b. *Aspergillus* spp. (*A. fumigatus, A. flavus*)	Septate, hyaline, dichotomously 45° angle branching of uniform width (3–12 μm); occasional conidial heads.
	c. *Geotrichum* spp.	Hyphae (4–12 μm) and rectangular arthroconidia are present and sometimes rounded.
	d. *Penicillium* spp.	Most species resemble other hyaline filamentous fungi in morphology.
	P. marneffei (dimorphic)	Forms characteristic cells which divide by a central septum in tissue; there is no budding. Most cells in biopsy material are intracellular small oval structures (resemble *Histoplasma capsulatum*); occasional large, banana-shaped 'bullet' cells may be seen (Fig. 9.13).
	e. Other hyaline filamentous fungi 1. *Acremonium* (cases other than mycetoma) 2. *Fusarium* spp. 3. *Paecilomyces* 4. *Scedosporium sp.* (cases other than mycetoma)	Septate regular branched hyaline hyphae (2–4 μm width), occasional intercalary chlamydospores (*Scedosporium sp.* hyphae are very thin and may be light brown in colour).
B. Dematiaceous septate hyphae	*Bipolaris* spp. *Cladosporium* spp. *Curvularia* spp. *Drechslera* spp. *Exophiala* spp. *Exserohilum* spp.	Septate, branched, regular, brown hyphae (2–6 μm width); budding cells with single septum and chains of swollen rounded cells often present; in infection due to *Exophiala* and *Phialophora* spp., aggregates are sometimes seen.

Table B.4 *Continued*

Morphological form found	Fungi	Direct microscopic appearance
	Phialophora spp. *Wangiella dermatitidis* *Phaeoannellomyces* (*Exophiala*) *werneckii*	Large numbers of frequently branched hyphae with budding cells seen.
C. Aseptate hyphae	Zygomycetes a. *Mucor, Rhizopus* (common) b. *Absidia, Syncephalastrum*	Broad, thin-walled, infrequently septate or aseptate hyaline hyphae, 6–25 μm wide, with non-parallel contours and random branches; often appear bizarre and vacuolated (smaller hyphae may be confused with those of *Aspergillus* spp., especially *A. flavus*).
D. Yeast and pseudohyphae or hyphae	a. *Candida* spp.	Yeast cells (3–4 μm diameter) usually exhibit single buds, pseudo-hyphae (5–10 μm) are constricted at the ends; hyphae are septate.
	b. *Malassezia* spp. (in tinea versicolor)	Short, curved, occasionally branched hyphal fragments (2–4 μm) usually present with round yeast cells (3–8 μm) in compacted clusters ('spaghetti and meatballs' appearance).
E. Yeast-like tissue phase of some dimorphic fungi	a. *Blastomyces dermatitidis* (dimorphic)	Spherical to oval, multinucleate, large (8–15 μm) cells with thick walls (doubly refractile) and a single broad-based bud.
	b. *Cryptococcus neoformans* (not dimorphic)	Pleomorphic cells (2–20 μm), spherical or oval, surrounded by mucin-positive capsules and single or multiple narrow-based buds (thin necks).
	c. *Histoplasma capsulatum* (dimorphic)	Spherical to oval, budding (narrow necks), small (2–4 μm) cells, often clustered in mononuclear cells.
	d. *Histoplasma duboisii*	Large, spherical to ovoid '*duboisii*' yeast cells of varying size (7–15 μm), which are uninucleate, with irregularly distributed cytoplasm and thick, double-contoured walls.
	e. *Paracoccidioides brasiliensis* (dimorphic)	Large (10–60 μm) spherical to ovoid thick-walled cells with multiple buds attached by narrow necks ('steering wheel' forms).

Table B.4 *Continued*

Morphological form found	Fungi	Direct microscopic appearance
	f. *Sporothrix schenckii* (dimorphic)	Pleomorphic, medium-sized (2–10 μm), spherical to oval, 'cigar-shaped' yeast forms, that produce single (rarely multiple) buds, with irregular-stained cytoplasm. 'Asteroid bodies' may be seen.
F. Spherules	a. *Coccidioides immitis* (dimorphic)	Vary in size; may contain endospores or be empty (endospores show no budding); young spherule (sporangium) has a clear centre with peripheral cytoplasm and a prominent thick wall.
	b. *Rhinosporidium seeberi*	Large, thick-walled sporangia (100–350 μm) with sporangiospores (6–8 μm); mature sporangia are larger than spherules of *C. immitis*; hyphae may be found in cavitary lesions.
G. Sclerotic bodies	*Cladosporium carrionii* *Fonsecaea compactum* *Fonsecaea pedrosoi* *Phialophora verrucosa* *Rhinocladiella aquaspersa*	Brown, round to pleomorphic thick-walled cells (5–20 μm) with transverse septations; usually a tetrad of cells (due to two fission planes) is seen either extracellularly or within giant cells; occasionally, branched septate hyphae may be found with sclerotic bodies (these are more likely to occur close to the surface of the tissue).
H. Granules (in mycetoma)	a. White granules	In eumycotic mycetoma, the grains are composed of broad (2–5 μm) septate hyphae which may develop large cells at the periphery of the grain.
	1. *Acremonium* (*A. falciforme, A. kiliense, A. recifei*)	White, soft granules (200–300 μm); no cement-like matrix.
	2. *Aspergillus nidulans*	White, soft granules (65–160 μm); no cement-like matrix.
	3. *Fusarium* (*F. moniliforme, F. solani*)	White, soft granules (200–600 μm) with cement-like matrix.
	4. *Neotestudina rosatii*	White, soft granules (300–600 μm) with cement-like matrix at periphery.
	5. *Scedosporium apiospermum*	White, soft granules (200–300 μm) composed of hyphae and swollen cells at periphery with cement-like matrix.

Table B.4 *Continued*

Morphological form found	Fungi	Direct microscopic appearance
	b. Black granules	
	1. *Curvularia (C. geniculata, C. lunata)*	Black, large (500–1000 μm) hard grains with cement-like matrix at periphery.
	2. *Exophiala (E. jeanselmei)*	Black, soft, small (200–300 μm) granules, vacuolated, no cement-like matrix, dark hyphae and swollen cells seen.
	3. *Leptosphaeria*	*L. senegalensis* has large (400–600 μm), black, hard granules with cement-like matrix. *L. tompkinsii* has large (500–1000 μm) black, hard granules; periphery composed of polygonal swollen cells and centre of hyphal network.
	4. *Madurella*	*M. grisea*: black, soft granules (350–500 μm), no cement-like matrix, periphery with swollen cells and centre with hyphal network. *M. mycetomatis*: black to brown hard granules (200–900 μm), which may be compact and filled with cement-like matrix or filled with numerous vesicles; cement-like matrix in periphery and central area of light-coloured hyphae.
	5. *Pyrenochaeta romeroi*	Black, soft granules (300–600 μm), no cement-like matrix, polygonal swollen cells at periphery, network of hyphae at centre.
I. Filamentous bacteria	a. *Actinomadura (A. madurae, A. pelletieri)*	Gram-positive thin branching filaments, 0.5–1 μm in diameter (some *Nocardia* spp. are partially acid-fast when stained with modified Ziehl–Neelsen stain).
	b. *Streptomyces (S. somaliensis, S. paraguayensis)*	
	c. *Nocardia (N. brasiliensis, N. otitidis-caviarum, N. asteroides)*	
	d. *Actinomyces (A. israelii)*	
	e. Grains in actinomycotic mycetoma	In actinomycotic mycetoma, the grains are composed of Gram-positive bacterial filaments, 1 μm or less in diameter.

Table B.4 *Continued*

Morphological form found	Fungi	Direct microscopic appearance
	1. *N. asteroides*	Small (< 1000 μm), white to yellow, soft, with or without clubs.
	2. *N. brasiliensis*	Small (< 1000 μm), white to yellow, soft, with or without clubs.
	3. *N. otitidis-caviarum*	Small (< 1000 μm), white to yellow, soft, with or without clubs.
	4. *A. madurae*	Large (1000–10 000 μm), white to yellow, soft, with or without clubs.
	5. *A. pelletieri*	Small (< 500 μm), bright red, firm, smooth border.
	6. *S. somaliensis*	1000–2000 μm, yellow to brown, hard, round, smooth borders.
	7. *S. paraguayensis*	Small (< 500 μm), black, firm, clubs at periphery.
J. Piedra		
a. Black piedra	*Piedraia hortae*	Hard nodules found over and around the hair shaft; consist of tightly packed, cemented, dark brown hyphae. Mature nodules have numerous asci, each containing 2–8 fusiform, single-celled ascospores.
b. White piedra	*Trichosporon beigelii*	Nodules of variable size noted on surface of hair shaft; soft and easily separated from hair shaft. Nodules contain hyphae, arthroconidia and blastoconidia. Hyphae separate out into round to rectangular or oval arthroconidia (2–4 μm).

Sensitivity testing of fungi

Tests designated to ascertain the minimum amount of drug needed to inhibit the growth of fungal strains in culture (minimal inhibitory concentrations or MICs) are often assumed to be the most dependable means of determining the relative efficacy of different antifungal agents. However, interlaboratory reproducibility may not always be achieved, due to variations arising out of inoculum size, composition and pH of medium, temperature and duration of incubation and endpoint determination (Galgiani *et al.*, 1993; Cormican and Pfaller, 1993).

Sensitivity tests currently performed for yeasts and mycelial fungi are broth-based (broth dilution method) or agar-based (agar dilution and disc- or well-diffusion techniques). The selection of a medium depends on the drug being tested.

Broth media used include unbuffered yeast-nitrogen base (YNB) for flucytosine (5FC), antibiotic culture medium 3 FDA for polyenes and casein-yeast extract-glucose (CYG) broth or YNB for imidazoles. The National Committee for Clinical Laboratory Standards (NCCLS, 1997) of the USA has recently released an approved document (M27A) for sensitivity testing of yeasts; the recommended test medium is RPMI 1640 buffered to pH 7.0 with morpholinepropane sulphonic acid (MOPS) (NCCLS, 1997). Buffered YNB at pH 7.0 in a microtitre plate format was reported to be useful for obtaining results within 48 h when testing *Cryptococcus neoformans* (Ghannoum *et al.*, 1996). The RPMI 1640 medium has also been found to be suitable for adequate growth of filamentous fungi, the reading being taken visually after 48 h incubation at 37°C (Pfaller, 1997).

Agar media used include unbuffered yeast morphology agar (YMA) for 5FC, antibiotic culture medium 12, buffered YMA or Kimmig Agar for polyenes, and CYG or Kimmig agar for azoles. Buffered YNB (for broth tests) and buffered YMA (for agar tests) were reported to be useful for all three groups of compounds (Shadomy *et al.*, 1988).

Inocula are prepared from 24 to 48 h-old cultures in YNB and adjusted to contain 1,000,000 cfu/ml. Conidial suspensions of culture blocks containing hyphae and spores are used as the inocula for mycelial fungi. The variability in inocula preparation inherent in using mycelial growth has been removed by making use of spore suspensions (adjusted by spectrophotometric readings to contain 10,000 cfu/ml) and estimating the concentration of the antifungal agent required to inhibit the germination of these conidia or sporangiospores (Pfaller *et al.*, 1997).

Drugs commonly tested include 5FC, ketoconazole, miconazole, fluconazole, itraconazole and amphotericin B: expected MICs for *Candida albicans* to be sensitive are 0.5, 0.1, 0.1, 0.3, 0.1 and 0.5 mg/l respectively. The MIC for each imidazole can vary widely, especially for *Candida sp.* and other yeasts, so that sensitivity tests are useful. The essential features of the recommendations of the NCCLS M27A method are the use of the broth macrodilution format (final volume 1 ml), a defined culture medium (RPMI 1640), buffered to pH 7.0 with MOPS, and inoculum standardised by spectrophotometric reading to yield 500 to 2500 cells/ml and incubation at 35°C for 48 h for *Candida sp.* and 72 h for *C. neoformans*; endpoint determination for amphotericin B is the lowest concentration at which no growth is visible while for 5FC and the azoles, inhibition of at least 80% of growth is accepted as the endpoint. Since microbroth dilution testing is easier to perform, cheaper and more rapid, this method was evaluated in 96 well microtitre plates (final volume 200 μl) and found to give reliable, reproducible and comparable results. Adherence to the NCCLS method is reported to provide >90% intralaboratory and interlaboratory reproducibility, while use of the recommended quality control isolates (*Candida parapsilosis* ATCC 22019; *Candida krusei* ATCC 6528) ensures reliable test performance (NCCLS, 1997). Fluconazole resistance, due to active efflux from the cell common for all imidazoles, is well-recognized in AIDS patients.

Although some degree of interlaboratory reproducibility has been achieved in antifungal susceptibility testing of mycelial fungi (van Cutsem *et al.*, 1994), the predictive clinical value of such tests still has to be unequivocally demonstrated. In this respect, the NCCLS M27A method has been a useful starting point for the development of a standard method for susceptibility testing of filamentous fungi, especially *Aspergillus* (Rattan, 1999). Odds *et al.* (1998) evaluated antifungal suscep-tibilities of 9 isolates of filamentous fungi in vitro (determined by the NCCLS method in 11 different laboratories) and antifungal treatment outcomes in animal infection models; these workers concluded that only a limited association between MIC and treatment outcome was seen due to the limitations of the models used.

Agar diffusion systems have become very popular for antifungal susceptibil-ity testing of yeasts. In spite of limitations (difficulty in estimating size of inhibitory zone, deterioration of amphotericin B and azoles when stored in diluted form or discs, poor diffusion of azoles except fluconazole in such a system), a good correlation between MIC determination in YNB and diameter of zones of inhibition of growth of strains around a 50 µg fluconazole disc on Yeast Nitrogen Agar has been demonstrated (Rattan, 1999).

The E-test (AB Biodisk, Solna, Sweden) is a patented commercial method for determination of MIC which is similar to the disc diffusion test except that instead of a disc, a calibrated plastic strip impregnated with a concentration gradient of the antifungal agent is used. E-test results compare well with those obtained by the NCCLS method for *Candida sp.*, but a marked disparity exists between the E-test and broth dilution MIC for fluconazole when testing *C. neofor-mans* (Rattan, 1999). E-test technology has recently been evaluated for testing isolates of *Aspergillus, Fusarium* and *Rhizopus*. Another new method for testing the MIC for *Aspergillus niger* is the Bio-Cell Tracer (van Cutsem *et al.*, 1994).

Synergy testing can be performed but satisfactory in vitro results may not yield clinical success. In particular, amphotericin B + 5FC has been successful for cryptococcal infection. Amphotericin B + fluconazole has been shown to be additive for candidosis in murine studies, but amphotericin + ketoconazole or itraconazole has been shown to be antagonistic in animal models of aspergillosis.

Acanthamoeba

Skin and wound biopsies should be inoculated directly on to non-nutrient agar, made up in Page's amoebal saline (Page, 1988). This involves use of modified

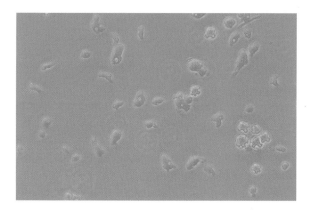

Figure B.13:
Trophozoites and
cysts of *Acanthamoeba*
spp. cultured on non-
nutrient amoebal
saline agar, spread
with bacteria, with
phase-contrast
microscopy and a
green filter (×200).

Neff's amoebal saline (AS). A separate stock solution of each component is made up by dissolving in 100 ml glass-distilled water: NaCl 1.20 g, $MgSO_4.7H_2O$ 0.04 g, $CaCl_2.2H_2O$ 0.04 g, Na_2HPO_4 1.42 g, KH_2PO_4 1.36 g. The final dilution is prepared by adding 10 ml of each stock solution to 950 ml glass-distilled water to make 1 litre in total of AS. To prepare the non-nutrient amoebal agar, 15 g of plain agar is added to 1 l of AS, which is autoclaved and dispensed into 100-ml bottles or smaller. This can be stored at room temperature. It should be boiled before use and fresh plates poured of hot agar. In this way fungal conta-mination can be avoided. The agar plates should be spread with live *Klebsiella* spp. or *E. coli* as a food source (Penland and Wilhelmus, 1997), which is more effective than the traditional use of a killed organism. This should be prepared in advance by culturing *Klebsiella* spp. or *E. coli* on nutrient agar plates and then washing the bacteria off into normal sterile saline. A swab is used to spread the live bacteria over the non-nutrient agar plate as a lightly turbid suspension.

These prepared AS agar plates are then inoculated directly from skin and wound material. The plate is incubated at 32°C for 4 weeks, wrapped up in clean disposable plastic bags. Fresh agar should not be kept for more than 24 hours. The material on the plate should be inspected with an inverted micro-scope for the presence of typical trophozoites (Figs B.13 and B.14), rounded-up pre-cysts (Fig. B.15) or cysts of *Acanthamoeba* (Figs B.13 and B.16). If facilities for culture are not available, skin and wound material may be mailed in sterile containers with saline to a suitable laboratory.

Amoebae will usually, but not always, be visible by low-power light microscopy after 1 week; after 2 weeks, the whole plate is covered by the typical double-walled, star-shaped cysts (Fig. B.16). Each point of the star is the ostiole (Fig. B.17) through which the internalized amoeba communicates with the outside world; it is normally plugged with mucopolysaccharide.

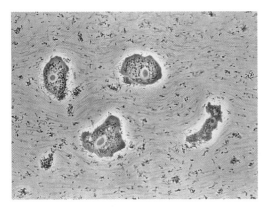

Figure B.14: Trophozoites of *Acanthamoeba* in a bacterial biofilm (Simmons PA, Tomlinson A, Seal DV. *Optom Vis Sci* 1998, 75, 860-66) (× 200).

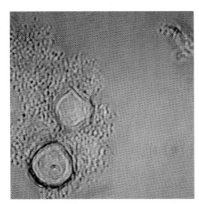

Figure B.15: Rounded-up 'pre-cysts' of *Acanthamoeba* (× 400).

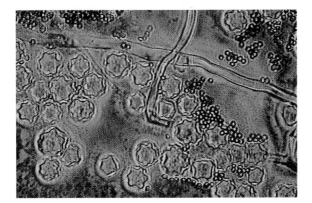

Figure B.16: Typical cysts of *Acanthamoeba* on agar (× 200).

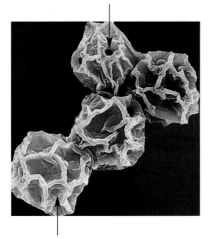

Figure B.17: Scanning electron microscopy of ostioles of *Acanthamoeba* cysts.

Sensitivity testing

For drugs to be effective, they have to penetrate to the internalized amoeba within the cyst through either the ostioles or pores within the cyst wall. For *in vitro* drug sensitivity testing, trophozoites and cysts of *Acanthamoeba* can either be cultured axenically in proteose peptone glucose (PPG) solution (Page, 1988) or on amoebal saline agar plates. A method has been described for ocular isolates, which could be used for skin isolates, when dilutions of drugs were carried out in microtitre plates and *Acanthamoeba* cultures of trophozoites and cysts were added (Hay *et al.*, 1994b). The plates are incubated at 32°C and the concentrations of dilutions with surviving cells are recorded. This assesses the minimum trophozoiticidal amoebicidal concentration (MTAC), and the minimum cysticidal concentration (MCC). If this is not possible, isolates should be sent to a reference laboratory.

Serology

Testing serum for the presence of antibody to the organism is useful for aiding recognition of: brucellosis by agglutination and radioimmunoassay tests; of syphilis (in its diverse forms) using both non-specific cardiolipid (reagin) tests such as the Venereal Disease Research Laboratory (VDRL) test and a specific treponemal test such as the *Treponema pallidum* immobilization (TPI), fluorescent treponemal antibody (FTA) or *Treponema pallidum* haemagglutination (TPHA); of borreliosis causing Lyme's disease with an ELISA test and toxoplasmosis using the Sabin–Feldman dye test or latex or ELISA tests. Serology testing for *S. pyogenes* and *S. aureus* is given on p. 225.

Appendix C
IDENTIFICATION AND CULTURE FOR VIRUSES AND MOLECULAR BIOLOGY

Laboratory diagnosis of viruses

Certain viruses can infect the skin, including representatives from DNA, RNA and retroviruses. Standard methods for viral detection rarely require much adaptation for use in skin infection. The procedures are available in standard works of virology.

There are four basic approaches to laboratory diagnosis of virus infections. These are:

1. Direct examination of fluid, cells or tissue samples (Woods and Walker, 1996).
2. Virus isolation using tissue culture.
3. Serology.
4. Molecular methods, especially the polymerase chain reaction (PCR).

Table C.1 lists tests for direct examination, virus isolation and serological methods.

Molecular methods

Molecular biology methods have revolutionized diagnostic laboratory procedures and are playing an increasingly important role in the diagnosis of dermatological infectious disease. This is especially true of the polymerase chain reaction (PCR) method. Comprehensive accounts of the basic science of molecular biology are available, as are books with basic molecular biological methods. PCR technology is comprehensively described (Rapley, 1996). Methods have been collated for use of molecular biology as a tool for diagnostic molecular microbiology (Persing *et al.*, 1995).

The PCR method permits amplification of DNA in a cell-free system in a single incubation tube. Amplification of target sequences can be achieved using small quantities of oligonucleotide primers, which bind specifically to DNA immediately surrounding the target area, together with nucleotides and polymerase enzyme. This can be achieved even if the target DNA is in an impure state or is denatured. The technique, being extremely sensitive, requires interpretation relative to negative controls, since false positive results can and do

Table C.1 Tests for direct examination, isolation and serological methods

Virus	Direct examination	Virus isolation	Serological methods
DNA viruses			
Herpes simplex[a]	Multinucleated giant cells	Inoculation into HeLa cells	Complement fixation (CF)`, haemagglutination, neutralization
	Cytopathogenic effects (CPEs)	Chorioallantoic membrane of embryonated hen's egg	Not always present in recurrence
		Susceptible cell culture detection by immunofluorescence (IF), CPEs	Positive with HSV-2
HSV-1 [HHV-1]	Cowdry type A intranuclear inclusions	Intracerebral suckling mice	Four-fold increase in antibody titre between paired sera
HSV-2 [HHV-2]	IF using monoclonal antibodies, in situ hybridization of cells		Of limited value
Varicella zoster	Multinucleated giant cells	Inoculation into:	CF best
VZV [HHV-3]	Lipschutz bodies (IF)	Diploid cell lines in human cell cultures + CPE (amnion [best] or embryonic lungs or kidneys)	Increase in heterotypic antibody titre to VSV antigen can occur in persons with HSV with previous VSV infection.
		No growth in hen's eggs or laboratory animals	
	IF for VZV antigens	Not as sensitive as primary monkey kidney cells	
	Tranmission electron microscopy (TEM)		
Epstein–Barr virus (EBV) [HHV-4]	–	Fresh umbilical cord blood lymphocytes Immortalization at 6–8 weeks	Paul–Bunnell, Monospot test IF

Table C.1 *Continued*

Virus	Direct examination	Virus isolation	Serological methods
		EBV nAg–IF	Increased antibody titre against EBV early antigen with continuing viral replication
		EBV DNA-nucleic acid hybridization CPEs	
Cytomegalo-virus [HHV-5]	Intranuclear ('owl eye' cells) and occasional cytoplasmic inclusions	Human fibroblast cell cultures	CF, haemagglutination, neutralization
		Standard laboratory cultures (HeLa, Hep-2, MKC) not susceptible CPE depends on viral count (1–3 weeks for small numbers)	Fourfold increase in CF antibody titre
Adenovirus	Intranuclear inclusion bodies (not pathognomic for adenovirus)	HeLa cells or primary cultures of human embryonic cell lines	CF, haemagglutination, neutralization
	IF, IP for early infection and rapid diagnosis	Human embryonic kidney (HEK) – 7 days to CPE	Fourfold increase in CF antibody titre indicative of adenovirus infection Neutralization for serotyping
Poxviruses Orf	TEM	Fibroblast mono-layers from sheep embryo skin and muscle with CPEs Primate cells Human amnion cells No growth in eggs	–
Vaccina, (Small pox)	TEM	Chicken egg allantoic membrane	–
Molluscum contagiosum	Metterson–Patterson or molluscum bodies TEM	Many ways non-transmissible Cytopathic changes in different species with no production of infectious	–

Table C.1 *Continued*

Virus	Direct examination	Virus isolation	Serological methods
Human papilloma-virus (HPV)	TEM	progeny viruses No growth in eggs None available	—

RNA viruses

Virus	Direct examination	Virus isolation	Serological methods
Picornaviruses Coxsackie, ECHO, polio	TEM, Light microscopy of limited use IF of viral antigens	Cell culture system: primary monkey kidney cells, human cell culture Virus heat sensitive (grows at 30–34°C) CPEs	Coxsackie B group IgM test and poliovirus tests only
Coxsackie A24 variant virus	IF of viral antigens	Primary human embryonic lung cell culture	—
Measles virus	Giant intranuclear inclusions IFA staining	Difficult and time consuming Use primary human or simian cells	Haemagglutination inhibition
Mumps virus	Immunofluorescent antibody (IFA) staining	Embryonated hens egg Primary chick embryo fibroblast cells CPEs	Haemagglutination inhibition; neutralization CF on paired sera
Rubella	Limited value	Limited value	Haemagglutination inhibition ELISA IFA Detection of specific anti-Rubella IgM for rapid diagnosis
Arboviruses, retroviruses and HIV	Refer to textbook of virology		

[a]The Surecell *Herpes simplex* virus (HSV) kit is a test for HSV antigen using a monoclonal antibody-based immunoassay. It has been evaluated and found to have a 70% sensitivity and 100% specificity in the detection of HSV antigen compared to tissue culture (Asbell *et al.*, 1995). The test kit requires no special equipment and can be carried out in the clinic.
CF = complement fixation; CPE = cytopathic effect; HEK = human embryo kidney; HeLa = Helen Lane; HHV = human herpes virus; HSV = *Herpes simplex* virus; IF = immuno and fluorescence; IP = intraperitoneal; Lm = light microscopy; mAb = monoclonal antibody; MKC = monkey kidney cells; RI = radio-immunoassay; TEM = transmission electron microscopy; VZV = Varicella zoster virus.

occur. Measures must be taken to ensure that contamination of the target sequence by extraneous DNA is obviated.

The PCR technique is being applied to diagnosis of dermatological infectious disease. In virology, the PCR technique has been used extensively for viral detection in body fluids and tissues. Other applications include detection of: *M. leprae* (van Beers *et al.*, 1994); *Necator americanus* and *Ancylostoma duodenale* (Monti *et al.*, 1998); *Chlamydia trachomatis* (Fan *et al.*, 1993); *Mycobacterium tuberculosis* (Kotake *et al.*, 1994); *Toxoplasma gondii* (Norrie *et al.*, 1996); *Borrelia burgdorferi* using a specific gene from cerebrospinal fluid and vitreous in Lyme disease (Karma *et al.*, 1995); and for a DNA fragment with sequence specificity for the 16S rRNA gene of *Tropheryma whippelii* in an AIDS patient (Maiwald *et al.*, 1995).

Rochalimaea henselae, the possible aetiological agent of cat-scratch disease, was identified by PCR in a patient with Parinaud's oculoglandular syndrome in whom culture was unhelpful (Le *et al.*, 1994). PCR, using appropriate primers, can be applied to tissue containing *Histoplasma capsulatum* or to *Toxoplasma gondii* in paraffin-embedded sections (Brezin *et al.*, 1990), by a technique which involves *in situ* hybridization. This technique can similarly be used to identify mycoses in tissue, including *Fusarium* spp. (Alexandrakis *et al.*, 1996). The limitation of the PCR method is a failure to distinguish between live and dead organisms. PCR has been used to relate human Papillomavirus 16 to squamous cell carcinoma in AIDS patients (Maclean *et al.*, 1996).

Molecular methods, including Southern blotting, have been used in laboratory practice in recent years. These techniques essentially include extraction of nucleic acids (DNA and RNA) from intact or disrupted microbial cells, the cloning of specific fragments of the DNA in bacteria, the determination of the precise sequence of bases of the DNA fragment (the process of sequencing) and the accurate detection of a specific DNA fragment within a complete genome by use of a labelled probe (the process of hybridization). Molecular typing of this nature can also be achieved using an analogous method termed 'random amplification of polymorphic DNA' (RAPD); this approach has been used, for example, to type strains of *C. trachomatis* (Scieux *et al.*, 1993).

Mitochondrial DNA fingerprinting by restriction fragment length polymorphism (RFLP) of *Acanthamoeba* spp. has been used to compare clinical and environmental isolates (Gautom *et al.*, 1994). Genus- and subgenus-specific oligonucleotide probes for *Acanthamoeba* spp. have been developed using the fluorescent *in situ* hybridization (FISH) technique (Stothard *et al.*, 1999). An 18S rDNA PCR method has been developed for identification of genus and genotype of *Acanthamoeba* spp. using both clinical and environmental isolates (Schroeder *et al.*, 2000).

Appendix D
A SIMPLE SCHEME FOR ASSESSING AND MANAGING WOUNDS
Jackie Middleton

It is important to record details of wound care management in order to be sure that adequate healing is taking place. This is especially needed for care of pressure sores in the elderly or immobile patient in whom there can be further erosion of tissue without healing over several months. By charting the progress of each wound, it is soon obvious whether healing is progressing or failing. Failure to heal needs to be recognized early and the reasons investigated whether it be malnutrition in the patient or a type of antiseptic dressing that is deleterious for the wound.

A suggested scheme is given for assessing wounds which involves the physician, nurse and pharmacist. The form should be completed as accurately as possible, initially and after each dressing change. The following notes (*) are to assist completion of the form:

Location of wound:	position of wound on the body *viz.* dorsal surface left forearm
Type of wound:	burn, pressure sore, leg ulcer, surgical wound, trauma etc.
Grade of wound:	**1a** red or blistered area that may break down
	1b healed area covered by a scab
	2 superficial break in skin *viz.* graze
	3 destruction of skin but no cavity visible
	4 destruction of skin and underlying tissue with cavity

A **primary dressing** is applied directly to the wound; a **secondary dressing** holds it in place.

Skin care management of the elderly and immobile patient is important 'around the clock' to prevent the formation of pressure sores. This involves nursing care turning the patient frequently and use of the various types of pressure-changing beds.

Wound treatment chart

Patient Label (name, age, address)	Sensitivities/allergies Ward
Consultant	Date Weight of patient
Location of wound*	Type of wound* Grade of wound*
Wound assessed by	Nurse responsible Pharmacist responsible
Dressing(s) selected Primary* Secondary*	Trade name Cost
Dressing changes recommended	.... times per day .... times per week

| Dressing change Number | 1 | 2 | 3 | 4 | 5 | 6 |
| | 7 | 8 | 9 | 10 | 11 | 12 |
	13	14	15	16	17	18
Date						
Time						
Length of wound (mm)						
Width of wound (mm)						
Depth of wound (mm)						
Operator						

Accurate assessment of healing is essential in wound care management. A multi-disciplinary approach between practitioners ensures the most effective care can be achieved for the patient. Following careful assessment of the wound and the level of tissue repair, the most appropriate dressing can be selected from the wide range currently available (Appendix E). The characteristics of the optimum dressing have been described by many authors, but fundamentally, an ideal dressing should allow a wound to heal naturally and provide protection from further damage and infection.

The process of healing is dependent on a variety of factors and circumstances which must be considered at the initial wound assessment. Factors which affect wound healing have been described in many text books and include infection, poor hydration, mobility and nutritional status. Good nutrition and wound hydration are of particular importance and McLaren (1992) has stated that if these factors are not properly addressed, healing may not take place.

Wound classification methods are often based on the assessment of tissue loss. Wounds with minimal tissue loss, such as a surgical incision, heal by first intention. Wounds with extensive tissue loss such as pressure sores and leg ulcers heal by second intention. In the latter case, more granulation tissue is needed to occupy the wound cavity and healing is often prolonged. Chronic wounds are defined as those of long duration with slow healing and a likelihood of recurrence (Dealey, 1999). These wounds are often contaminated with micro-organisms and the risk of infection is high. Although the healing process is slow, careful and regular assessments are still essential to recognise early signs of complications.

An holistic approach to wound care ensures that nurses assess *all* the patients' needs, including nutrition, mobility, pain control and anxiety as the resolution of all these issues will contribute to successful wound healing.

Appendix E
WHICH DRESSING? A PHARMACOPOEIA OF POSSIBILITIES

A flow diagram for assessing which type of dressing to place on an open wound is given in Fig. E.1 (Which dressing?). This diagram considers the possibilites of infectious versus non-infectious discharge and the 'wet' and 'dry' wound. Details of individual techniques and products are given below, including instructions when *not* to use them.

The Wound Chart (Appendix D) is used to monitor the progress of a wound and should be kept with the care plans including the type of dressing prescribed. When a patient is discharged from hospital, the Wound Chart should be filed in the patient's notes for future reference.

Leg ulcers and other lesions below the knee

These wounds often have a complex aetiology including vascular insufficiency, and need specialist treatment. Advice must be given by the physician or surgeon before any treatment is undertaken.

General wound cleansing

Gentle irrigation with warmed normal saline (0.9%) is the method of choice. Avoid the use of cotton wool or gauze where possible as these products adhere to the wound as foreign body particles and interfere with structured tissue regeneration (see Chapter 6).

When a detergent or antiseptic action is needed, chlorhexidine gluconate 0.05% (pink solution in sachets – e.g. Unisept) may be used. Avoid using in the eyes and middle ear.

It is important to ensure that the wound remains moist at all times as moist wounds heal more rapidly than dry wounds and with less scarring.

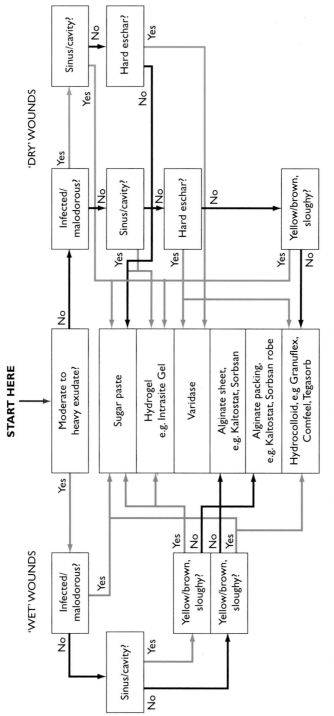

Figure E.1: Which dressing? Examine the wound carefully and assess the level of exudate. Use the flow diagram above to choose the most appropriate dressing.

Dressings for infected / malodorous wounds

If it is thought that a wound is infected, it must be swabbed for microbial culture and antibiotic sensitivities; antibiotic therapy is indicated only if there is surrounding cellulitis.

Hydrogel dressings

A typical gel, such as Intrasite (formerly Scherisorb) gel, consists of a modified carmellose co-polymer, water and propylene glycol. It is a thick, translucent paste and is presented premixed in sachets.

Indications

Intrasite gel is recommended for use on wet and dry wounds. It can also be used to soften and hydrate an eschar (the thick, black, dry 'leather' material) found on some wounds. It will absorb excess exudate from a wound and it can also be used for instillation into sinuses.

Method of use

Squeeze the gel directly on to the wound and smooth to a depth of approximately 5 mm (1/4 in.).

Cover with a low-adherent secondary dressing (such as Melolin) and tape in place or use a semipermeable film dressing (such as Opsite or Tegaderm). The use of a film dressing is particularly important if there is a possibility of contamination, for example, with faeces.

Frequency of dressing change

For sloughing and dry wounds change daily. When wounds are granulating a change of dressing every 3 days should suffice.

Sugar paste

Sugar paste consists of finely ground powdered sugar (sucrose) and polyethylene glycol 400 (refer to Chapter 6). It is available in thin and thick formulations and is presented in plastic screw-capped containers. It should be stored in the refrigerator and warmed to body temperature before use. It needs to be prepared in controlled clean conditions (instructions given in Chapter 6 and available from Dr K Middleton, Principal Pharmacist, Northwick Park Hospital, Harrow, Middlesex, HA1 3UJ, UK).

Indications

Sugar paste is the treatment of choice for infected and malodorous wounds. It has also been used with good effect on sloughy and granulating wounds. The thin paste is suitable for instillation into abscess cavities with narrow openings or sinuses. The thick paste can be used for packing into deep wounds, including pressure sores, or applying to flat open wounds (refer to Chapter 6).

Sugar paste is not suitable for the treatment of wounds with a hard eschar.

Method of use

Thin paste. Warm the container of sugar paste to body temperature and stir thoroughly to ensure even mixing. To apply, remove the plunger from a syringe and pour the sugar paste directly into the barrel of the syringe. Reinsert the plunger and apply the paste directly to the wound. Alternatively, for application to a sinus attach a Kwill (fine plastic tubing) to the end of the syringe before instillation.

Cover immediately with non-adherent secondary dressing and tape in place. If possible, use a semipermeable film dressing such as Opsite or Tegaderm where contamination due to faeces etc. is likely.

Thick paste. Warm the sugar paste in its original container to body temperature. To pack a cavity, remove the paste from the container with a gloved hand and fill the wound to overflowing (refer to Chapter 6). For a surface wound, apply a layer approximately 12– 25 mm (1/2–1 in.) thick. Cover immediately with a non-adherent dressing and tape in place. If possible, use a semipermeable film dressing (such as Opsite) where contamination such as from faeces is likely.

Frequency of dressing change

For the best effect, apply sugar paste twice daily – this is particularly important for infected and malodorous wounds as the paste breaks down and liquefies. If necessary, cleanse the wound with normal saline (warmed) before redressing.

Note: Sugar paste can be used safely in diabetic patients – any sucrose that may be absorbed from a wound will be excreted unchanged in the urine. The sucrose in sugar paste is not split to glucose and fructose as the necessary enzyme is only found in the gastrointestinal tract and not in wounds, skin or systemically.

Varidase

Varidase is a biological debriding agent that contains two enzymes, streptokinase and streptodornase, whose combined effects lead to the liquefaction of the main viscous substances resulting from inflammatory or infective processes. Varidase has no effect on collagen or healthy tissue. The Varidase Topical combi-pack contains a vial of dry sterile powder, a 20-ml vial of sterile normal saline and a sterile transfer needle.

Varidase can be used to cleanse necrotic and infected wounds and is of particular value in aiding the removal of hard black eschar and thick dry slough.

Method of use

Reconstitution: add 20 ml normal saline slowly to the vial of dry Varidase powder using the transfer needle provided. Shake very gently and avoid frothing – vigorous shaking will destroy the enzymes in Varidase. The resulting clear solution can be withdrawn into a syringe. Any unused solution may be stored in a refrigerator for up to 24 hours, after which time it must be discarded.

To aid in the removal of hard eschar the preferred methods of application are:

1. to cross-hatch the area into approximately 3–5-mm squares using a sterile scalpel and to a sufficient depth to allow penetration of the enzyme solution to the underlying material. Soak a piece of gauze in the Varidase solution and apply directly to the wound. Cover the wound with a semipermeable film dressing such as Opsite or Tegaderm to prevent drying.
2. to inject Varidase with a syringe and needle into the area beneath the eschar. Take care not to inject too much, as this will increase pressure beneath the eschar and cause pain. Cover with a semipermeable film dressing.

The eschar will invariably loosen after a few days of such treatment and can often be removed mechanically.

Other methods of applying Varidase are:

1. presoak a piece of gauze with Varidase and apply directly to the wound. To prevent drying, cover with a semipermeable film dressing (such as Opsite or Tegaderm).
2. pack the wound lightly with gauze and then soak with Varidase. To prevent drying cover with a semipermeable film dressing (such as Opsite or Tegaderm).
3. dissolve the contents of a vial of Varidase in 5 ml sterile water and mix thoroughly with 15 ml sterile lubricating jelly (such as K-Y jelly) and apply directly to the wound. This method may be beneficial when the use of other dressings is not possible or is undesirable.

Frequency of dressing changes

Varidase treatment should be repeated once or twice daily. Continue therapy until granulation tissue begins to form and re-epithelialization has begun (usually 1–2 weeks).

Other treatments available for infected wounds

Povidone-iodine ointment (Betadine) is useful for some wounds but must not be used for prolonged therapy. Povidone-iodine is more toxic for polymorphonuclear cells than for bacteria (Broek and Furth, 1980) so that it can delay wound healing and should only be used with caution.

Acetic acid 3% can be used on wounds infected with *Pseudomonas* spp., which are particularly susceptible to it.

Phenoxyethanol 2.2% solution is good for wounds known to be contaminated with *Pseudomonas* spp. and *Proteus* spp. but not very effective against other micro-organisms.

Dressings for non-infected wounds

Alginate dressings

There are many products within this group and the gelling characteristics vary according to the product used. Some products have limited gelling capacity and form a partially gelled sheet that can be easily lifted off whilst others form an amorphous gel that can be rinsed off with normal saline.

Indications

These dressings are ideal for the management of bleeding wounds, including lacerations and nosebleeds. Alginate dressings are also suitable for application to exuding (wet) wounds.

Contraindications

Alginate dressings should not be used on dry wounds or those covered with hard necrotic tissue. In addition, alginates are not recommended for use on dirty or infected wounds.

Method of use

First cleanse the wound – warmed normal saline is the solution of choice – and place the dressing lightly on the wound surface. Cover with a low-adherent secondary dressing such as Melolin or, if the wound is very wet, an absorbent pad, and tape in place.

Alginate 'rope' is suitable for packing cavities and large sinuses, but it should not be placed into narrow sinuses nor packed tightly as removal may be difficult. Cover the area with an appropriate secondary dressing such as Melolin and tape in place.

Removal of alginate fibres is facilitated by irrigation with warmed normal saline.

Frequency of change

Heavily exuding wounds require daily changes of the dressing. Wounds producing less exudate will require less frequent changes, typically every 2–3 days.

Hydrocolloid dressings

These include Granuflex, Comfeel and Tegasorb. They invariably consist of a thin plastic film on to which is bonded a mixture of materials, usually natural products including gelatin, pectin and carboxymethylcellulose. They are presented as sheets or wafers and interact with wound exudate to form a viscous yellowish gel.

Indications

Hydrocolloids are suitable for the treatment of a wide range of wound types ranging from dry wounds to those with a moderate level of exudate. They are also of value in the treatment of wounds covered with dry, black necrotic tissue (eschar) as often found on the heels and elbows of bedridden patients.

Contraindications

Hydrocolloids should not be used on clinically infected wounds or on heavily exuding wounds.

Method of use

Remove the dressing from the backing paper and press gently into position over the wound. To ensure good adhesion of the dressing to the surrounding skin it is essential to allow an overlap of at least 3 cm from the margin of the wound. As the dressing warms to body heat adhesion will improve.

265

A secondary dressing is not usually required over a hydrocolloid. However there are occasions when the dressing may slide over the wound, for instance when applied to the sacral area, and in these circumstances it may be advisable to secure the edge of the dressing with a secondary adhesive dressing. Hypafix or Mefix may be suitable for this purpose in many patients but should not be used where the skin is fragile or delicate.

Note: This type of dressing, when in contact with a wound, liquefies to produce a yellow pus-like material which has a strong odour. Both the patient and the nurse should be aware that this is not pus and does not indicate the presence of infection.

Care must be taken to avoid disturbing the margins of the wound when removing hydrocolloid dressings. The wound should be cleaned carefully with warmed normal saline before application of the next dressing.

Frequency of dressing change

As the matrix of the dressing absorbs exudate it forms a yellowish mass which is visible through the back of the dressing. When the area of the yellow mass is the same as that of the wound the dressing should be changed. On heavily exuding wounds this process may take only 1 day (in which case it would be advisable to reconsider the choice of dressing), but on drier wounds the dressing may need changing as infrequently as every 7 days.

Wound treatments to avoid

The following dressings have been shown to be either ineffective or deleterious to wounds and the granulation process. They are not recommended for use unless chemical *debridement* is required, such as for heavily contaminated war wounds when Eusol or related products are relevant in the early management.

- Topical antibiotics in gauze (tulle) dressing – Fucidin (fusidic acid) Tulle (Intertulle), framycetin sulphate 1% (Sofra-Tulle), Cicatrin (neomycin/bacitracin) (hospital pharmacy produced):
  - cell-mediated hypersensitivity/allergic reactions may occur;
  - antibiotic resistance may develop;
  - there may be adherence to granulation tissue and damage when removed.
- Eusol (Chlorinated Lime and Boric Acid Solution BP 1993) and related products, such as Dakin's solution (Surgical Chlorinated Soda Solution BPC 1973 [0.5% available chlorine in sterile water]) and Chloramine-T (1 in 250 dilution of powder lethal to most bacteria):
  - extremely toxic to all skin cells, leucocytes and bacteria;
  - impairs blood flow to wounds.

- Cetrimide in Travasept, Tisept, cetrimide cream:
  - extremely toxic to all wound tissues and leucocytes even at very low concentrations.
- Chlorhexidine paraffin tulle – Bactigras:
  - tends to adhere to wounds;
  - chlorhexidine is poorly released from ointments (this does not apply to creams).
- Debrisan (dextranomer beads, paste and pads):
  - not particularly effective;
  - often difficult to remove from wounds;
  - very expensive.
- Dyes, for example gentian violet, brilliant green, mercurochrome:
  - not very effective;
  - potentially very toxic.
- Proflavine – usually presented as a cream or emulsion:
  - poor antibacterial activity as the proflavine is not released from the emulsion base;
  - mutagenic.
  - stains bright yellow.
- Metronidazole gel:
  - should only be used to treat rosacea;
  - antibiotics/antibacterials given systemically should not be used topically; metronidazole is best used orally (400 mg three times daily) to aid the management of malodorous wounds along with sugar paste applied topically.
- Gauze packing:
  - Highly undesirable as the new granulation tissue will grow into the mesh of the packing material and be destroyed as the dressing is removed (refer to Chapter 6).

The table below (E.1) compares the prices of various recommended products as sold for a single treatment regimen.

Table E.1 Price guide.

	Size	Price (UK£)
Granuflex wafers	10 × 10 cm	2.18
	15 × 20 cm	4.48
	20 × 30 cm	11.15
Granuflex paste	30 g	2.68
Kaltostat sheets	7.5 × 12 cm	1.62
	15 × 25 cm	6.40
Kaltostat 'rope'	2 g	3.00
Sugar paste	250 g	3.60
Varidase	1 vial	8.57

REFERENCES

Adachi J, Endo K, Fukuzumi T et al. (1998) Increasing incidence of streptococcal impetigo in atopic dermatitis. *J Dermatol Sci*, **17**, 45–53.

Adam RD, Hunter G, Di Tomasso J et al. (1994) Mucormycosis: emerging prominence of cutaneous infections. *Clin Infect Dis*, **19**, 67–76.

Aebi C, Ahmed A, Ramilo O (1996) Bacterial complications of primary varicella in children. *Clin Infect Dis*, **23**, 698–705.

Ajello L, McGinnis M (1984) Nomenclature of human pathogenic fungi. In: Weufen W, Berencsi G, Groschel D et al. (eds) *Grundlagen der Antiseptik*, vol. 1, part 4. Verlag Volk und Gesundheit: Berlin, 365–77.

Alexandrakis G, Sears M, Gloor P (1996) Postmortem diagnosis of *Fusarium* panophthalmitis by the polymerase chain reaction. *Am J Ophthalmol*, **121**, 221–5.

Allen AM, Taplin D, Twigg L (1971) Cutaneous streptococcal infections in Vietnam. *Arch Dermatol*, **104**, 271–80.

Ambrose U, Middleton K, Seal DV (1991) In vitro studies of water activity and bacterial growth inhibition of Sucrose-Polyethylene Glycol 400-Hydrogen Peroxide and Xylose-Polyethylene Glycol 400-Hydrogen Peroxide pastes used to treat infected wounds. *Antimicrob Agents Chemother*, **35**, 1799–803.

Amin SB, Ryan RM, Metlay LA et al. (1998) *Absidia corymbifera* infections in neonates. *Clin Infect Dis*, **26**, 990–2.

Anandi V, Jeya M, Subramaniyan CS et al. (1997) Actinomycotic mycetoma of the thumb. *Indian J Med Microbiol*, **15**, 43–4.

Anonymous (editorial) (1991) Healing of cavity wounds. *Lancet*, **337**, 1010–11.

Arbuthnott J, Furman B (eds) (1998) *European Conference on Toxic Shock Syndrome.* International Congress and Symposium Series 229. Royal Society of Medicine, London: 1–216.

Archer H, Middleton K, Seal D et al. (1987) Toxicity of topical sugar. *Lancet*, **i**, 1485–6.

Archer H, Middleton K, Seal D et al. (1990) A controlled model of moist wound healing: comparison between semi-permeable film, antiseptics and sugar paste. *J Exp Path*, **71**, 155–70.

Arsura EL, Kilgore WB, Caldwell JW et al. (1998) Association between facial cutaneous coccidiomyocosis and meningitis. *West J Med*, **169**, 13–16.

Asbell PA, Torres MA, Kamenar T et al. (1995) Rapid diagnosis of ocular *Herpes simplex* infections. *Br J Ophthalmol*, **79**, 473–5.

Attapattu MC (1997a) Human mycotic infections in Sri Lanka: new trends and challenges. In: Srivastava OP, Srivastava AK, Shukla PK (eds) *Advances in Medical Mycology*, vol. 2. Evoker Research Perfecting Co., Lucknow, India: 77–89.

Attapattu MC (1997b) Chromoblastomycosis – a clinical and mycological study of 71 cases from Sri Lanka. *Mycopathologia*, **137**, 145–51.

Bargman H (1995) Successful treatment of cutaneous sporotrichosis with liquid nitrogen: report of three cases. *Mycoses*, **38**, 285–7.

Barker F, Leppard B, Seal DV (1987) Streptococcal necrotizing fasciitis: comparison between histological and clinical features. *J Clin Pathol*, **40**, 335–41.

Barrios NJ, Kirkpatrick DV, Murciano A *et al.* (1990) Successful treatment of disseminated *Fusarium* infection in an immunocompromised child. *Am J Paediatr Haematol Oncol*, **12**, 319–24.

Begovac J, Morton E, Lisic M *et al.* (1990) Group A beta-haemolytic streptococcal toxic shock-like syndrome. *Pediatr Inf Dis J*, **9**, 369–70.

Belani K, Schlievert PM, Kaplan EL *et al.* (1991) Association of exotoxin-producing group A streptococci and severe disease in children. *Pediatr Infect Dis J*, **10**, 351–4.

Bentur Y, Shupak A, Ramon Y *et al.* (1998) Hyperbaric oxygen therapy for cutaneous soft-tissue zygomycosis complicating diabetes mellitus. *Plast Reconstr Surg*, **102**, 822–4.

Bergdoll MS (1990) Toxic shock syndrome from surgical infections. In: Wadstrom T, Eliasson I, Holder I, Ljungh A (eds) *Pathogenesis of Wound and Biomaterial-Associated Infections*. Springer-Verlag, London: 121–8.

Bessen DE, Sotir CM, Readdy TL *et al.* (1996) Genetic correlates of throat and skin isolates of group A streptococci. *J Infect Dis*, **173**, 896–900.

Bhatti N, Larson E, Seal DV *et al.* (1990) Encephalitis due to Epstein–Barr virus. *J Infect*, **20**, 69–72.

BHIVA Guidelines Co-ordinating Committee (1997) British HIV Association guidelines for antiretroviral treatment of HIV seropositive individuals. *The Lancet*, **349**, 1086–92.

Bodemer C, Panhans A, Chretien-Marquet B *et al.* (1997) Staphylococcal necrotizing fasciitis in the mammary region in childhood: a report of five cases. *J Pediatr*, **131**, 466–9.

Boffa MJ, Wilkinson SM, Beck MH (1996) Screening for corticosteroid hypersensitivity. *Contact Dermatitis*, **33**, 149–51.

Bonifaz A, Martinez-Soto E, Carrasco-Gerard E *et al.* (1997) Treatment of chromoblastomycosis with itraconazole, cryosurgery and a combination of both. *Int J Dermatol*, **36**, 542–7.

Booth LV, Lang DA, Athersuch R (1990) Isolation of *Vibrio cholerae* non-01 from a Somerset farmworker and his tropical fish tank. *J Infect*, **20**, 55–7.

Borges AS, Ferreira MS, Silvestre MT *et al.* (1997) Histoplasmosis in immunodepressed patients; study of 18 cases seen in Unberlandia, MG, Brazil. *Rev Soc Bras Med Trop*, **30**, 119–24.

Bourrel P, Andreu JM, Cazenave B (1989) Mycetoma of the hand. Apropos of ten cases. *Ann Chir*, **43**; 814–23.

Brennan SS, Leaper DJ (1985) The effect of antiseptics on the healing wound: a study using the rabbit ear chamber. *Br J Surg* **72**, 780–2.

Brewer GE, Meleney FL (1926) Progressive gangrenous infection of the skin and subcutaneous tissues, following operation for acute perforative appendicitis. *Ann Surg*, **84**, 438–50.

Brezin AP, Equga CE, Burnier M *et al.* (1990) Identification of *Toxoplasma gondii* in paraffin-embedded sections by the polymerase chain reaction. *Am J Ophthalmol*, **110**, 599–604.

Broek PJ van den, Furth R van (1980) Interaction between Betadine solution, cells and micro-organisms. In: The Proceedings of the World Congress on Antisepsis. HP Publishing, New York: 25-7.

Brook I (1988) Pathogenicity of capsulate and non-capsulate members of *Bacteroides fragilis* and *B. melaninogenicus* groups in mixed infections with *Escherichia coli* and *Streptococcus pyogenes*. *J Med Microbiol*, **27**, 191–8.

Brook I (1996) Aerobic and anaerobic microbiology of necrotizing fasciitis in children. *Pediatr Dermatol*, **13**, 281–4.

Brook I, Frazier EH (1995) Clinical and microbiological features of necrotizing fasciitis. *J Clin Microbiol*, **33**, 2382–7.

Brook MG, Bannister BA (1988) Scarlet fever can mimic toxic shock syndrome. *Postgrad Med J*, **64**, 965–7.

Brun-Buisson C (1998) Methicillin-resistant *Staphylococcus aureus*: evolution et epidemiologie. *Pathol Biol*, **46**, 227–34.

Bryceson ADM, Hay RJ (1998) Parasitic worms and protozoa. In: Champion RH, Burton JL, Burns DA, Breathnach SM (eds) *Rook, Wilkinson & Ebling's Textbook of Dermatology*. Blackwell Science, London: 1377–1422.

Campbell CK (1987) *Polycytella hominis* gen. et sp. nov., a cause of human pale grain mycetoma. *J Med Vet Mycol*, **25**, 301–5.

Cao L, Chen DL, Lee C *et al.* (1998) Detection of specific antibodies to an antigenic mannoprotein for diagnosis of *Penicillium marneffei* penicilliosis. *J Clin Microbiol*, **36**, 3028-31.

Castro LGM, Salebian A, Sotto MN (1990) Hyalohyphomycosis by *Paecilomyces lilacinus* in a renal transplant patient and a review of human *Paecilomyces* species infections. *J Med Vet Mycol*, **28**, 15–26.

Chakrabarti A, Kumar P, Padhye AA *et al.* (1997) Primary cutaneous zygomycosis due to *Saksenaea vasiformis* and *Apophysomyces elegans*. *Clin Infect Dis* **24**, 580–3.

Chanarin I, Stephenson E (1988) Vegetarian diet and cobalamin deficiency: their association with tuberculosis. *J Clin Pathol* **41**, 759–62.

Chariyalestsak S, Sirisanthana T, Supparatpinyo K *et al.* (1996) Seasonal variation of disseminated *P. marneffei* infections in northern Thailand: a clue to the reservoir. *J Infect Dis*, **173**, 1490–3.

Chen CH, Shih JF, Hsu YT (1991) Disseminated coccidioidomycosis with skin, lung and lymph node involvement of a case. *J Formos Med Assoc*, **90**, 788–92.

Chirife J, Herszage L, Joseph A *et al.* (1983a) In vitro studies of bacterial growth inhibition in concentrated sugar solutions: microbiological basis for the use of sugar in treating infected wounds. *Antimicrob Agents Chemother*, **23**, 766–73.

Chirife J, Herszage L, Joseph A *et al.* (1983b) In vitro antibacterial activity of concentrated polyethylene glycol 400 solutions. *Antimicrob Agents Chemother*, **24**, 409–12.

Chodorowska G, Lecewicz-Torun B (1996) Long-term observation of a case of cutaneous blastomycosis in Poland treated with fluconazole. *Mycoses*, **39**, 283–7.

Chomarat M, Chapuis C, Lepape *et al.* (1990) Two cases of severe infection with beta-haemolytic group A streptococci associated with a toxic-shock-like syndrome. *Eur J Clin Microbiol Infect Dis*, **9**, 901–3.

Choong KY, Roberts LJ (1996) Ritual Samoan body tattooing and associated sporotrichosis. *Australas J Dermatol*, **37**, 50–3.

Cole GW, Silverberg NL (1986) The adherence of *Staphylococcus aureus* to human corneocytes. *Arch Dermatol*, **122**, 166–72.

Cone LA, Woodard DR, Schlievert PM *et al.* (1987) Clinical and bacteriological observations of a toxic-shock like syndrome due to *Streptococcus pyogenes*. *N Engl J Med*, **317**, 146–9.

Cooper RA, Molan PC, Harding KG (1999) Antibacterial activity of honey against strains of *Staphylococcus aureus* from infected wounds. *J Roy Soc Med*, **92**, 283–5.

Cormican MG, Pfaller MA (1993) Standardisation of antifungal susceptibility testing. *J Antimicrob Chemother*, **38**, 561–78.

Cuadros RG, Vidotto V, Bruatto M (1990) Sporotrichosis in the metropolitan area of Cusco, Peru, and its region. *Mycoses*, **33**, 231–40.

Cuce LC, Wroclawski EL, Sampaio SA (1980) Treatment of paracoccidioidomycosis, candidiasis, chromomycosis, lobomycosis and mycetoma with ketoconazole. *Int J Dermatol*, **19**, 405–8.

Darmstadt GL (1997) Staphylococcal and streptococcal skin infections. In: Harahap M (ed.) *Diagnosis and Treatment of Skin Infections*. Blackwell Science, London: 7–115.

Davies RR, Spencer H, Wakelin PO (1964) A case of human protothecosis. *Trans R Soc Trop Med Hyg*, **58**, 448–51.

Davson J, Jones DM, Turner L (1988) Diagnosis of Meleney's synergistic gangrene. *Br J Surg*, **75**, 267–71.

Deeks SG, Smith M, Holodniy M *et al.* (1997) HIV-1 protease inhibitors. *JAMA*, **277**, 145–53.

Deng Z, Yun M, Ajello L (1986) Human penicilliosis marneffei and its relation to the bamboo rat (*Rhizomys pruinosus*). *J Med Vet Mycol*, **24**, 383–9.

Desai AP, Pandit AA, Gupte PD (1997) Cutaneous blastomycosis: report of a case with diagnosis by fine needle aspiration cytology. *Acta Cytol*, **41** (Suppl 4), 1317–19.

Desakorn V, Smith MD, Walsh AL *et al.* (1999) Diagnosis of *Penicillium marneffei* infection by quantitation of urinary antigen by using an enzyme immunoassay. *J Clin Microbiol*, **37**, 117–21.

Develoux M, Ndiaye B, Dieng MT (1995) Mycetomas in Africa. *Sante*, **5**, 211–17.

Dewsnup DH, Galgiani JN, Graybill JR *et al.* (1996) Is it ever safe to stop azole therapy for *Coccidioides immitis* meningitis? *Ann Intern Med*, **124**, 305–10.

Diaz M, Puente R, de Hoyos LA *et al.* (1991) Itraconazole in the treatment of coccidioidomycosis. *Chest*, **100**, 682–4.

Dickinson M, Kalayanamit T, Yang CA *et al.* (1998) Cutaneous zygomycosis (mucormycosis) complicating endotracheal intubation; diagnosis and successful treatment. *Chest*, **114**, 340–2.

DiSalvo AF (1987) Mycotic morbidity – an occupational risk for mycologists. *Mycopathologia*, **99**, 147–53.

Dismukes WE, Bradsher RW, Cloud GC *et al.* (1992) Itraconazole therapy for blastomycosis and histoplasmosis. *Am J Med*, **93**, 489–97.

Dixon DM, Polak-Wyss A. (1991) The medically important dematiaceous fungi and their identification. *Mycoses*, **34**, 1–18.

Duong TA (1996) Infection due to *Penicillium marneffei*, an emerging pathogen: review of 155 reported cases. *Clin Infect Dis*, **23**, 125–30.

Edwards-Jones V, Foster HA (1994) The effect of topical antimicrobial agents on the production of toxic shock syndrome toxin-1. *J Med Microbiol*, **41**, 408–13.

Edwin C (1989) Structure–function analysis of toxic shock syndrome toxin 1. *Rev Inf Dis*, **11**(Suppl 1), 137–9.

Eisfelder M, Okumoto S, Toyoma K (1993) Experience with 241 sporotrichosis cases in China/Japan. *Hautarzt*, **44**, 524–8.

Emmons CW, Binford CH, Utz JP *et al.* (1977) *Medical Mycology*. Lea & Febiger, Philadelphia.

Evans MRW, Etuaful SN, Amofah G *et al.* (1999) Squamous cell carcinoma secondary to Buruli ulcer. *Trans Roy Soc Trop Med Hyg*, **93**, 63–4.

Fan J, Zhang WH, Wu YY *et al.* (1993) Detection of infections of the eye with *Chlamydia trachomatis* by the polymerase chain reaction. *Int Ophthalmol*, **17**, 327–30.

Farmer BA, Bradley JS, Smiley PW (1985) Toxic shock syndrome in a scald burn victim. *J Trauma*, **25**, 1004–6.

Ferguson MWJ, Leigh IM (1998) Wound healing. In: Champion RH, Burton JL, Burns DA, Breathnach SM (eds) *Rook, Wilkinson & Ebling's Textbook of Dermatology*. Blackwell Science, London: 337–56.

Ferris BD, Goldie B, Weir W (1987) An unusual presentation of tuberculosis – injury tuberculosis. *Injury*, **18**, 347–9.

Ficker L, Ramakrishnan M, Seal DV *et al.* (1991) Role of cell-mediated immunity to staphylococci in blepharitis. *Am J Ophthalmol*, **111**, 473-9.

Frame JD, Eve MD, Hackett MEJ *et al.* (1985) The toxic-shock syndrome in burned children. *Burns*, **11**, 234–41.

Frankel DH, Rippon JW (1989) *Hendersonula toruloidea* infection in man: index cases in the non-endemic American host, and a review of the literature. *Mycopathologia*, **105**, 175–86.

Frean J, Blumberg L, Woolf M (1993) Disseminated blastomycosis masquerading as tuberculosis. *J Infect*, **26**, 203–6.

Friedman GD (1994) *Primer of Epidemiology*, 4th edn. McGraw-Hill, New York.

Fuchs J, Milbradt R, Pecher SA (1990) Lobomycosis: case reports and overview. *Cutis*, **46**, 227–34.

Fujisawa H, Kohda H (1998) Necrotizing fasciitis caused by *Vibrio vulnificus* differs from that caused by streptococcal infection. *J Infect*, **36**, 313–16.

Galgiani B (1991) Coccidioidomycosis. In: Gatti F, de Vroey C, Persi A (eds) *Human Mycoses in Tropical Countries*, 13th edn. OCSI, Bologna: 197–201.

Galgiani JN (1993) Susceptibility testing of fungi: current status of the standardisation process. *Antimicrob Ag Chemother*, **37**, 2517–21.

Gaunt PN, Seal DV (1987) Group G streptococcal infection. *J Infect*, **15**, 5–20.

Gautom RK, Lory S, Seyedirashti S *et al.* (1994) Mitochondrial DNA fingerprinting of *Acanthamoeba* spp. isolated from clinical and environmental sources. *J Clin Microbiol*, **32**, 1070–3.

Ghannoum MA, Rex JH, Galgiani JN (1996) Susceptibility testing of fungi: current status of correlation of in vitro data with clinical outcome. *J Clin Microbiol*, **34**, 489–95.

Gordon H, Middleton K, Seal D *et al.* (1985) Sugar and wound healing. *Lancet*, **ii**, 663–4.

Grant SM, Clissold SP (1989) Itraconazole: a review of its pharmacodynamic and pharmacokinetic properties and therapeutic use in superficial and systemic mycoses. *Drugs*, **37**, 310–44.

Graybill JR, Stevens DA, Galgiani JN *et al.* (1990) Itraconazole treatment of coccidioidomycosis. *Am J Med*, **89**, 282–90.

Gubler DJ (1998) Dengue and dengue haemorrhagic fever. *Clin Microbiol Rev*, **11**, 480–96.

Guerrant RL (1986) Amebiasis: introduction, current status and research questions. *Rev Infect Dis*, **8**, 218–27.

Gugnani HC, Nzelibe FK, Osunkoo IC (1986) Onychomycosis due to *Hendersonula toruloidea* in Nigeria. *J Med Vet Mycol*, **24**, 239–41.

Gugnani HC, Ezeanolue BC, Khalil M *et al.* (1995) Fluconazole in the therapy of deep mycoses. *Mycoses*, **38**, 485–8.

Hajjeh R, McDonnell S, Reef S *et al.* (1997) Outbreak of sporotrichosis among tree nursery workers. *J Infect Dis,* **176**, 499–504.

Hallas G (1985) The production of pyrogenic exotoxins by group A streptococci. *J Hyg Camb,* **95**, 47–57.

Halow KD, Harner RC, Fontenelle LJ *et al.* (1996) Primary skin infections secondary to *Vibrio vulnificus*: the role of operative intervention. *J Am Coll Surg*, **183**, 329–34.

Hammar H, Wanger L (1977) Erysipelas and necrotizing fasciitis. *Br J Dermatol,* **96**, 409–19.

Hampp EG, Mergenhagen SE (1963) Experimental intracutaneous fusobacterial and fusospirochaetal infections. *J Infect Dis*, **112**, 84–99.

Harvey Wood K, Raine P, Seal DV *et al.* (1998) Five-year study of TSS in children with burns: value of screening. In: Arburthnott J, Furman B (eds) *European Conference on Toxic Shock Syndrome*. International Congress and Symposium Series 229. Royal Society of Medicine, London: 22–3.

Hay J, Kirkness CM, Seal DV *et al.* (1994) Drug resistance and *Acanthamoeba* keratitis: the quest for alternative antiprotozoal chemotherapy. *Eye*, **8**, 555–63.

Hay J, Seal DV (1996a) Ornamental fish: look but do not touch! *J R Soc Med*, **89**, 359.

Hay J, Seal DV (1996b) BSE: cow politics revisited. *J R Soc Med*, **89**, 659–60.

Hay RJ, Moore MK (1984) Clinical features of superficial fungal infections caused by *Hendersonula toruloidea* and *Scytalidium hyalinum*. *Br J Dermatol*, **110**, 677–83.

Hay RJ, Estrada Castenon R, Alarcon H *et al.* (1994) Wastage of family income on skin disease – a study of skin infection in Guerrero, Mexico. *BMJ*, **309**, 848–9.

Hay RJ, Moore MK (1998) Mycology. In: Champion RH, Burton JL, Burns DA, Breathnach SM (eds) *Rook, Wilkinson & Ebling's Textbook of Dermatology*. Blackwell Science, London: 1277–376.

Helm TN, Longworth PL, Hall GS *et al.* (1990) Case report and review of resolved fusariosis. *J Am Acad Dermatol*, **23**, 393–8.

Hemashettar BM, Patil CS (1989) Chronic paronychia and onychomycosis associated with *Fusarium solani* and *Trichosporon beigelii*. *J Sci Soc*, **16**, 3–6.

Herszage L, Montenegro JR, Joseph AL (1980) Tratamiento de las heridas supuradas con azucar granulado comercial. *Biol Trab Soc Argent*, **41**, 315–30.

Holm SE (1995) Epidemiology and pathogenesis of invasive group A streptococcal infections in Sweden. *Can J Infect Dis*, **6**(Suppl C), 235c [Abstract 0312].

Holt PA, Armstrong AM, Norfolk GA *et al.* (1987) Toxic-shock syndrome due to staphylococcal infection of a burn. *Br J Clin Pract*, **41**, 582–3.

Huerre M, Ravisse P, Solomon H *et al.* (1993) Human protothecosis and environment. *Bull Soc Pathol Exot*, **86**, 484–8.

Hutchinson JJ, Lawrence JC (1991) Wound infection under occlusive dressings. *J Hosp Infect*, **17**, 83–94.

Ijima S, Takase T, Otsuka F (1995) Treatment of chromomycosis with oral high dose of amphotericin B. *Arch Dermatol*, **131**, 399–401.

Imwidthaya P (1994a) Human pythiosis in Thailand. *Postgrad Med J*, **70**, 558–60.

Imwidthaya P (1994b) Systemic fungal infections in Thailand. *J Med Vet Mycol*, **32**, 395–9.

Imwidthaya P, Srimuang S (1992) Immunodiffusion test for diagnosing basidiobolomycosis. *Mycopathologia*, **118**, 127–31.

Jayanetra P, Nitiyanant P, Ajello L *et al.* (1984) Penicilliosis marneffei in Thailand; report of five human cases. *Am J Trop Med Hyg*, **33**, 637–44.

Jeddar A, Kharsany A, Ramsaroop K *et al.* (1985) The antibacterial action of honey: an in vitro study. *S Afr Med J*, **67**, 257–8.

Jha V, Sree Krishna V, Chakrabarti A *et al.* (1996) Subcutaneous phaeohyphomycosis in a renal transplant recipient: a case report and review of the literature. *Am J Kidney Dis*, **28**, 137–9.

Johnson LP, L'Italien JJ, Schlievert PM (1986) Streptococcal pyrogenic exotoxin type A (scarlet fever toxin) is related to *S. aureus* enterotoxin B. *Mol Gen Genet*, **203**, 354–6.

Joynt GM, Gomersall CD, Lyon DJ (1999) Severe necrotising fasciitis of the extremities caused by Vibrionaceae: experience of a Hong Kong tertiary referral hospital. *Hong Kong Med J*, **5**, 63–8.

Kalter DC (1986) The epidemiology of *Trichosporon beigelii* infection in Houston, Texas. *Br J Dermatol*, **115**(Suppl 30), 15.

Kamalam A, Thambiah AS (1979) Adiaspiromycosis of human skin caused by *Emmonsia crescens*. *Sabouraudia*, **17**, 377–81.

Kameswaran S (1991) Rhinosporidiosis. In: Gatti F, de Vroey C, Persi A (eds) *Human Mycoses in Tropical Countries*, 13th edn. OCSI, Bologna: 151–7.

Kanazaki H, Ueda M, Morishita Y *et al.* (1997) Producibility of exfoliative toxin and staphylococcal coagulase types of *S. aureus* strains isolated from skin infections and atopic dermatitis. *Dermatology*, **195**, 6–9.

Kantipong P, Panich V, Pongsurachet V *et al.* (1998) Hepatic penicilliosis in patients without skin lesions. *Clin Infect Dis*, **26**, 1215–17.

Kao TW, Hung CC, Hsueh PR *et al.* (1997) Microbiologic and histologic diagnosis of histoplasmosis in Asia. *J Formos Med Assoc*, **96**, 374–8.

Karma A, Seppala I, Mikkila H *et al.* (1995) Diagnosis and clinical characteristics of ocular Lyme borreliosis. *Am J Ophthalmol*, **119**, 127–35.

Kauffman CA (1995) Old and new therapies for sporotrichosis. *Clin Infect Dis*, **21**, 981–5.

Kauffman CA, Carver PL (1997) Use of azoles for systemic antifungal therapy. *Adv Pharmacol* **39**, 143–89.

Kauffman CA, Pappas PG, McKinsey DS *et al.* (1996) Treatment of lymphocutaneous and visceral sporotrichosis with fluconazole. *Clin Infect Dis*, **22**, 46–50.

Kaul R, McGeer A, Low DE *et al.* (1997) Population-based surveillance for group A streptococcal necrotizing fasciitis: clinical features, prognostic indicators and microbiologic analysis of 77 cases. Ontario Group A Streptococcal Study. *Am J Med*, **103**, 18–24.

Kennedy H, Seal DV (1996) Influence of inoculum, medium and serum on the in-vitro susceptibility of coagulase-negative staphylococci to teicoplanin and vancomycin. *J Antimicrob Chemother*, **37**, 1103–9.

Khaitan BK, Lakhanpal S, Banerjee U *et al.* (1998) Sporotrichosis in an unusual location – geographically and dermatologically. *Indian J Pathol Microbiol*, **41**, 461–3.

Kingston D, Seal DV (1990) Current hypotheses on synergistic microbial gangrene. *Br J Surg* **77**, 260–4.

Knutson RA, Merbitz LA, Creekmore MA *et al.* (1981) Use of sugar and povidone-iodine to enhance wound healing: five years' experience. *South Med J*, **74**, 1329–35.

Kotake S, Kimura K, Yoshikawa K *et al.* (1994) Polymerase chain reaction for the detection of *Mycobacterium tuberculosis* in ocular tuberculosis. *Am J Ophthalmol*, **117**, 805–6.

Krishnan SGS, Senthamilselvi G, Kamalam A *et al.* (1998) Entomophthoromycosis in India: a four-year study. *Mycoses*, **41**, 55–8.

Kullavanijaya P, Rojanavanich V (1995) Successful treatment of chromoblastomycosis due to *Fonsecaea pedrosoi* by the combination of itraconazole and cryotherapy. *Int J Dermatol*, **34**, 804–7.

Kumar B, Kaur I, Chakrabarti A *et al.* (1991) Treatment of deep mycoses with itraconazole. *Mycopathologia*, **115**, 169–74.

Kuo TT, Hseuh S, Wu JL *et al.* (1987) Cutaneous protothecosis: a clinicopathologic study. *Arch Pathol Lab Med*, **111**, 737–40.

Kusuhara M, Hachisuka H, Sasai Y (1988) Statistical survey of 150 cases of sporotrichosis. *Mycopathologia*, **102**, 129–33.

Kwangsukstith C, Vanittanakom N, Khanjanasthiti P *et al.* (1990) Cutaneous sporotrichosis in Thailand: first reported case. *Mycoses*, **33**, 513–17.

Lal S, Garg BR, Rao RS *et al.* (1984) Chromomycosis caused by *Exophiala jeanselmei*. *Indian J Dermatol Venereol Leprol*, **50**, 119–21.

Lasch EE, Frankel V, Vardy PA *et al.* (1971) Epidemic glomerulonephritis in Israel. *J Infect Dis*, **124**, 141–7.

Lawrence JC (1996) Dressings for burns. In: Settle JAD (ed.) *Principles and Practice of Burns Management*. Churchill Livingstone, London: 259–69.

Lawrence DN, Ajello L (1986) Lobomycosis in western Brazil: report of a clinical trial with ketoconazole. *Am J Trop Med*, **35**, 162–6.

Le HH, Palay DA, Anderson B *et al.* (1994) Conjunctival swab to diagnose ocular cat scratch disease. *Am J Ophthalmol*, **118**, 249–50.

Leff JA, Repine JE (1993) Neutrophil-mediated tissue injury. In: Abramson JS, Wheeler JG (eds) *The Neutrophil*. Oxford University Press, New York: 229–62.

Li YH, Toh CL, Khoo C *et al.* (1997a) Necrotising fasciitis – an old enemy or a new foe. *Ann Acad Med Singapore*, **26**, 175–8.

Li H, Zhang Y, Zhang Y (1997b) An epidemiological investigation report of sporotrichosis in Zhaodong area of Heilongjiang province. Abstracts of the 1st Congress of the Asia-Pacific Society for Medical Mycology, Nusa Dua-Bali, Indonesia, 4–7 December, p. 68.

Lima NS, Texeira G, Miranda J *et al.* (1977) Treatment of paracoccidioidomycosis with miconazole by the oral route: an on-going study. *Proc R Soc Med*, **70**(Suppl 1), 35–9.

Lin CS, Cheng SH (1998) *Aeromonas hydrophila* sepsis presenting as meningitis and necrotizing fasciitis in a man with alcoholic liver cirrhosis. *J Formos Med Assoc*, **97**, 498–502.

Linder N, Keller N, Huri C *et al.* (1998) Primary cutaneous mucormycosis in a premature infant: a case report and review of the literature. *Am J Perinatol*, **15**, 35–8.

Low DE (1995) Current concepts and future strategies to treat invasive streptococcal infections. *Can J Infect Dis*, **6**(Suppl C), 235c [Abstract 0314].

McAnally T, Parry EL (1985) Cutaneous protothecosis presenting as recurrent chromomycosis. *Arch Dermatol*, **121**, 1066–9.

McCullough CJ (1977) Tuberculosis as a late complication of total hip replacement. *Acta Orthop Scand*, **48**, 508–10.

Macdonald JB, Sutton RM, Knoll ML *et al.* (1956) The pathogenic components of an experimental fusospirochaetal infection. *J Infect Dis*, **98**, 15–20.

McGinnis MR (1996) Mycetoma. *Dermatol Clin*, **14**, 97–104.

Maclean H, Dhillon B, Ironside J (1996) Squamous cell carcinoma of the eyelid and the acquired immunodeficiency syndrome. *Am J Ophthalmol*, **121**, 219–21.

MacLennan JD (1943) Anaerobic infections of war wounds. *Lancet*, **ii**, 63–6, 94–9, 123–6.

Mahe A, Prual A, Konate M *et al.* (1995) Skin diseases of children in Mali: a public health problem. *Trans Roy Soc Trop Med Hyg*, **89**, 467–70.

Mahgoub ES (1989) Mycetoma. In: Hay RJ (ed.) *Tropical Fungal Infections*. Baillière's Clinical Tropical Medicine and Communicable Diseases, vol. 4, no. 1, 321–44.

Maiti PK, Haldar PK (1998) Mycetomas in exposed and non-exposed parts of the body: a study of 212 cases. *Indian J Med Microbiol*, **16**, 19–22.

Maiwald M, Meier-Willersen H, Hartmann M *et al.* (1995) Detection of *Tropheryma whippelii* DNA in a patient with AIDS. *J Clin Microbiol*, **33**, 1354–56.

Maresca B, Ali AI, Kobayashi GS (1987) Incidence of histoplasmin skin reactivity in Somalia: an epidemiological study. *Mycopathologia*, **98**, 77–81.

Marples RR, Richardson JF, Seal DV *et al.* (1985) Adhesive tapes in the special care baby unit. *J Hosp Infect*, **6**, 398–405.

Marshall J, Leeming JP, Holland KT (1987) The cutaneous microbiology of normal human feet. *J Appl Bacteriol*, **62**, 139–46.

Masri Fridling GD (1996) Dermatophytosis of the feet. *Dermatol Clin*, **14**, 33–40.

Matsumoto Y, Shibata M, Adachi A *et al.* (1996) Two cases of protothecosis in Nagoya, Japan. *Australas J Dermatol*, **37**(Suppl 1), 542–3.

Meleney FL (1924) Hemolytic streptococcus gangrene. *Arch Surg*, **9**, 317–64.

Mendoza L, Kaufman L, Mandy W *et al.* (1997) Serodiagnosis of human and animal pythiosis using enzyme-linked immunosorbent assay. *Clin Diagn Lab Immunol*, **4**, 715–18.

Middleton KR, Seal DV (1985) Sugar as an aid to wound healing. *Pharm J*, **235**, 757–8.

Mirelman D (1987) Ameba–bacterium relationship in amebiasis. *Microbiol Rev*, **51**, 272–84.

Monteil M, Hobbs J, Citron K (1987) Selective immunodeficiency affecting staphylococcal response. *Lancet,* **ii**, 880-83.

Monti JR, Chilton NB, Qian BZ *et al.* (1998) Specific amplification of *Necator americanus* or *Ancylostoma duodenale* DNA by PCR using markers in ITS-1 rDNA, and its implications. *Mol Cell Probes*, **12**, 71–8.

Moore MK (1986) *Hendersonula toruloidea* and *Scytalidium hyalinum* infections in London, England. *J Med Vet Mycol*, **24**, 219–30.

Mukherjee AK, Mukherjee D, Mukhopadhayay M (1986) Histoplasmosis in India: a clinicopathological review with a report of a case in a child. *Indian J Pathol Microbiol*, **29**, 263–70.

Mukhopadhyay D, Ghosh LM, Thammayya A *et al.* (1995) Entomophthoromycosis caused by *Conidiobolus coronatus*: clinicomycological study of a case. *Auris Nasus Larynx*, **22**, 139–42.

Murdoch I, Abiose A, Babalola O *et al.* (1994) Ivermectin and onchocercal optic neuritis: short-term effects. *Eye*, **8**, 456–61.

Naidu J, Singh SM (1997) Medical mycology in India: retrospectives and perspectives. In: Srivastava OP, Srivastava AK, Shukla PK (eds) *Advances in Medical Mycology*, vol. 2. Evoker Research Perfecting Co., Lucknow, India: 91–110.

Nasta P, Donisi A, Cattane A *et al.* (1997) Acute histoplasmosis in Spelunkers returning from Mato Grosso, Peru. *J Travel Med*, **4**, 176–8.

Nather A, Wong FYH, Balasubramaniam P *et al.* (1987) Streptococcal necrotizing myositis: a rare entity. A report of 2 cases. *Clin Orthop*, **215**, 206–11.

National Committee for Clinical Laboratory Standards (1997) Reference method for broth dilution antifungal susceptibility testing of yeasts. Approved standard M27A. Wayne, USA: NCCLS.

Negroni R, Rubinstein P, Hermmann A *et al.* (1997) Results of miconazole therapy in twenty-eight patients with paracoccidioidomycosis. *Proc R Soc Med*, **70**, (Suppl. 1): 24–8.

Ng KH, Siar CH (1996) Review of oral histoplasmosis in Malaysians. *Oral Surg Oral Med Oral Pathol Oral Radiol Endod*, **81**, 303–7.

Noble WC (1997) Staphylococcal carriage and skin and soft tissue infection. In: Crossley KB, Archer GL (eds) *The Staphylococci in Human Disease*. Churchill Livingstone, New York: 401–12.

Noble WC, Hope YM, Midgley G *et al.* (1986) Toewebs as a source of Gram-negative bacilli. *J Hosp Infect*, **8**, 248–56.

Norrie K, Tokushima T, Yano A (1996) Quantitative polymerase chain reaction in diagnosing ocular toxoplasmosis. *Am J Ophthalmol*, **121**, 441–2.

Nouira R, Denguezli M, Skhiri S *et al.* (1994) Cutaneopulmonary blastomycosis. *Ann Dermatol Venereol*, **121**, 180–2.

Odds FC, van Gerven F, Espinel-Ingroff A *et al.* (1998) Evaluation of possible correlations between antifungal susceptibilities of filamentous fungi in vitro and antifungal treatment outcomes in animal infection models. *Antimicrob Ag Chemother*, **42**, 282–8.

O'Grady F, Lambert H, Finch RG *et al.* (eds) (1997) *Antibiotic and Chemotherapy*, 7th edn. Churchill Livingstone, London.

Onderdonk AB, Kasper DL, Mansheim BJ *et al.* (1979) Experimental animal models of anaerobic infections. *Rev Infect Dis*, **1**, 291–301.

Otoyama K, Tomizawa N, Niguchi I *et al.* (1989) Cutaneous protothecosis: a case report. *J Dermatol*, **16**, 496–9.

Oyeka CA, Gugnani HC (1992) Isoconazole nitrate versus clotrimazole in foot and nail infections due to *Hendersonula toruloidea*, *Scytalidium hyalinum* and dermatophytes. *Mycoses*, **35**, 357–61.

Padhye AA, Pathak AA, Katkar VJ *et al.* (1994) Oral histoplasmosis in India: a case report and an overview of cases reported during 1968–1992. *J Med Vet Mycol*, **32**, 93–103.

Page FC (1988) A new key to freshwater and soil gymnamoebae. Culture collection of algae and protozoa. Fresh Water Biological Association, Cumbria, UK.

Paraskaki I, Lebessi E, Legakis NJ (1996) Epidemiology of community-acquired *Pseudomonas aeruginosa* infections in children. *Europ J Clin Microbiol Infect Dis*, **15**, 782–6.

Parra G, Rodriguez-Iturbe B, Batsford S *et al.* (1998) Antibody to streptococcal zymogen in the serum of patients with acute glomerulonephritis: a multicentric study. *Kidney Int*, **54**, 509–17.

Paul C, Dupont B, Pialoux G *et al.* (1991) Chromoblastomycosis with malignant transformation and cutaneous-synovial secondary localisation. The potential therapeutic role of itraconazole. *J Med Vet Mycol*, **29**, 313–15.

Peerapur BV, Inamadar AC (1997) Mycetoma of the scalp due to *Nocardia brasiliensis*. *Indian J Med Microbiol*, **15**, 85–6.

Penland RL, Wilhelmus KR (1997) Comparison of axenic and monoxenic media for isolation of *Acanthamoeba*. *J Clin Microbiol*, **35**, 915–22.

Penman AD, Lanier DC, Avara WT *et al.* (1995) *Vibrio vulnificus* wound infections from the Mississippi Gulf coastal waters: June to August 1993. *South Med J*, **88**, 531–3.

Persing DH, Smith TF, Tenover FC *et al.* (eds) (1995) *Diagnostic Molecular Microbiology. Principles and Applications.* American Society for Microbiology, USA.

Pfaller MA, Rex JH, Rinaldi MG (1997) Antifungal susceptibility testing: technical advances and potential clinical applications. *Clin Infect Dis*, **24**, 776–84.

Pierard GE, Rurangirwa A, Arrese-Estrada J *et al.* (1990) Cutaneous protothecosis treated with itraconazole. *Ann Soc Belge Med Trop*, **70**, 105–12.

Polak A (1990) Melanin as a virulence factor in pathogenic fungi. *Mycoses*, **33**, 215–24.

Poon-King T, Potter EV, Svartman M *et al.* (1973) Epidemic acute nephritis with reappearance of M type 55 streptococci in Trinidad. *Lancet*, **i**, 475–9.

Porter CB, Hinthorn DR, Couchonnal G *et al.* (1981) Simultaneous *Streptococcus* and *Picornavirus* infection – muscle involvement in acute rhabdomyolysis. *JAMA*, **245**, 1545–7.

Pradinaud R (1991) Lobomycosis. In: Gatti F, de Vroey C, Persi A (eds) *Human Mycoses in Tropical Countries*, 13th edn. OCSI, Bologna: 141–9.

Quieroz-Telles F, Purim KS, Fillus JN *et al.* (1992) Itraconazole in the treatment of chromoblastomycosis due to *Fonsecaea pedrosoi*. *Int J Dermatol*, **31**, 805–12.

279

Quimby SR, Connolly SM, Winkelmann RK (1992) Clinicopathologic specturm of specific cutaneous lesions of disseminated coccidioidomycosis. *J Am Acad Dermatol*, **26**, 79–85.

Radford SA, Johnson EM, Warnock DW (1997) In vitro studies of activity of voriconazole (UK 109, 496), a new triazole antifungal agent against emerging and less common mould pathogens. *Antimicrob Agents Chemother*, **41**, 841–3.

Rajendran C, Ramesh V, Misra RS *et al.* (1990) Sporotrichosis in Nepal. *Int J Dermatol*, **29**, 716–18.

Rapley R (ed.) (1996) *PCR Sequencing Protocols*. Humana Press, London.

Rattan A (1999) Antifungal susceptibility testing. *Indian J Med Microbiol*, **17**, 125–28.

Regev A, Weinberger M, Fishman M *et al.* (1998) Necrotizing fasciitis caused by *Staphylococcus aureus*. *Europ J Clin Microbiol Infect Dis*, **17**, 101–3.

Restrepo A (1994) Treatment of tropical mycoses. *J Am Acad Dermatol*, **31**(3, part 2): S91–102.

Restrepo A, Gonzales A, Gomez I *et al.* (1988) Treatment of chromoblastomycosis with itraconazole. *Ann N Y Acad Sci*, **544**, 504–16.

Richardson MD, Warnock DW (1993) *Fungal Infection: Diagnosis and Management*. Blackwell Scientific, Oxford.

Ridley DS, Jopling WH (1966) Classification of leprosy according to immunity; a five-year group system. *Int J Lepr*, **34**, 255–73.

Rietschel RL, Conde-Salazar L, Goossens A *et al.* (1999) *Atlas of Contact Dermatitis*. Martin Dunitz, London: 77, 117.

Rippon JW (1988) *Medical Mycology: The Pathogenic Fungi and the Pathogenic Actinomycetes*, 3rd edn. WB Saunders, London.

Ritz HL, Kirkland JJ, Band GG *et al.* (1984) Association of high levels of serum antibody to staphylococcal toxic shock antigen with nasal carriage of toxic shock antigen-producing strains of *S. aureus*. *Infect Immunol*, **43**, 954–8.

Rodriguez G, Barrera GP (1997) The asteroid body of lobomycosis. *Mycopathologia*, **136**, 71–4.

Rollman O, Johansson S (1987) *Hendersonula toruloidea* infection: successful response of onychomycosis to nail avulsion and topical ciclopiroxalmine. *Acta Derm Venereol*, **67**, 506–10.

Sapico FL, Ginunas VJ, Thornhill-Joynes M *et al.* (1986) Quantitative microbiology of pressure sores in different stages of healing. *Diagn Microbiol Infect Dis*, **5**, 31–8.

Schlievert P (1998) Trends within the pyrogenic toxin superantigen family. In: Arbuthnott J, Furman B (eds) *European Conference on Toxic Shock Syndrome*. International Congress and Symposium Series 229. Royal Society of Medicine, London: 79–84.

Schneller FR, Gulati SC, Cunningham IB *et al.* (1990) *Fusarium* infections in patients with haematologic malignancies. *Leuk Res*, **14**, 961–6.

Schreider F, Chatoo M (1997) Another cause of necrotizing fasciitis? *J Infect*, **35**, 177–8.

Schroeder JM, Booton GC, Hay J *et al.* (2000) Use of subgenic 18S rDNA PCR for genus and genotype identification of *Acanthamoeba* from human keratitis and sewage sludge. *Paper submitted*.

Scieux C, Grimont F, Regnault B *et al.* (1993) Molecular typing of *Chlamydia trachomatis* by random amplification of polymorphic DNA. *Res Microbiol*, **144**, 395–404.

Seal DV (1995) Necrotizing fasciitis and 'flesh-eating virus syndrome'. *J Infect*, **30**, 179–80.

Seal DV (1996) Incidence of necrotizing fasciitis – true or false? *J Hosp Infect*, **33**, 230–31.

Seal DV, Amos H (1982) Current concepts in antisepsis. *Br J Clin Pract*, Suppl 25: 1–88.

Seal DV, Clarke RP (1990) Electronic particle counting for evaluating the quality of air in operating theatres: a potential basis for standards. *J Appl Bacteriol*, **68**, 225–30.

Seal DV, Kingston D (1988) Streptococcal necrotizing fasciitis: development of an animal model to study its pathogenesis. *Brit J Exp Path*, **69**, 813–31.

Seal DV, Lightman S (1987) Immunodeficiency, immunity and staphylococcal infection. *Lancet*, **ii**, 1522.

Seal DV, Middleton K (1991) Healing of cavity wounds with sugar. *Lancet*, **338**, 571–2.

Seal DV, Stephenson ML, Geary NW *et al.* (1988) Aerobic pathogenic flora of the diabetic foot and its relationship to neuropathy and gangrene. *Microb Ecol in Health and Dis*, **1**, 39–44.

Seal DV, Ficker L, Wright P *et al.* (1991a) The case against thiomersal. *Lancet*, **338**, 315–16.

Seal DV, Wilkins E, Colman G (1991b) Pyoderma in Israel due to *Streptococcus pyogenes* M type 'Potter C'. *Trans R Soc Trop Med Hyg*, **85**, 306–7.

Seal DV, Wright P, Ficker L (1995) Placebo controlled trial of fusidic acid gel and oxytetracycline for recurrent blepharitis and rosacea. *Br J Ophthalmol*, **79**, 42–5.

Seal DV, Bron AJ, Hay J (1998) *Ocular Infection – Investigation and Treatment in Practice.* Martin Dunitz, London: 1–275.

Sellers BJ, Woods ML, Morris SE *et al.* (1996) Necrotizing group A streptococcal infections associated with streptococcal toxic shock syndrome. *Am J Surg*, **172**, 523–7.

Selwyn S, Durodie J (1985) In: Simatos D, Multon JL (eds) *Properties of Water in Foods.* Martinus Nijhoff, Amsterdam, Holland: 293.

Sen SK, Talley P, Zua M (1997) Blastomycosis: report of a case with non-invasive rapid diagnosis of dermal lesions by the Papanicolaou technique. *Acta Cytol*, **41**(Suppl 4), 1399–401.

Senhamilselvi G, Kamalam A, Ajithadas K *et al.* (1998) Scenario of chronic dermatophytosis: an Indian study. *Mycopathologia*, **140**, 129–35.

Serrano JA, Novo-Montero D, Mejia MA *et al.* (1994) Mycetoma in Venezuela. Series of cases in the state of Lara (1976–1994). Multidisciplinary family-case comparison, epidemiologic study (1994–1996). In: Debabov VG, Dudnik YW, Dahilenko VN (eds). Proc. IX Symposium Int Biol Actinomicetos. Moscu, Russia: Biotechnology, 7–8, 289–293.

Serrano JA, Mejia MA, Garcia E *et al.* (1998a) *Streptomyces somaliensis* as an aetiologic agent of actinomycetoma in Lara State, Venezuela. *J Mycol Med*, **8**, 97–104.

Serrano JA, Pisani ID, Lopez FA (1998b) Black grain minimycetoma caused by *Pyrenochaeta mackinnonii*: the first clinical case of eumycetoma reported in Barinas state, Venezuela. *J Mycol Med*, **8**, 34–9.

Settle JAD (1996) General management. In: Settle JAD (ed.) *Principles and Practice of Burns Management.* Churchill Livingstone, London: 223–41.

Shadomy S, Shadomy HJ (1988) Standardisation of anti-fungal susceptibility tests against filamentous fungi. In: Torres Rodriguez J (ed.) *Proceedings of the X Congress of the International Society for Human and Animal Mycology*, JR Praus, Barcelona: 213–17.

Shafei H, McCormick CS, Donnelly RJ (1992) Madura foot of the chest wall: cure after radical excision. *Thorac Cardiovasc Surg*, **40**, 198–200.

Shanahan EM (1997) Cutaneous infection in meat workers. *Occupational Medicine*, **47**, 197–202.

Shawcross S, Edwards-Jones V, Foster H (1998) The effect of silver sulphadiazine on the position of tst in the *S. aureus* genome. In: Arbuthnott J, Furman B (eds) *European Conference on Toxic Shock Syndrome*. International Congress and Symposium Series 229. Royal Society of Medicine, London: 131–3.

Shinefield HR, Ribble JC, Boris M *et al.* (1972) Bacterial interference. In: Cohen JO (ed.) *The Staphylococci*. Wiley-Interscience, New York: 503–15.

Shulman ST (1993) Invasive group A streptococcal infections and streptococcal toxic shock syndrome. *Pediatr Infect Dis J*, **12**, S21–4.

Shulman JA, Nahmias AJ (1972) Staphylococcal infection: clinical aspects. In: Cohen JO (ed.) *The Staphylococci*. Wiley-Interscience, New York: 457–82.

Simmons PA, Tomlinson A, Seal DV (1998) The role of *Pseudomonas aeroginosa* biofilm in the attachment of *Acanthamoeba* to four types of hydrogel contact lens materials. *Optom Vis Sci*, **75**, 860-66.

Singh G, Ray P, Sinha SK *et al.* (1996) Bacteriology of necrotizing infections of soft tissues. *Aust N Z J Surg*, **66**, 747–50.

Singh PN, Ranjana K, Singh YI (1999) Indigenous disseminated *Penicillium marneffei* infection in the state of Maipur, India; report of 4 autochthonous cases. *J Clin Microbiol,* **37**, 2699-2702.

Sirisanthana T (1997) Infection due to *Penicillium marneffei. Ann Acad Med Singapore*, **26**, 701–4.

Slater CA, Sickel JZ, Visvesvara GS *et al.* (1994) Brief report: successful treatment of disseminated *Acanthamoeba* infection in an immunocompromised patient. *N Engl J Med* **331**, 85–7.

Smith GR, Till D, Wallace LM, Noakes DE (1989) Enhancement of the infectivity of *Fusobacterium necrophorum* by other bacteria. *Epidemiol Infect*, **102**, 447–58.

Smith JMB, Marples MJ (1965) Dermatophyte lesions in the hedgehog as a reservoir of penicillin-resistant staphylococci. *J Hyg Camb*, **63**, 293–302.

Stevens DA (1995) Coccidioidomycosis. *N Engl J Med*, **332**, 1077–82.

Stevens DL, Tanner MH, Winship J *et al.* (1989) Severe group A streptococcal infections associated with a toxic shock-like syndrome and scarlet fever toxin A. *N Engl J Med* **321**, 1–7.

Stevens FA (1927) The occurrence of *Staphylococcus aureus* infection with a scarlatiniform rash. *JAMA,* **88**, 1957–8.

Stolz SJ, Davis JP, Vergeront JM *et al.* (1985) Development of serum antibody to toxic shock toxin among individuals with toxic shock syndrome in Wisconsin. *J Infect Dis*, **151**, 883–9.

Stothard DR, Hay J, Schroeder-Diedrich JM *et al.* (1999) Fluorescent oligonucleotide probes for the clinical and environmental detection of *Acanthamoeba* and the T4 18S rDNA sequence type. *J Clin Microbiol*, **37**, 2687–93.

Streeton CL, Hanna JN, Messer *et al.* (1995) An epidemic of post-streptococcal glomerulonephritis among aboriginal children. *J Paediatr Child Health*, **31**, 245–8.

Sugar AM (1997) Combination antifungal therapy. Abstracts of 20th International Chemotherapy Conference, Sydney 29 June–3 July, 65, abstract 3017.

Supparatpinyo K, Khamwan C, Baosoung V et al. (1994) Disseminated *Penicillium marneffei* infection in Southeast Asia. *Lancet*, **344**, 110–13.

Supparatpinyo K, Perriens J, Nelson KE et al. (1998) A controlled trial of itraconazole to prevent relapse of *Penicillium marneffei* infection in patients infected with human immunodeficiency virus. *N Engl J Med*, **339**, 1739–43.

Sutton DA, Fothergill AW, Rinaldi MG (1998) *Guide to Clinically Significant Fungi*. Williams & Wilkins, Baltimore.

Tang WY, Lo KK, Lam WY et al. (1995) Cutaneous protothecosis: report of a case in Hong Kong. *Br J Dermatol*, **133**, 479–82.

Taylor HR, Nutman TB (1996) Onchocerciasis. In: Pepose JS, Holland GN, Wilhelmus KR (eds) *Ocular Infection and Immunity*. Mosby Year Book, Chicago: 1481–504.

Thianprasit M, Chaiprasert A, Imwidthaya P (1996) Human pythiosis. *Curr Top Med Mycol*, **7**, 43–54.

Thomas PA (1994) Mycotic keratitis: an under-estimated mycosis. *J Med Vet Mycol*, **32**, 235–56.

Toborda PR, Toborda VA, McGinni MR (1999) *Lacazia loboi* gen. Nov., comb. Nov., the etiologic agent of lobomycosis. *J Clin Microbiol,* **37**, 2031-3.

Todd J, Fishaut M, Kapral F et al. (1987) Toxic-shock syndrome associated with phage-group I staphylococci. *Lancet*, **ii**, 1116–18.

Topham JD (1992) In a Zanzibar factory. *Pharm J,* **241**, 191–2.

Torres-Martinez C, Mehta D, Butt A et al. (1992) Streptococcus-associated toxic shock. *Arch Dis Child*, **67**, 126–30.

Trouillet JL, Chastre J, Fagon JV et al. (1985) Use of granulated sugar in treatment of open mediastinitis after cardiac surgery. *Lancet*, **ii**, 180–3.

Trouillet J, Chastre J, Gilbert C (1988) Use of granulated sugar in the treatment of mediastinal infection after surgery: a four year experience. *Cardiac Surg,* **2**, 501–9.

Tsuji K, Hirohara J, Fukui Y et al. (1993) Prototothecosis in a patient with systemic lupus erythematosus. *Intern Med*, **32**, 540–2.

Tuft S, Kemeney M, Seal D et al. (1992) Role of *S. aureus* in chronic allergic conjunctivitis. *Ophthalmology*, **99**, 180–4.

Ulbricht H, Worz K (1994) Therapy with ciclopirox lacquer of onychomycoses caused by moulds. *Mycoses*, **37**, 97–100.

van Beers SM, Izumi S, Madjid B et al. (1994) An epidemiology study of leprosy infection by serology and polymerase chain reaction. *Int J Lepr*, **62**, 1–9.

van Burik J-AH, Colven R, Spach DH (1998) Cutaneous aspergillosis. *J Clin Microbiol*, **36**, 3115–21.

van Cutsem J, Kurata H, Matsuoka H et al. (1994) Anti-fungal drug susceptibility testing. *J Med Vet Mycol*, **32**(Suppl. 1), 267–76.

van den Eeden SK, Habel LA, McKnight B et al. (1998) Risk factors for incident and recurrent condylomata acuminata among men. A population-based study. *Sex Transm Dis*, **25**, 278–84.

van Gelderen de Komaid A, Duran EL (1995) Histoplasmosis in northwestern Argentina: prevalence of histoplasmosis capsulati and paracoccidioidomycosis in the

283

population south of Chuscha, Gonzalo and Potrero in the province of Tucuman. *Mycopathologia*, **129**, 17–23.

van Tyle JH (1984) Ketoconazole. Mechanism of action, spectrum of activity, pharmacokinetics, drug interactions, adverse reactions and therapeutics. *Pharmacotherapy*, **4**, 343–73.

van der Werf TS, Van der Werf Winette TA, Groothuis DG *et al.* (1989) *Mycobacterium ulcerans* infection in Ashanti region, Ghana. *Trans Roy Soc Trop Med Hyg*, **83**, 410–13.

Waldvagel FA (1990) *Staphylococcus aureus* (including toxic shock syndromes). In: Mandell GL, Gordon Douglas R, Bennett JE (eds) *Principles and Practices of Infectious Diseases*, 3rd edn. Churchill Livingstone, London:

Weiss SJ (1989) Tissue destruction by neutrophils. *N Engl J Med*, **320**, 365–76.

Wen FQ, Sun YD, Watanabe K *et al.* (1996) Prevalence of histoplasmin sensitivity in healthy adults and tuberculosis patients in southwest China. *J Med Vet Mycol*, **34**, 171–4.

White MI, Noble WC (1980) Skin response to protein A. *Proc Roy Soc Edinburgh*, **79B**, 43–6.

Wiesenthal AM, Todd JK (1984) Toxic shock syndrome in children aged 10 years or less. *Pediatrics*, **74**, 112–7.

Wilkinson SM, English JSC (1991) Hydrocortisone sensitivity: a prospective study into the value of tixocortol-21-pivalate and hydrocortisone acetate as patch test markers. *Contact Dermatitis*, **25**, 132–3.

Wilson CG, Thomas NW (1984) Interaction of tissues with polyethylene glycol vehicles. *Pharm Int*, **5**, 94–7.

Winter GD (1962) Formation of the scab and the rate of epithelialisation of superficial wounds in the skin and the young domestic pig. *Nature*, **193**, 293–4.

Winter GD, Scales JT (1963) Effect of air drying and dressings on the surface of a wound. *Nature*, **197**, 91–2.

Wirth F, Perry R, Eskenazi A *et al.* (1997) Cutaneous mucormycosis with subsequent visceral dissemination in a child with neutropaenia: a case report and review of the paediatric literature. *J Am Acad Dermatol*, **36**, 336–41.

Woods GL, Walker DH (1996) Detection of infection or infectious agents by use of cytologic and histologic stains. *Clin Microbiol Rev*, **9**, 382–404.

Yip KM, Fung KS, Adeyemi-Doro FA (1996) Necrotizing fasciitis of the foot caused by an unusual organism, *Vibrio vulnificus*. *J Foot Ankle Surg*, **35**, 222–4.

Yoshizuka N, Abe K, Sasaki O *et al.* (1997) *Aeromonas hydrophila* necrotizing fasciitis and gas gangrene in a diabetic patient on haemodialysis. *Nephrol Dial Transplant*, **12**, 1730–4.

Youssef N, Wyborn CHE, Holt G *et al.* (1979) Ecological effects of antibiotic production by dermatophyte fungi. *J Hyg Camb*, **82**, 301–7.

Yu R (1995) Successful treatment of chromoblastomycosis with itraconazole. *Mycoses*, **38**, 79–83.

Zafar AB, Butler RC, Reese DJ *et al.* (1995) Use of 0.3% triclosan (Bacti-Stat) to eradicate an outbreak of methicillin-resistant *Staphylococcus aureus* in a neonatal nursery. *Am J Infect Control*, **23**, 200–8.

FURTHER READING

Arbuthnott J, Furman B (eds) (1998) European Conference on Toxic Shock Syndrome. International Congress and Symposium Series 229. Royal Society of Medicine, London: 1–216.

Ayliffe GAJ, Lowbury EJL, Geddes AM *et al.* (1992) *Control of Hospital Infection. A Practical Handbook*, 3rd edn. Chapman & Hall, London.

Baran R, Hay R, Haneke E, Tosti A, Piraccini BM (1999) *Onychomycosis: the Current Approach to Diagnosis and Therapy*. Martin Dunitz, London.

Barrow GI, Feltham RKG (1993) *Cowan and Steel's Manual for the Identification of Medical Bacteria*, 3rd edn. Cambridge University Press, Cambridge.

Bos JD (ed.) (1989) *Skin Immune System*. CRC Press, Boca Raton, Fla: 1–501.

Bryceson ADM, Hay RJ (1998) Parasitic worms and protozoa. In: Champion RH, Burton JL, Burns DA, Breathnach SM (eds) *Rook, Wilkinson & Ebling's Textbook of Dermatology*. Blackwell Science, London: 1377–1422.

Coggon D, Rose G, Barker DJP (1996) *Epidemiology for the Uninitiated*, 3rd edn. BMJ Publishing Group, London.

Cohen IK, Diegelmann RF, Lindblad WJ (eds) (1995) *Wound Healing – Biochemical and Clinical Aspects*. Saunders, Philadelphia: 1–630.

Crossley KB, Archer GL (eds) (1997) *The Staphylococci in Human Disease*. Churchill Livingstone, New York.

Dealey C (1999) *The Care of Wounds: a Guide for Nurses*, 2nd edn, Blackwell, Oxford.

Ferguson MWJ, Leigh IM (1998) Wound healing. In: Champion RH, Burton JL, Burns DA, Breathnach SM (eds) *Rook, Wilkinson & Ebling's Textbook of Dermatology*. Blackwell Science, London: 337–356.

Friedman GD (1994) *Primer of Epidemiology*, 4th edn. McGraw-Hill, New York.

Gawkrodger DJ (1998) Mycobacterial infections. In: Champion RH, Burton JL, Burns DA, Breathnach SM (eds) *Rook, Wilkinson & Ebling's Textbook of Dermatology*. Blackwell Science, London: 1181–214.

Harahap M (ed.) (1997) *Diagnosis and Treatment of Skin Infections*. Blackwell Science, London: 1–463.

Harahap M (ed.) (1989) *Mycobacterial Skin Diseases*. Kluwer Academic Publishers, Lancaster: 1–142.

Hay J, Adriaans B (1998) Bacterial infections. In: Champion RH, Burton JL, Burns DA, Breathnach SM (eds) *Rook, Wilkinson & Ebling's Textbook of Dermatology*. Blackwell Science, London: 1097–180.

Hay RJ, Moore M (1998) Mycology. In: Champion RH, Burton JL, Burns DA, Breathnach SM (eds) *Rook, Wilkinson & Ebling's Textbook of Dermatology*. Blackwell Science, London: 1277–376.

James MT, Harwood RF (1969) *Herms's Medical Entomology*, 6th edn. Macmillan, London.

Lorian V (ed.) (1996) *Antibiotics in Laboratory Medicine*, 3rd edn. Williams & Wilkins, Baltimore.

McCulloch JM, Kloth LC, Feedar JA (1995) *Wound Healing – Alternatives in Management*. Davis, Philadelpha: 1–442.

McLaren S (1992) Nutrition and wound healing. *J Wound Care*, **1**, 45–55.

Matthews DE, Farewell VT (1996) *Using and Understanding Medical Statistics*, 3rd edn. Karger, Basel.

Morison M, Moffatt C, Bridel-Nixon J, Bale S (1997) *Nursing Management of Chronic Wounds*. Mosby, London: 1–298.

O'Grady F, Lambert H, Finch RG *et al*. (1997) (eds) Antibiotic and Chemotherapy, 7th edn. Churchill Livingstone, London.

Parish WE, Breathnach SM (1998) Clinical immunology and allergy. In: Champion RH, Burton JL, Burns DA, Breathnach SM (eds) *Rook, Wilkinson & Ebling's Textbook of Dermatology*. Blackwell Science, London: 229–76.

Parish LC, Witkowski JA, Vassileva S (1995) *Color Atlas of Cutaneous Infections*. Blackwell Science, London: 1–177.

Puri BK (1996) *Statistics in Practice. An illustrated guide to SPSS*. Arnold, London.

Reese RE, Betts RF (eds) (1991) *A Practical Approach to Infectious Diseases*, 3rd edn. Little, Brown, Boston.

Rietschel RL, Conde-Salazar L, Goossens A *et al*. (1999) *Atlas of Contact Dermatitis*. Martin Dunitz, London: 1–325.

Rowntree D (1991) *Statistics without Tears*. Penguin, London.

Sanders CV, Nesbitt LT (eds) (1995) *The Skin and Infection*. Williams & Wilkins, Baltimore: 1–325.

Seal DV, Bron A, Hay J (1998) *Ocular Infection: Investigation and Treatment in Practice*. Martin Dunitz, London.

Settle JAD (1996) *Principles and Practice of Burns Management*. Churchill Livingstone, London.

Sterling JC, Kurtz JB (1998) Viral infections. In: Champion RH, Burton JL, Burns DA, Breathnach SM (eds) *Rook, Wilkinson & Ebling's Textbook of Dermatology*. Blackwell Science, London: 995–1096.

Stevens DL (ed.) (1995) Skin, soft tissue, bone and joint infections. In: Mandell GL (ed.) Vol. 2. *Atlas of Infectious Diseases*. Churchill Livingstone, Philadelphia.

INDEX

295